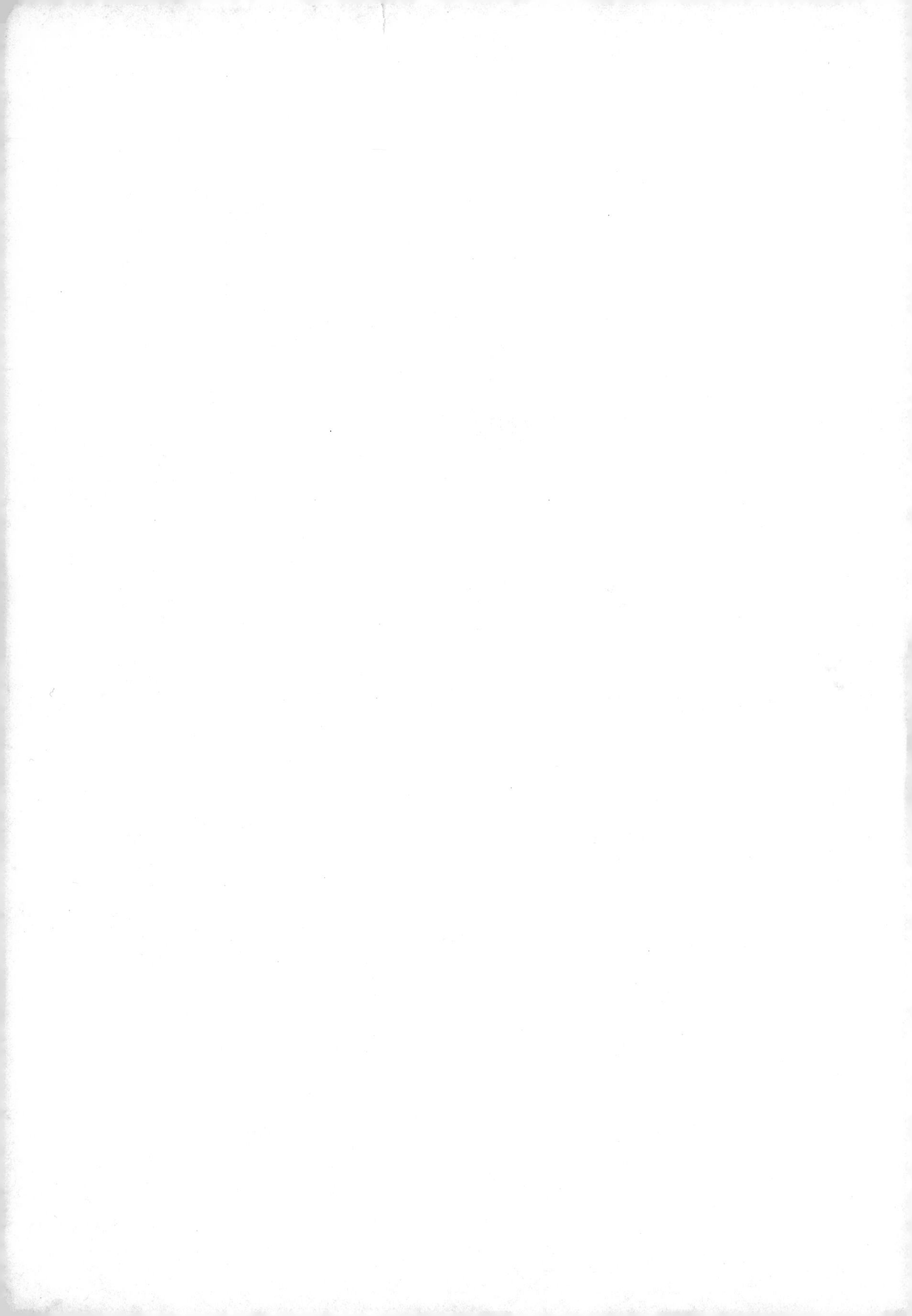

Applied Biopharmaceutics and Pharmacokinetics

SECOND EDITION

Applied Biopharmaceutics and Pharmacokinetics

Leon Shargel, Ph.D.
Associate Professor
Pharmacy and Pharmacology
Massachusetts College of Pharmacy and Allied Health Sciences
Boston, Massachusetts

Andrew B.C. Yu, Ph.D.
Senior Research Pharmacist
Product Development
Sterling Winthrop Research Institute
Rensselaer, New York

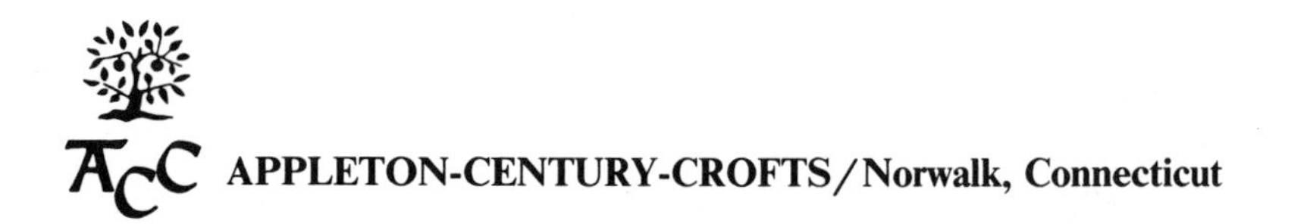

APPLETON-CENTURY-CROFTS/Norwalk, Connecticut

0-8385-0106-0

Notice: Our knowledge in clinical sciences is constantly changing. As new information becomes available, changes in treatment and in the use of drugs become necessary. The author(s) and the publisher of this volume have taken care to make certain that the doses of drugs and schedules of treatment are correct and compatible with the standards generally accepted at the time of publication. The reader is advised to consult carefully the instruction and information material included in the package insert of each drug or therapeutic agent before administration. This advice is especially important when using new or infrequently used drugs.

87 88 89/10 9 8 7 6 5

Prentice-Hall of Australia, Pty. Ltd., Sydney
Prentice-Hall Canada, Inc.
Prentice-Hall Hispanoamericana, S.A., Mexico
Prentice-Hall of India Private Limited, New Delhi
Prentice-Hall International, Inc., London
Prentice-Hall of Japan, Inc., Tokyo
Prentice-Hall of Southeast Asia (Pte.) Ltd., Singapore
Whitehall Books Ltd., Wellington, New Zealand
Editora Prentice-Hall do Brasil Ltda., Rio de Janeiro

Library of Congress Cataloging in Publication Data

Shargel, Leon, 1941–
Applied biopharmaceutics and pharmacokinetics.

Bibliography: p.
Includes index.
1. Biopharmaceutics. 2. Pharmacokinetics. I. Yu, Andrew B.C., 1945– . II. Title. [DNLM: 1. Biopharmaceutics. 2. Kinetics. 3. Pharmacology. QV 38 S531a]
RM301.4.S52 1985 615′.7 85-1356
ISBN 0-8385-0106-0

Design: Jean M. Sabato-Morley

PRINTED IN THE UNITED STATES OF AMERICA

Contents

Preface to the Second Edition

This revised edition reflects the expanding interest in biopharmaceutics and pharmacokinetics. The format is similar to that of the first edition—basic concepts are presented with an emphasis on the practical applications of biopharmaceutic and pharmacokinetic principles. Along with the theoretical discussions are practice problems with complete and annotated solutions. Furthermore, tables and figures have been added to illustrate and further clarify the fundamental biopharmaceutic and pharmacokinetic relationships.

Many chapters have been expanded by including more examples and applications to amplify the theoretical principles. Chapter 6, "Biopharmaceutic Aspects of Drug Products," Chapter 10, "Hepatic Elimination," and Chapter 15, "Application of Pharmacokinetics in Clinical Situations" have been completely revised to reflect the increasing body of knowledge in these areas. Chapter 19, "Controlled Release Drug Products" has been added to this edition and is comprised of all new material.

In writing the second edition we have tried to maintain our objective of presenting basic theoretical principles that have practical applications in biopharmaceutics and pharmacokinetics. We have therefore concentrated mainly on those theoretical principles that are widely accepted and used. Moreover, we have tried to present these principles on a level fundamental enough for students trying to learn and understand the basic concepts in biopharmaceutics and pharmacokinetics.

We would like to thank our students, colleagues, and friends for their valuable criticisms and suggestions.

Leon Shargel
Andrew B.C. Yu

Preface to the First Edition

The main objective of this book is to present basic concepts in practical bioparmaceutics and pharmacokinetics to students with at least a minimal skill in mathematics. The primary emphasis is on application and understanding of concepts. Basic theoretical discussions of the principles of biopharmaceutics and pharmacokinetics are provided, along with illustrative examples designed to help clarify these concepts. Additional practice problems and their solutions are also included to help the student gain skill in applying theories in practical problem solving. These problems range from the very simple to the fairly difficult in order to challenge the more advanced students.

This book was written with a series of learning objectives in mind. After reading this book the student should be able to:

1. Define the basic concepts in biopharmaceutics and pharmacokinetics.
2. Use raw data and derive the pharmacokinetic models and parameters that best describe the process of drug absorption, distribution, and elimination.
3. Critically evaluate biopharmaceutic studies involving drug product equivalency and unequivalency.
4. Design and evaluate dosage regimens of drugs, using pharmacokinetic and biopharmaceutic parameters.
5. Detect potential clinical pharmacokinetic problems and apply basic pharmacokinetic principles to solve them.

This text is primarily intended for the undergraduate student of pharmacy and the allied health professions. However, graduate students in pharmacology, medicine, clinical pharmacy, and other biomedical areas should also find it useful. This book may be used either independently or as a supplementary text in conjunction with a more extensive textbook. Students whose lack of training in mathematics has made them hesitant to study pharmacokinetics should encounter little difficulty in using this book.

Biopharmaceutics and pharmacokinetics constitute a rapidly growing discipline. For those who desire more in-depth treatment, references for specific subject areas are provided at the ends of the chapters.

This book was initiated by our students, who felt that there was a need for a textbook with a special emphasis on explanations and examples. To answer this need, we have deviated from the "treatise" approach and have presented our subject with more generous coverage of areas that students find especially difficult. We have received numerous suggestions from students and have incorporated them into this publication. We hope that this book will be particularly helpful for students who have heretofore found biopharmaceutics and pharmacokinetics difficult and unapproachable.

Leon Shargel
Andrew B.C. Yu

Applied Biopharmaceutics and Pharmacokinetics

CHAPTER ONE

Review of Mathematical Fundamentals

The mathematics presented here is for review purposes only. For a more complete discussion of fundamental principles, a suitable textbook in mathematics should be consulted.

EXPONENTS AND LOGARITHMS

Exponents

In the expression

$$N = b^x \tag{1.1}$$

x is the exponent and b^x is the xth power of the base b. For example,

$$1000 = 10^3$$

whereby 3 is the exponent and 10^3 is the third power of the base 10, or 1000.

Laws of Exponents	*Example*
$a^x \cdot a^y = a^{x+y}$	$10^2 \cdot 10^3 = 10^5$
$(a^x)^y = a^{xy}$	$(10^2)^3 = 10^6$
$\dfrac{a^x}{a^y} = a^{x-y}$	$\dfrac{10^2}{10^4} = 10^{-2}$
$\dfrac{1}{a^x} = a^{-x}$	$\dfrac{1}{10^2} = 10^{-2}$
$\sqrt[y]{a} = a^{1/y}$	$\sqrt[3]{a} = a^{1/3}$

Logarithms

The logarithm of a positive number N to a given base b is the exponent or the power x to which the base must be raised to equal the number N. Therefore, if

$$N = b^x \tag{1.2}$$

then

$$\log_b N = x$$

For example, with common logarithms (log), or logarithms using base 10,

$$100 = 10^2$$
$$\log 100 = 2$$

The number 100 is considered the *antilogarithm* of 2.

Natural logarithms (ln) use the base e, the value of which is 2.718282. To relate natural logarithms to common logarithms, the following equation is used:

$$2.303 \log N = \ln N \tag{1.3}$$

Exponential Expression	*Logarithmic Statement*
$10^3 = 1000$	$\log 1000 = 3$
$10^2 = 100$	$\log 100 = 2$
$10^1 = 10$	$\log 10 = 1$
$10^0 = 1$	$\log 1 = 0$
$10^{-1} = 0.1$	$\log 0.1 = -1$
$10^{-2} = 0.01$	$\log 0.01 = -2$
$10^{-3} = 0.001$	$\log 0.001 = -3$

Laws of Logarithms

$$\log ab = \log a + \log b$$

$$\log \frac{a}{b} = \log a - \log b$$

$$\log a^x = x \log a$$

$$-\log \frac{a}{b} = +\log\left(\frac{b}{a}\right)$$

Of special interest is the following relationship:

$$\ln e^{-x} = -x \tag{1.4}$$

Equation 1.4 can be compared with the following example:

$$\log 10^{-2} = -2$$

It should be noted that a logarithm has no units. A logarithm is dimensionless and is considered a real number.

PRACTICE PROBLEMS

1. Find the log of 35.

Solution

Write out the exponential form of 35, 3.5×10. The mantissa for the numerical part is 5441 (see Appendix, Table 1). For the determination of logs in scientific notation, the numerical part is always a number between 1 and 10. Therefore, the mantissa from the log table is its logarithm. The characteristic is zero, since these numbers expressed in scientific notation are expressed as the number times 10^0. Therefore,

$$\begin{aligned}\log(3.5 \times 10) &= \log 3.5 + \log 10\\ &= 0.5441 + 1.0\\ &= 1.5441\\ 35 &= 10^{1.5441}\end{aligned}$$

2. Find the log of 0.028.

Solution

$$\begin{aligned}\log 0.028 &= \log(2.8 \times 10^{-2})\\ &= \log 2.8 + \log 10^{-2}\\ &= 0.4472 + (-2)\\ &= -1.5528\end{aligned}$$

3. Find the log of 0.0031.

Solution

$$\begin{aligned}\log 0.0031 &= \log(3.1 \times 10^{-3})\\ &= \log 3.1 + \log 10^{-3}\\ &= 0.4914 + (-3)\\ &= -2.5086\end{aligned}$$

This can also be written as

$$\bar{3}.4914 \text{ or } 7.4914 - 10$$

4. The process for finding an antilog is the reverse of finding a log. The antilog is the number that corresponds to the logarithm, such that the antilog for 3 (in base 10) is 1000 (or 10^3).

a. Find the antilog of 2.3820.

Solution

Evaluate the mantissa 0.3820 on the log table (Appendix, Table 1) and find the number that corresponds to it, which in this case is 2.41. The mantissa is given as a number between 1 and 10. The characteristic is 2. Thus, the antilog of 2.3820 is

$$2.41 \times 10^2 = 241$$

b. Find the antilog of $\bar{3}.6345$.

Solution

Look up the mantissa 6345 in the log table and find the number that corresponds to it: 431. The characteristic is -3. Therefore, the antilog of $\bar{3}.6345$ is

$$4.31 \times 10^{-3}$$

5. Exponential functions.

a. Evaluate $e^{-1.3}$

Solution

In Table 3 of the Appendix, find the number corresponding to 1.3 in the column marked e^{-x}: the number is 0.2725. Therefore,

$$e^{-1.3} = 0.2725$$

b. Find the value of K in the following expression:

$$25 = 50e^{-4K}$$

Solution

$$e^{-4K} = \frac{25}{50} = 0.50$$

Find the value in the column e^{-x} that corresponds to 0.50. In this case 0.4966 is the closest value, which is equal to $e^{-0.70}$. Therefore,

$$e^{-4K} = e^{-0.70}$$
$$-4K = -0.70$$
$$K = \frac{0.70}{4} = 0.175$$

c. A very common problem in pharmacokinetics is to evaluate an expression such as

$$C_p = C_p^0 e^{-kt}$$

For example, find the value of C_p in the following equation when $t = 2$:

$$C_p = 35e^{-0.15t}$$

$$C_p = 35e^{-0.15(2)} = 35e^{-0.30}$$

Solution

From Table 3 in the Appendix (Exponential Functions),

when $x = 0.30$, $e^{-x} = 0.7408$

Therefore,

$$C_p = 35(0.7408) = 25.9$$

Since $e^{-x} = 1/e^{x}$, as the value for x becomes larger, then the value for e^{-x} becomes smaller.

CALCULUS

Since in pharmacokinetics drugs in the body are considered to be in a dynamic state, calculus is an important tool for analyzing drug movement quantitatively.

Differential Calculus

Differential calculus is a branch of calculus that involves finding the rate at which a variable quantity is changing. For example, a specific amount of drug X is placed in a beaker of water to dissolve. The rate at which the drug dissolves is expressed by *Fick's law*:

$$\text{Dissolution rate} = \frac{dX}{dt} = \frac{PA}{l}(C_1 - C_2)$$

where d = denotes a very small change; X = drug X; t = time; P = permeability constant; A = surface area of drug; l = length of diffusion layer; C_1 = concentration of drug in the diffusion layer; and C_2 = concentration of drug in the solvent. The derivative dX/dt may be interpreted as a change in X (or a derivative of X) with respect to a change in t.

In pharmacokinetics the amount of drug in the body is a variable quantity, and time is considered to be an independent variable. Thus, we consider the amount of drug to vary with respect to time.

EXAMPLE

The concentration C of a drug changes as a function of time t:

$$C = f(t) \tag{1.5}$$

Consider the following data:

Plasma Concentration of Drug C (μg/ml)	*Time (hr)*
12	0
10	1
8	2
6	3
4	4
2	5

The concentration of drug C in the plasma is declining by 2 μg/ml for each hour of time. We can therefore express the rate of change in the concentration of the drug with respect to time (i.e., derivative of C) as:

$$\frac{dC}{dt} = 2 \mu g/\text{ml hr} \tag{1.6}$$

Here $f(t)$ is a mathematical equation that describes how C changes, expressed as

$$C = 12 - 2t \tag{1.7}$$

Integral Calculus

Integration is the reverse of differentiation and is considered as the summation of $f(x) \cdot dx$; the integral sign $\int$ implies summation. For example, given the function $y - ax$, plotted in Figure 1-1, the integration would be $\int ax \cdot dx$. The integration process here is actually a summing up of the small individual pieces under the graph. When x is specified and is given boundaries from a to b, then the expression becomes a definite integral, i.e., summing up of the area from $x = a$ to $x = b$.

A *definite* integral of a mathematical function may be thought of as the sum of individual areas under the graph of that function. There are several reasonably accurate numerical methods for approximating an area. These methods can be programmed into a computer for rapid calculation. The *trapezoidal rule* is a numerical method frequently used in pharmacokinetics to calculate the area under the plasma–drug time curve, called area under the curve (AUC). For example, Figure 1-2 contains a curve depicting the elimination of a drug from the plasma after a single intravenous injection. The drug plasma levels and the corresponding time intervals plotted in Figure 1-2 are as follows:

Time (hr)	*Plasma Drug Level (μg/ml)*
0.5	38.9
1.0	30.3
2.0	18.4
3.0	11.1
4.0	6.77
5.0	4.10

The area between time intervals can be calculated with the following formula:

$$[\text{AUC}]_{t_{n-1}}^{t_n} = \frac{C_{n-1} + C_n}{2}(t_n - t_{n-1}) \tag{1.8}$$

where [AUC] = area under the curve; t_n = time of observation of drug concentration

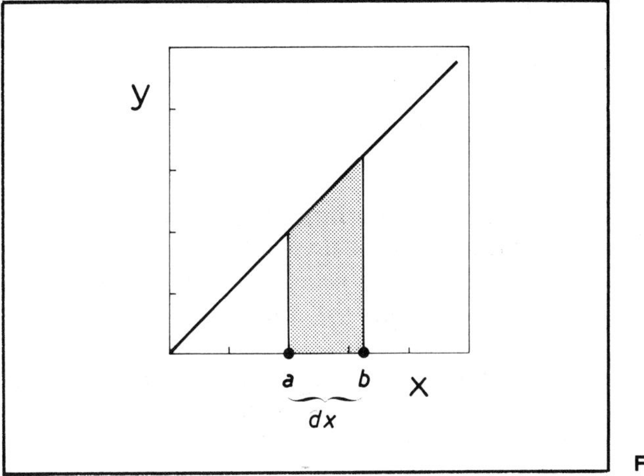

Figure 1-1. Integration of $y = ax$.

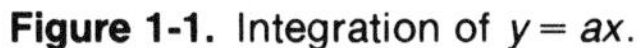

C_n; and t_{n-1} = time of prior observation of drug concentration corresponding to C_{n-1}.

To obtain the AUC from 1 to 4 hr in Figure 1-2, each portion of this area must be summed. The AUC between 1 and 2 hr is found by proper substitution into Equation 1.8:

$$[\text{AUC}]_{t_1}^{t_2} = \frac{30.3 + 18.4}{2}(2 - 1) = 24.35 \ \mu\text{g hr/ml}$$

Similarly, the AUC between 2 and 3 hr is calculated as 14.75 μg hr/ml and the AUC between 3 and 4 hr is calculated as 8.94 μg hr/ml. The total AUC between 1

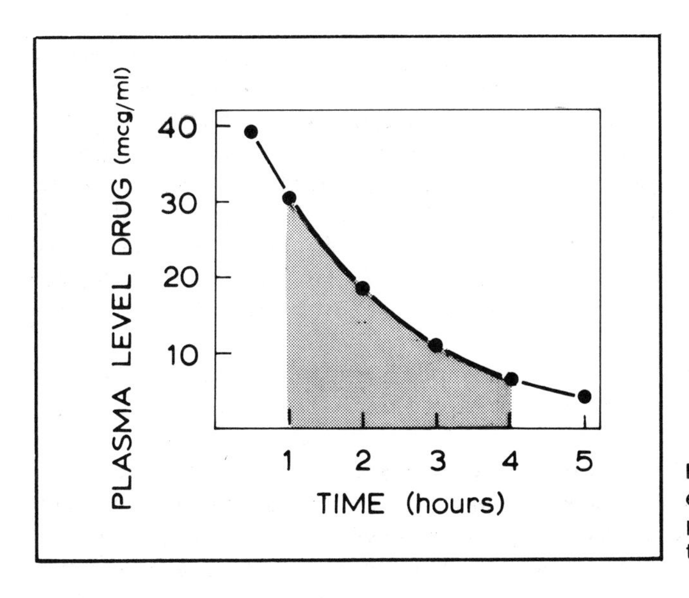

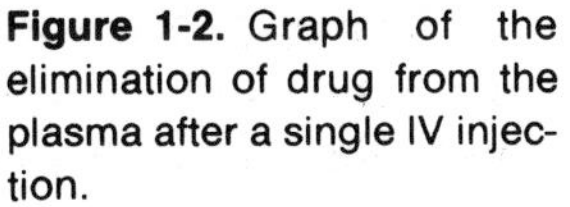

Figure 1-2. Graph of the elimination of drug from the plasma after a single IV injection.

and 4 hr is obtained by adding the three smaller AUC values together.

$$\begin{aligned}[\text{AUC}]_{t_1}^{t_4} &= [\text{AUC}]_{t_1}^{t_2} + [\text{AUC}]_{t_2}^{t_3} + [\text{AUC}]_{t_3}^{t_4} \\ &= 24.35 + 14.75 + 8.94 \\ &= 48.04\ \mu\text{g hr/ml}\end{aligned}$$

The total area under the plasma drug level versus time curve (Fig. 1-2) is obtained by summation of each individual area between two consecutive time intervals using the trapezoidal rule. The value on the y axis when time equals zero is estimated by back extrapolation of the data points using a log linear plot (i.e., log y versus x).

This numerical method of obtaining the AUC is fairly accurate if sufficient data points are available. As the number of data points increase, the trapezoidal method of approximating the area becomes more accurate.

The trapezoidal rule assumes a linear or straight-line function between data points. If the data points are spaced widely, then the normal curvature of the line will cause a greater error in the area estimate.

At times the area under the plasma level time curve is extrapolated to $t = \infty$. In this case the residual area $[\text{AUC}]_{t_n}^{t_\infty}$ is calculated as follows:

$$[\text{AUC}]_{t_n}^{t_\infty} = \frac{C_{\text{p}_n}}{k} \tag{1.9}$$

where C_{p_n} = last observed plasma concentration at t_n and k = slope obtained from the terminal portion of the curve.

GRAPHS

The construction of a curve or straight line by plotting observed or experimental data on a graph is an important method of visualizing relationships between variables. By general custom, the values of the independent variable (x) are placed on the horizontal line in a plane, or on the abscissa (x axis), whereas the values of the dependent variable are placed on the vertical line in the plane, or on the ordinate (y axis), as demonstrated in Figure 1-3. The values are usually arranged so that they increase from left to right and from bottom to top. The values may be spaced arbitrarily along each axis to optimize any observable relationships between the two variables. In pharmacokinetics, time is usually plotted on the abscissa and drug concentrations on the ordinate.

Two types of graph paper is usually used in pharmacokinetics. These are Cartesian or rectangular coordinate graph paper (Fig. 1-4) and semilog graph paper (Fig. 1-5).

Semilog paper is available with one, two, three, or more cycles per sheet, each cycle representing a 10-fold increase in the numbers, or a single $\log_{10}$ unit. This paper allows placement of the data at logarithmic intervals so that the numbers need not be converted to their corresponding log values prior to plotting on the graph.

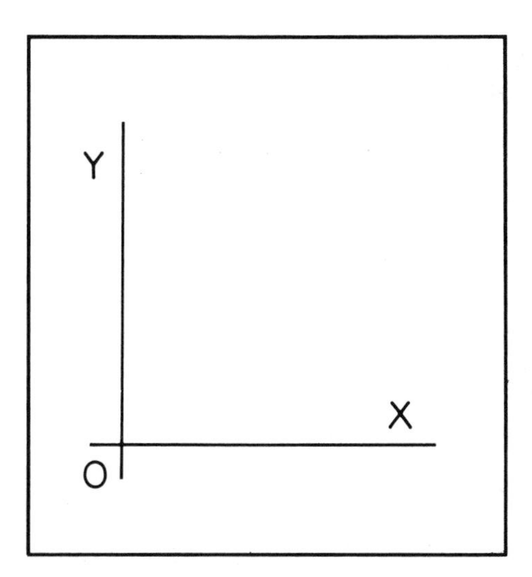

Figure 1-3. Standard arrangement of independent (x) and dependent (y) variables on a graph.

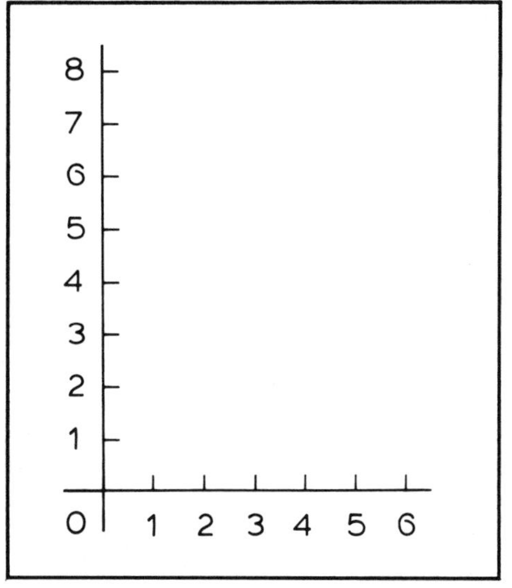

Figure 1-4. Rectangular coordinates.

Curve Fitting

Fitting a curve to the points on a graph implies that there is some sort of relationship between the variables x and y, such as dose of drug versus pharmacologic effect (e.g., lowering of blood pressure). Moreover, the relationship is not confined to isolated points but is a continuous function of x and y. In many cases a hypothesis is made concerning the relationship between the variables x and y. Then

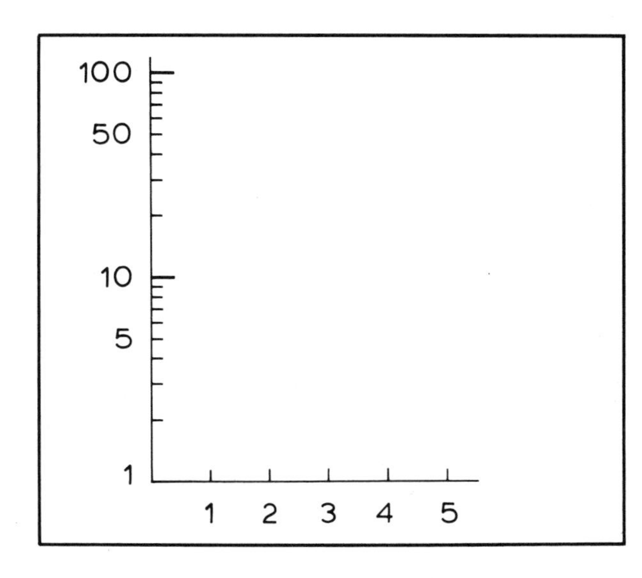

Figure 1-5. Semilog coordinates.

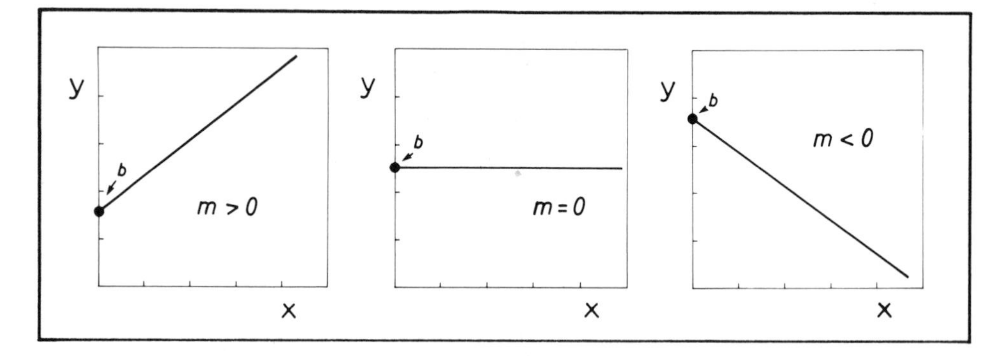

Figure 1-6. Graphic demonstration of variations in slope (m).

an empirical equation is formed that best describes the hypothesis. This empirical equation must satisfactorily fit the experimental or observed data.

Physiologic variables are not always linearly related. However, it may be possible to arrange or transform the data to express the relationship between the variables as a straight line. Straight lines are very useful for accurately predicting values for which there are no experimental observations. The general equation of a straight line is

$$y = mx + b \tag{1.10}$$

where $m =$ slope and $b = y$ intercept. Equation 1.10 could yield any one of the graphs shown in Figure 1-6, depending on the value of m. It should be noted that the absolute magnitude of m gives some idea of the steepness of the curve. For example, as the value of m approaches 0, the line becomes more horizontal. As the absolute value of m becomes larger, the line slopes further upward or downward, depending on whether m is positive or negative, respectively. For example, the equation

$$y = -15x + 7$$

would indicate a slope of -15 and a y intercept at $+7$. The negative sign indicates that the curve is sloping downward from left to right.

Determination of the Slope

Slope of a Straight Line on a Rectangular Coordinate Graph. The value of the slope may be determined from any two points on the curve. The slope of the curve is equal to $\Delta y/\Delta x$, as shown in the following equation:

$$\text{Slope} = \frac{y_2 - y_1}{x_2 - x_1} \tag{1.11}$$

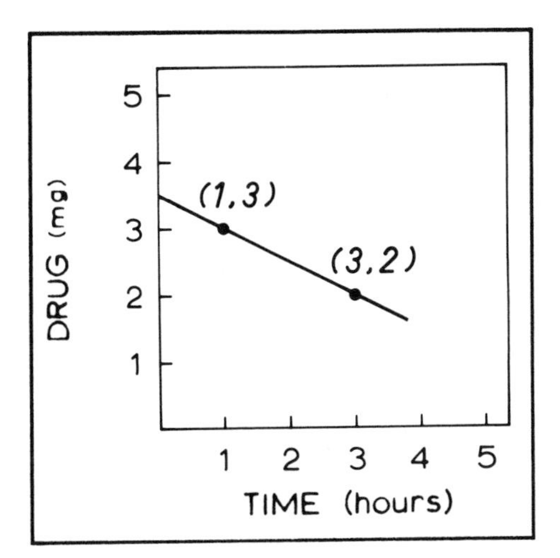

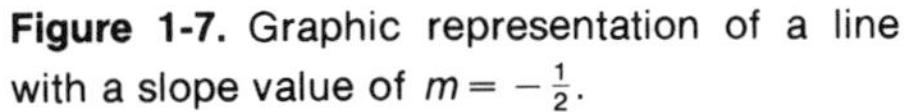
Figure 1-7. Graphic representation of a line with a slope value of $m = -\frac{1}{2}$.

The slope of the line plotted in Figure 1-7 would be

$$m = \frac{2-3}{3-1} = \frac{-1}{2}$$

Since the y intercept is equal to 3.5, the equation for the curve by substitution into Equation 1.10 would be

$$y = -\tfrac{1}{2}x + 3.5$$

Slope of a Straight Line on a Semilog Graph. When using semilog paper, the y values are plotted on a logarithmic scale without performing actual logarithmic conversions, whereas the corresponding x values are plotted on a linear scale. Therefore, in order to determine the slope of a straight line on semilog graph paper, it is necessary to convert the y values to logarithms, as shown in the following equation:

$$\text{Slope} = \frac{\log y_2 - \log y_1}{x_2 - x_1} \tag{1.12}$$

Least-Squares Method. Very often an empirical equation is calculated to show the relationship between two variables. Experimentally, data may be obtained that suggest a linear relationship between an independent variable x and a dependent variable y. The straight line that characterizes the relationship between the two variables is called a *regression line*. In many cases the experimental data may have some error and therefore show a certain amount of scatter or deviations from linearity. The least-squares method is a useful procedure for obtaining the line of best fit through a set of data points. In using this method, it is assumed that there is, in fact, a linear relationship between the variables. Statistical tests for linearity are available in most standard statistical textbooks.

PRACTICE PROBLEMS

1. Plot the following data and obtain the equation for the line that best fits the data by (a) using a ruler and (b) using the method of least squares.

x (mg)	*y (hr)*	*x (mg)*	*y (hr)*
1	3.1	5	15.3
2	6.0	6	17.9
3	8.7	7	22.0
4	12.9	8	23.0

Solution

a. Ruler
Place a ruler on a straightedge over the data points and draw the best line that can be observed. Take any two points and determine the slope by the slope formula given in Equation 1.11 and the y intercept. This method can give a reasonably quick approximation if there is very little scatter in the data.

b. Least-Squares Method
In the least-squares method the slope m and the y intercept b (Eq. 1.13) are calculated so that the average sum of the deviations squared is minimized. The deviation, d, is defined by

$$b + mx - y = d \tag{1.13}$$

If there are no deviations from linearity, then $d = 0$ and the exact form of Equation 1.13 is as follows:

$$b + mx - y = 0$$

To find the slope, m, and the intercept, y, the following equations are used:

$$m = \frac{\sum(x)\sum(y) - n\sum(xy)}{\left[\sum(x)\right]^2 - n\sum(x^2)} \tag{1.14}$$

where n = number of data points.

$$b = \frac{\sum(x)\sum(xy) - \sum(x^2)\sum y}{\left[\sum(x)\right]^2 - n\sum(x^2)} \tag{1.15}$$

where Σ is the sum of n data points.

Using the data above, tabulate values for x, y, x^2, and xy as shown below:

x	y	x^2	xy
1	3.1	1	3.1
2	6.0	4	12.0
3	8.7	9	26.1
4	12.9	16	51.6
5	15.3	25	76.5
6	17.9	36	107.4
7	22.0	49	154.0
8	23.0	64	184.0
$\Sigma x = 36$	$\Sigma y = 108.9$	$\Sigma x^2 = 204$	$\Sigma xy = 614.7$

Now substitute the values into Equations 1.14 and 1.15.

$$b = \frac{(36)(614.7) - (204)(108.9)}{(36)^2 - (8)(204)} = 0.257 \text{ mg}$$

$$m = \frac{(36)(108.9) - (8)(614.7)}{(36)^2 - (8)(204)} = 2.97 \text{ mg/hr}$$

Therefore, the linear equation that best fits the data is

$$y = 2.97x + 0.257$$

Although an equation for a straight line is obtained by the least-squares procedure, the reliability of the values should be ascertained. A *correlation coefficient*, r is a useful statistical term which indicates the relationship of the x, y data to a straight line. For a perfect linear relationship between x and y, $r = +1$ if the slope is ascending and -1 if the slope is descending. If $r = 0$, then no linear relationship between x and y exists. Usually, $r \geq 0.95$ demonstrates good evidence or a strong correlation that a linear relationship between x and y exists.

UNITS IN PHARMACOKINETICS

For an equation to be valid, the units or dimensions must be constant. In pharmacokinetics many different units are used, as listed in Table 1-1. For an accurate equation, both the integers and the units must balance. For example, a common expression for total body clearance is:

$$\text{Cl}_T = KV_\text{d}$$

After insertion of the proper units for each term in the above equation from Table 1.1,

$$\frac{\text{ml}}{\text{hr}} = \frac{1}{\text{hr}}\,\text{ml}$$

Thus, the above equation is valid as shown by the equality ml/hr = ml/hr.

An important rule in using equations with different units is that the units may be added, subtracted, divided, or multiplied as long as the final units are consistent and valid. When in doubt, check the equation by inserting the proper units. For example,

$$\text{AUC} = \frac{FD_0}{KV_d} = \text{Concentration} \times \text{Time}$$

$$\frac{\mu\text{g}}{\text{ml}}\ \text{hr} = \frac{1\ \text{mg}}{\text{hr}^{-1}\ \text{liter}} = \mu\text{g hr/ml}$$

Certain terms have no units. These terms include logarithms and ratios. Percent may have no units and is mathematically expressed as a decimal between 0 and 1 or 0 and 100%, respectively. On occasion, percent may indicate mass/volume, volume/volume, or mass/mass. Table 1-1 lists common pharmacokinetic parameters with their symbols and units.

Graphs should always have the axes (abscissa and ordinate) properly labeled with units. For example, in Figure 1-7 the amount of drug on the ordinate (y axis) is given in milligrams and the time on the abscissa (x axis) is given in hours. The equation that best fits the points on this curve is the equation for a straight line, or

TABLE 1-1. COMMON UNITS USED IN PHARMACOKINETICS

Parameter	Symbol	Unit	Example
Rate	$\frac{dD}{dt}$	$\frac{\text{Mass}}{\text{Time}}$	mg/hr
	$\frac{dc}{dt}$	$\frac{\text{Concentration}}{\text{Time}}$	μg/ml hr
Zero-order rate constant	K_0	$\frac{\text{Concentration}}{\text{Time}}$	μg/ml hr
		$\frac{\text{Mass}}{\text{Time}}$	mg/hr
First-order rate constant	K	$\frac{1}{\text{Time}}$	1/hr or hr^{-1}
Drug	D	Mass	mg
Concentration	C	$\frac{\text{Mass}}{\text{Volume}}$	μg/ml
Plasma drug concentration	C_p	$\frac{\text{Drug}}{\text{Volume}}$	μg/ml
Volume	V	Volume	ml or liters
Area under the curve	AUC	Concentration × time	μg hr/ml
Fraction of drug absorbed	F	No units	0–1
Clearance	Cl	$\frac{\text{Volume}}{\text{Time}}$	ml/hr
Half-life	$t_{1/2}$	Time	hr

$y = mx + b$. Since the slope $m = \Delta y/\Delta x$, then the units for the slope should be milligrams per hour. Similarly, the units for the y intercept b should be the same units as those for y, namely, milligrams.

UNITS FOR EXPRESSING BLOOD CONCENTRATIONS

Various units have been used in pharmacology, toxicology, and the clinical laboratory to express drug concentrations in blood, plasma, or serum. Drug concentrations or drug levels should be expressed as mass/volume. The expressions mcg/ml, μg/ml, and mg/L are equivalent and are commonly reported in the literature. Drug concentrations may also be reported as mg% or mg/dl, both of which indicate milligrams of drug per 100 ml (deciliter). Two older expressions for drug concentration occasionally used in veterinary medicine are the terms ppm and ppb, which indicate the number of parts of drug per million parts of blood (ppm) or per billion parts of blood (ppb). One ppm is equivalent to 1.0 μg/ml. The accurate interconversion of units is often necessary to prevent confusion and misinterpretation.

BIBLIOGRAPHY

Riggs DS: The Mathematical Approach to Physiological Problems. Baltimore, Williams and Wilkins, 1963

Thomas GB: Calculus and Analytic Geometry. Reading, Mass., Addison-Wesley, 1960

CHAPTER TWO

Rates and Orders of Reactions

RATE

The rate of a chemical reaction or process is the velocity with which it occurs. Consider the following chemical reaction:

$$\text{drug } A \rightarrow \text{drug } B$$

If the amount of drug A is decreasing with respect to time (that is, the reaction is going in a forward direction), then the rate of this reaction can be expressed as

$$-\frac{dA}{dt}$$

Since the amount of drug B is increasing with respect to time, the rate of the reaction can also be expressed as:

$$+\frac{dB}{dt}$$

Usually only the parent (or pharmacologically active) drug is measured experimentally. The metabolites of the drug or the products of the decomposition of the drug may not be known or may be very difficult to quantitate. The rate of a reaction is determined experimentally by measuring the disappearance of drug A at given time intervals.

RATE CONSTANT

The order of a reaction refers to the way in which the concentration of drug or reactants influences the rate of a chemical reaction or process.

Zero-order Reactions

If the amount of drug A is decreasing at a constant time interval t, then the rate of disappearance of drug A is expressed as

$$\frac{dA}{dt} = -K_0 \tag{2.1}$$

The term K_0 is the zero-order rate constant and is expressed in units of mass/time (e.g., mg/min). Integration of Equation 2.1 yields the following expression:

$$A = -K_0 t + A_0 \tag{2.2}$$

where A_0 is the amount of drug at $t = 0$. Based on this expression (Eq. 2.2), a graph of A versus t would yield a straight line (Fig. 2-1). The y intercept would be equal to A_0, and the slope of the line would be equal to K_0.

EXAMPLE

A pharmacist weighs exactly 10 g of a drug and dissolves it in 100 ml of water. The solution is kept at room temperature and samples are removed periodically and assayed for the drug. The pharmacist obtains the following data:

Drug Concentration (mg/ml)	*Time (hr)*
100	0
95	2
90	4
85	6
80	8
75	10
70	12

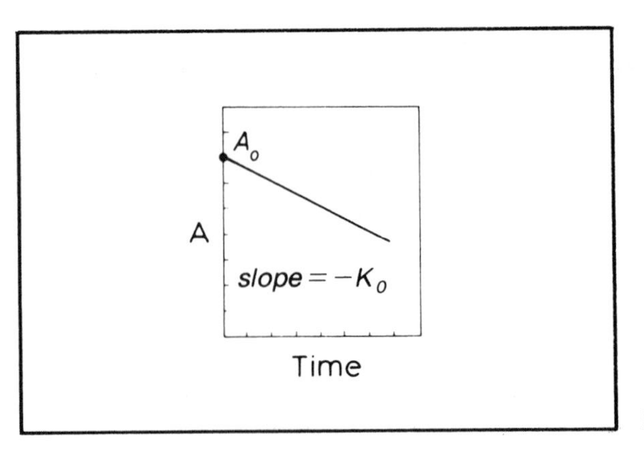

Figure 2-1. Graph of Equation 2.2.

From these data, a graph constructed by plotting the concentration of drug versus time will yield a straight line. Therefore, the rate of decline in drug concentration is of zero order.

The zero-order rate constant K_0 may be obtained from the slope of the line or by proper substitution into Equation 2-2.

If

$$A_0 = \text{concentration of } 100 \text{ mg/ml at } t = 0$$

and

$$A = \text{concentration of } 90 \text{ mg/ml at } t = 4 \text{ hr}$$

then

$$90 = -K_0(4) + 100$$

and

$$K_0 = 2.5 \text{ mg/ml hr}$$

Careful examination of the data will also show that the concentration of drug declines 5 mg/ml for each 2-hr interval. Therefore, the zero-order rate constant may be obtained by dividing 5 mg/ml by 2 hr:

$$K_0 = \frac{5 \text{ mg/ml}}{2 \text{ hr}} = 2.5 \text{ mg/ml hr}$$

First-Order Reactions

If the amount of drug A is decreasing at a rate that is proportional to the amount of drug A remaining, then the rate of disappearance of drug A is expressed as

$$\frac{dA}{dt} = -KA \tag{2.3}$$

where K is the first-order rate constant and is expressed in units of time^{-1} (e.g., hr^{-1}). Integration of Equation 2.3 yields the following expression:

$$\ln A = -Kt + \ln A_0 \tag{2.4}$$

Equation 2.4 may also be expressed as

$$A = A_0 e^{-Kt} \tag{2.5}$$

Since $\ln = 2.3 \log$, Equation 2.4 becomes

$$\log A = \frac{-Kt}{2.3} + \log A_0 \tag{2.6}$$

According to this equation, a graph of $\log A$ versus t would yield a straight line (Fig. 2-2).

The y intercept would be $\log A_0$, and the slope of the line would be equal to $-K/2.3$.

Half-life

Half-life ($t_{1/2}$) expresses the period of time required for the amount or concentration of a drug to decrease by one-half.

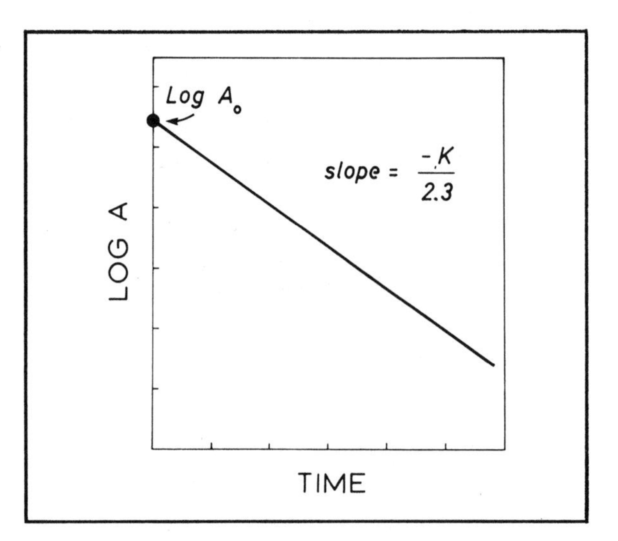

Figure 2-2. Graph of Equation 2.6.

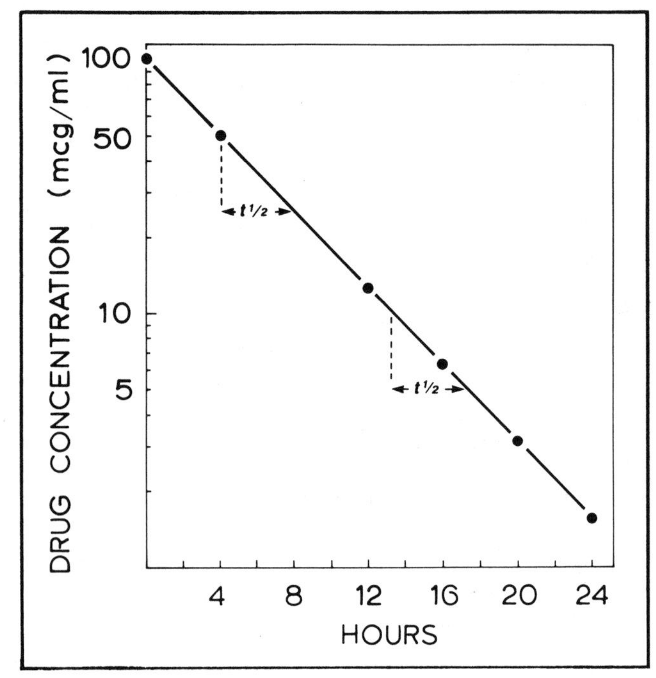

Figure 2-3. This graph demonstrates the constancy of the $t_{1/2}$ in a first-order reaction.

First-order Half-Life. The $t_{1/2}$ for a first-order reaction may be found by means of the following equation:

$$t_{1/2} = \frac{0.693}{K} \tag{2.7}$$

It is apparent from this equation that for a first-order reaction, $t_{1/2}$ is a constant. No matter what the initial amount or concentration of drug is, the time required for the amount to decrease by one-half is a constant (Fig. 2-3).

Zero-order Half-Life. In contrast to the first-order $t_{1/2}$, the $t_{1/2}$ for zero-order progress is not constant. The zero-order $t_{1/2}$ is proportional to the initial amount or concentration of the drug and is inversely proportional to the zero-order rate constant K_0:

$$t_{1/2} = \frac{0.5A_0}{K_0} \tag{2.8}$$

Since the $t_{1/2}$ changes periodically as drug concentrations decline, the zero-order $t_{1/2}$ has little practical value.

EXAMPLE

A pharmacist dissolves exactly 10 g of a drug into 100 ml of water. The solution is kept at room temperature and samples are removed periodically and assayed for the drug. The pharmacist obtains the following data:

Drug Concentration (mg / ml)	*Time (hr)*	*log Drug Concentration*
100.0	0	2.00
50.0	4	1.70
25.0	8	1.40
12.5	12	1.10
6.25	16	0.80
3.13	20	0.50
1.56	24	0.20

With these data, a graph constructed by plotting the logarithm of the drug concentrations versus time will yield a straight line on rectangular coordinates. More conveniently, the drug concentration values can be plotted directly at a logarithmic axis on semilog paper against time, and a straight line will be obtained (Fig. 2-3). The relationship of time versus drug concentration in Figure 2-3 indicates a first-order reaction.

The $t_{1/2}$ for a first-order process is constant and may be obtained from any two points on the graph that show a 50% decline in drug concentration. In this example, the $t_{1/2}$ is 4 hr. The first-order rate constant may be found by (a) obtaining the product of 2.3 times the slope or (b) by dividing 0.693 by the $t_{1/2}$, as follows:

(a) $$\text{Slope} = -\frac{K}{2.3} = \frac{\log y_2 - \log y_1}{x_2 - x_1}$$

$$-K = \frac{2.3(\log 50 - \log 100)}{4 - 0}$$

$$K = 0.173 \text{ hr}^{-1}$$

(b) $$K = \frac{0.693}{t_{1/2}}$$

$$K = \frac{0.693}{4} = 0.173 \text{ hr}^{-1}$$

QUESTIONS

1. Plot the following data on both semilog graph paper and standard rectangular coordinates.

Time (min)	*Drug A (mg)*
10	96
20	89
40	73
60	57
90	34
120	10
130	2.5

a. Does the decrease in the amount of drug *A* appear to be a zero-order or first-order process?
b. What is the rate constant *K*?
c. What is the half-life $t_{1/2}$?
d. Does the amount of drug *A* extrapolate to zero on the *x* axis?
e. What is the equation for the line produced on the graph?

2. Plot the following data on both semilog graph paper and standard rectangular coordinates.

Time (min)	*Drug A (mg)*
4	70
10	58
20	42
30	31
60	12
90	4.5
120	1.7

Answer questions a, b, c, d, and e set forth in the preceding problem.

3. A pharmacist dissolved a few milligrams of a new antibiotic drug into exactly 100 ml of distilled water and placed the solution in a refrigerator (5°C). At various time intervals the pharmacist removed a 10-ml aliquot from the solution and measured the amount of drug contained in each aliquot. The following data were obtained:

Time (hr)	*Antibiotic (μg/ml)*
0.5	84.5
1.0	81.2
2.0	74.5
4.0	61.0
6.0	48.0
8.0	35.0
12.0	8.7

   a. Is the decomposition of this antibiotic a first-order or zero-order process?
   b. What is the rate of decomposition of this antibiotic?
   c. How many milligrams of antibiotics were in the original solution prepared by the pharmacist?
   d. Give the equation for the line that best fits the experimental data.
4. A solution of a drug was freshly prepared at a concentration of 300 mg/ml. After 30 days at 25°C, the drug concentration in the solution was 75 mg/ml.
   a. Assuming first-order kinetics, when will the drug decline to one-half of the original concentration?
   b. Assuming zero-order kinetics, when will the drug decline to one-half of the original concentration?
5. How many half-lives ($t_{1/2}$) would it take for 99.9% of any initial concentration of a drug to decompose? Assume first-order kinetics.
6. If the half-life for decomposition of a drug is 12 hr, how long will it take for 125 mg of the drug to decompose 30%? Assume first-order kinetics and constant temperature.
7. Exactly 300 milligrams of a drug is dissolved into an unknown volume of distilled water. After complete dissolution of the drug, 1.0-ml samples were removed and assayed for the drug. The following results were obtained:

Time (hr)	*Concentration (mg/ml)*
0.5	0.45
2.0	0.3

   Assuming zero-order decomposition of the drug, what was the original volume of water in which the drug was dissolved?
8. For most drugs the overall rate of drug elimination is proportional to the amount of drug remaining in the body. What does this imply about the kinetic order of drug elimination?

CHAPTER THREE

Introduction to Pharmacokinetics

Biopharmaceutic and pharmacokinetic studies of drugs and drug products are useful in understanding the relationship between the physicochemical properties of the drug product and the pharmacologic or clinical effect. Figure 3-1 is a general scheme describing this dynamic relationship.

The study of *biopharmaceutics* entails investigation of the factors which influence the rate and amount of drug reaching the systemic circulation. Thus, biopharmaceutics involves factors that influence the release of drug from a drug product, the rate of dissolution of the drug, and the eventual bioavailability of drug. *Pharmacokinetics* involves the kinetics of drug absorption, distribution, and elimination (i.e., excretion and metabolism). The description of drug distribution and elimination if often termed drug *disposition*.

In the past, pharmacologists evaluated the relative availability of drugs by comparing specific pharmacologic, clinical, or possible toxic responses. For example, a drug such as isoproterenol causes an increase in heart rate when given intravenously but has no observable effect on the heart when given orally at the same dose level. Therefore, the systemic availability of drug may differ according to the route of administration. In addition, the dose of drug in one drug product may differ in bioavailability from the same dose in a second drug product, the obvious manifestation being a difference in therapeutic effectiveness between the two drugs. Thus, gross bioavailability differences can be observed by measuring therapeutic or toxic effects.

There are now sensitive, accurate, and precise analytical methods for the direct measurement of drugs in biological samples, such as plasma and urine. The pharmacokineticist is able to use these measurements of drug concentrations to describe more accurately the bioavailability differences among drugs and drug products.

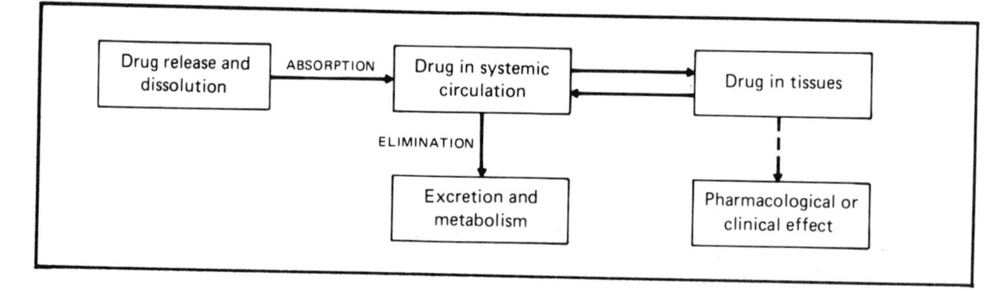

Figure 3-1. Scheme demonstrating the dynamic relationship between the drug, the drug product, and the pharmacologic effect.

PLASMA LEVEL–TIME CURVE

The plasma level–time curve is generated by measuring the drug concentration in plasma samples taken at various time intervals after a drug product is administered. The concentration of drug in each plasma sample is plotted on rectangular coordinate graph paper against the corresponding time at which the plasma sample was removed. As the drug reaches the general (systemic) circulation, plasma drug concentrations will rise up to a maximum. Usually absorption of a drug is more rapid than elimination. As the drug is being absorbed into the systemic circulation, the drug is distributed to all the tissues in the body and is also simultaneously being eliminated. Elimination of a drug can proceed by excretion or biotransformation or a combination of both.

The relationship of the drug level–time curve and various pharmacologic parameters for the drug is shown in Figure 3-2. MEC and MTC represent the *minimum effective concentration* and *minimum toxic concentration* of drug, respectively. For some drugs, such as those acting on the autonomic nervous system, it is useful to know the concentration of drug that will just barely produce a pharmacologic effect (i.e., MEC). Assuming the drug concentration in the plasma is in equilibrium with the tissues, the MEC reflects the minimum concentration of drug needed at the receptors to produce the desired pharmacologic effect. Similarly, the MTC represents the drug concentration needed to just barely produce a toxic effect. The *onset time* corresponds to the time required for the drug to reach the MEC. The *intensity* of the pharmacologic effect is proportional to the number of drug receptors occupied, which is reflected in the observation that higher plasma drug concentrations produce a greater pharmacologic response, up to a maximum. The *duration* of drug action is the difference between the onset time and the time for the drug to decline back to the MEC.

In contrast, the pharmacokineticist can also describe the plasma level–time curve in terms of such pharmacokinetic terms as peak plasma level, time for peak plasma level, and area under the curve, or AUC (Fig. 3-3). The *time of peak plasma level* is the time of maximum drug concentration in the plasma and is roughly proportional to the average rate of drug absorption. The *peak plasma level* or maximum drug concentration is usually related to the dose and the rate constants

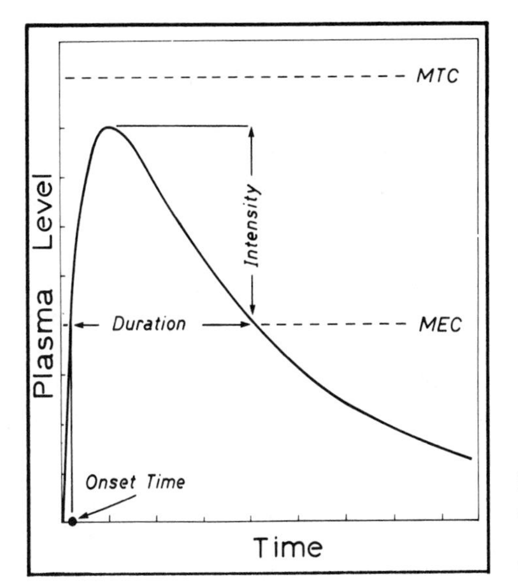

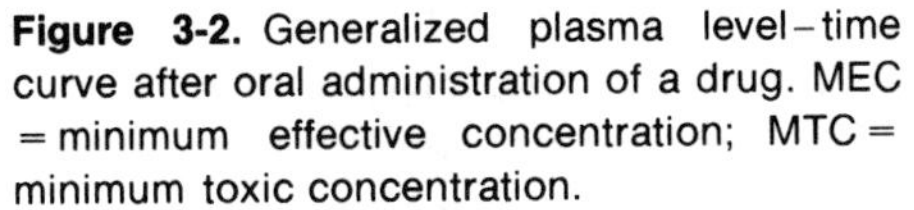
Figure 3-2. Generalized plasma level–time curve after oral administration of a drug. MEC = minimum effective concentration; MTC = minimum toxic concentration.

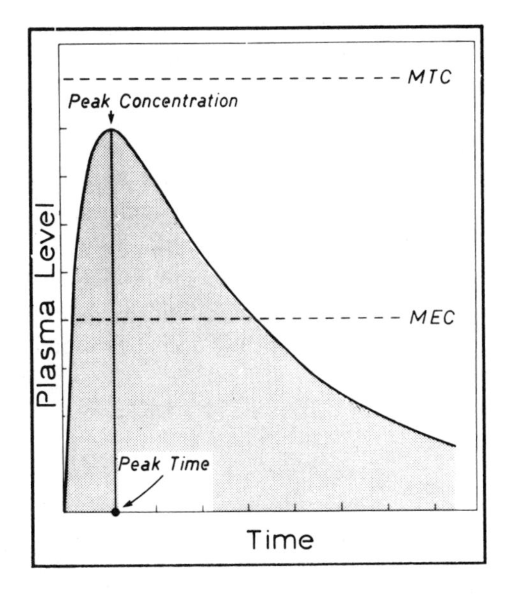

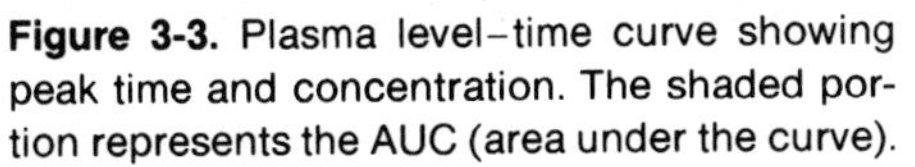
Figure 3-3. Plasma level–time curve showing peak time and concentration. The shaded portion represents the AUC (area under the curve).

for absorption and elimination of the drug. The AUC is related to the amount of drug absorbed systemically. These and other pharmacokinetic parameters are discussed in succeeding chapters.

The Significance of Measuring Plasma Drug Concentrations

The intensity of the pharmacologic or toxic effect of a drug is often related to the concentration of the drug at the receptor sites, usually located in the tissue cells. Since most of the tissue cells are richly perfused with tissue fluids or plasma, checking the plasma drug level is a responsive method of monitoring the course of therapy.

Clinically, individual variations in the pharmacokinetics of drugs are quite common. Monitoring the concentration of drugs in the blood or plasma ascertains that the calculated dose actually delivers the plasma level required for therapeutic effect. With some drugs, receptor sensitivity in individuals varies so that monitoring of plasma levels is needed to distinguish the patient who is receiving too much drug from the patient who is supersensitive to the drug. Moreover, the patient's physiologic functions may be affected by disease, nutrition, environment, concurrent drug therapy, and other factors. Pharmacokinetic models allow more accurate interpretation of the relationship between plasma drug levels and pharmacologic response. In the absence of pharmacokinetic information, plasma drug levels are relatively useless in dosage adjustment. For example, suppose a single blood sample from a patient was assayed and found to contain 10 μg/ml. According to the literature, the maximum safe concentration of this drug is 15 μg/ml. In order to apply this information properly, it is important to know when the blood sample was drawn, what dose of drug was given, and the route of administration. If the proper information is available the use of pharmacokinetic equations and models may describe the blood level–time curve accurately.

Monitoring of drug plasma concentrations allows for the adjustment of the drug dosage in order to individualize and optimize therapeutic drug regimens. In the presence of alteration in physiologic functions due to disease, monitoring plasma drug concentrations may provide a guide to the progress of the diseased state and enable the investigator to modify the drug dosage accordingly. Clinically, sound medical judgment and observation are most important. Therapeutic decisions should not be based solely on plasma drug concentrations.

PHARMACOKINETIC MODELS

Drugs are in a dynamic state within the body. In a biologic system drug events often happen simultaneously. In order to describe a complex biologic system, simplifying assumptions are made concerning the movement of drugs. A hypothesis or model is conceived using mathematical terms, which are a concise means of expressing quantitative relationships. Various mathematical models can be devised to simulate the rate processes of drug absorption, distribution, and elimination. These mathematical models make possible the development of equations to describe drug concentrations in the body as a function of time.

For example, assume a drug is given by intravenous injection and that it rapidly dissolves in the body fluids. A pharmacokinetic model that would describe this situation would be a tank containing a volume of fluid which is rapidly equilibrated with the drug. As in the human body, a fraction of the drug would be continually eliminated as a function of time (Fig. 3-4). The concentration of the drug in the tank after a given dose would be governed by two parameters: (1) the fluid volume of the tank and (2) the elimination of drug per unit of time. In pharmacokinetics these parameters are assumed to be constants. If a known set of drug concentrations in the tank were determined at various time intervals, then the volume of fluid in the tank and the rate of drug elimination would be established.

Since drug concentrations are dependent on time, the two variables in this example, drug concentration and time, are called *dependent* and *independent* variables, respectively. In practice, pharmacokinetic parameters are not measured directly but are determined experimentally from a set of dependent and independent variables collectively known as *data*. From these data a pharmacokinetic model is estimated and tested for validity and the pharmacokinetic parameters are obtained.

The number of parameters needed to describe the model depends on the complexity of the process and on the route of drug administration. In practice, there is a limitation on the amount of data that may be obtained. As the number of parameters that need to be evaluated increases, accurate estimation of these parameters becomes proportionately more difficult. With complex pharmacokinetic models, computer programs are used to estimate all the parameters. However, for the parameters to be valid, the number of data points should always exceed the number of parameters in the model.

Pharmacokinetic models are useful to:

1. Predict plasma, tissue, and urine drug levels with any dosage regimen.
2. Calculate the optimum dosage regimen for each patient individually.
3. Estimate the possible accumulation of drugs and/or metabolites.
4. Correlate drug concentrations with pharmacologic or toxicologic activity.
5. Evaluate differences in the rate or extent of availability between formulations (bioequivalence).
6. Describe how changes in physiology or disease affect the absorption, distribution, or elimination of the drug.
7. Explain drug interactions.

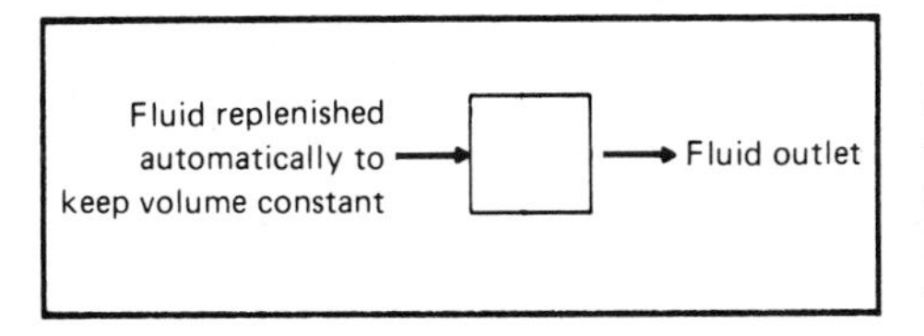

Figure 3-4. Tank with a constant volume of fluid equilibrated with drug. The volume of the fluid is 1.0 L. The fluid outlet is 10 ml/min. The fraction of drug removed per unit of time is 10/1000, or 0.01 min^{-1}.

Since a model is based on a hypothesis and simplifying assumptions which describe biologic systems in mathematical terms, a certain degree of caution is necessary when relying totally on the pharmacokinetic model to predict drug action. In practice, the model must be tested experimentally under a variety of study conditions. Usually, the simplest pharmacokinetic model is tested. Statistical criteria such as the use of the sum of squares of the deviations between the experimental data and the calculated values obtained from the model are used to determine how well the model fits the data. If the model does not fit accurately all the experimental observations, a new more complex model (hypothesis) may be proposed and subsequently tested. It is always important to realize that the pharmacokinetic data should not replace clinical observations in the patient and sound judgment by the clinician.

Compartment Models

The body can be represented as a series, or systems, of compartments that communicate reversibly with each other. A compartment is not a real physiologic or anatomic region but is considered as a tissue or group of tissues which have similar blood flow and drug affinity. Within each compartment the drug is considered to be uniformly distributed. Mixing of the drug within a compartment is rapid and homogeneous and is considered to be "well stirred" so that the drug concentration represents an average concentration and each drug molecule has an equal probability of leaving the compartment. Compartment models are based on linear assumptions using linear differential equations.

Conceptually, drugs move dynamically in and out of compartments. Rate constants are used to represent the overall rate processes of drug entry into and exit from the compartment. The model is an open system since drug can be eliminated from the system.

Mammillary Model. The mammillary model is the most common compartment model used in pharmacokinetics. The model consists of one or more peripheral compartments connected to a central compartment. The central compartment is assigned to represent plasma and highly perfused tissues which rapidly equilibrate with drug. The mammillary model may be considered as a strongly connected system since one can estimate the amount of drug in any compartment of the system after drug is introduced into a given compartment. When an intravenous dose of drug is given, the drug enters directly into the central compartment. Elimination of drug occurs from the central compartment since the organs involved in drug elimination, primarily kidney and liver, are well-perfused tissues.

Several types of compartment models are described in Figure 3-5. The pharmacokinetic rate constants are represented by the letter K. Compartment 1 repre-

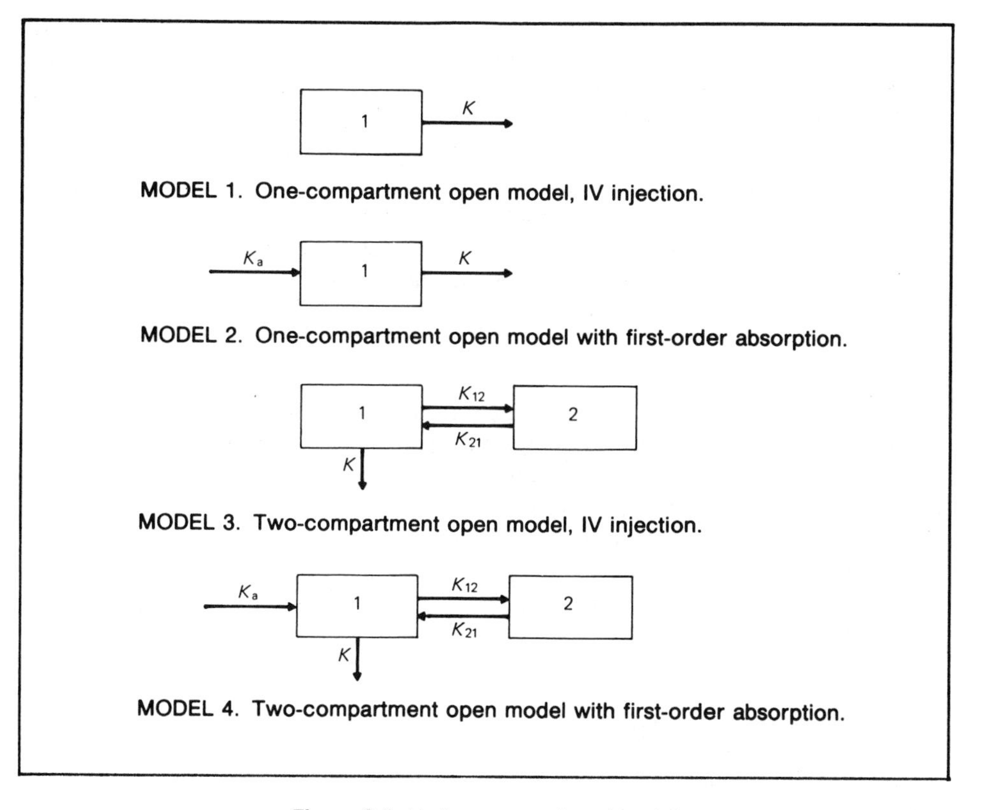

Figure 3-5. Various compartment models.

sents the plasma or central compartment, and compartment 2 represents the tissue compartment. The drawing of models has three functions. It (1) enables the pharmacokineticist to write differential equations to describe drug concentration changes in each compartment, (2) gives a visual representation of the rate processes, and (3) shows how many pharmacokinetic constants are necessary to describe the process adequately.

EXAMPLE

Two parameters are needed to describe model 1, Figure 3-5: the volume of the compartment and the elimination rate constant, K. In the case of model 4, Figure 3-5, the pharmacokinetic parameters consist of the volumes of compartments 1 and 2 and the rate constants—K_a, K, K_{12}, and K_{21}—for a total of six parameters.

In studying these models, it is important to know whether drug concentration data may be obtained directly from each compartment. For models 2 and 3, Figure 3-5, data concerning compartment 2 cannot be obtained easily because tissues are not easily sampled and may not contain homogenous concentrations of drug. If the amount of drug absorbed and eliminated per unit time is obtained by sampling compartment 1, then the amount of drug contained in the tissue can be estimated mathematically. The appropriate mathematical equations for describing these models and evaluating the various pharmacokinetic parameters are given in the succeeding chapters.

Caternary Model. In pharmacokinetics the mamillary model must be distinguished from another type of compartmental model called the *caternary* model. The caternary model consists of compartments joined to one another like the compartments of a train (Fig. 3-6). In contrast, the mammillary model consists of one or more compartments around a central compartment like satelites. Since the caternary model does not apply to the way most functional organs in the body are directly connected to the plasma, it is not used as often as the mammillary model.

Physiologic Model (Flow Model)

Physiologic models, also known as *blood flow* or *perfusion* models, are pharmacokinetic models based on known anatomic and physiologic data. The major differences between the perfusion model and the conventional compartment model are as follows.

First, no data fitting is required in the perfusion model. Drug concentrations in the various tissues are predicted by organ tissue size, blood flow, and experimentally determined drug tissue–blood ratios (i.e., partition of drug between tissue and blood).

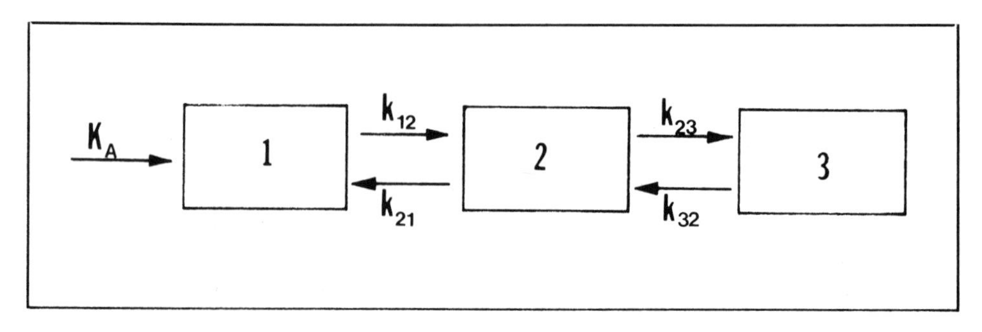

Figure 3-6. Example of caternary model.

Second, blood flow, tissue size, and the drug tissue–blood ratio may vary due to certain pathophysiologic conditions. Thus the effect of these variations on drug distribution must be taken into account in physiologic models.

Third, and most important of all, physiologically based pharmacokinetic models can be applied to several species, and with some drugs human data may be extrapolated. Extrapolation is not possible with the compartment models, since the volume of distribution in such models is a mathematical concept that does not relate simply to blood volume and blood flow. To date, numerous drugs (including digoxin, lidocaine, methotrexate, and thiopental) have been described with perfusion models. Tissue levels of some of these drugs cannot be predicted successfully with compartment models, although they generally describe blood levels well. An example of a perfusion model is shown in Figure 3-7.

The number of tissue compartments in a perfusion model varies with the drug. Typically, the tissues or organs that have no drug penetration are excluded from consideration. Thus, such organs as the brain, the bones, and other parts of the

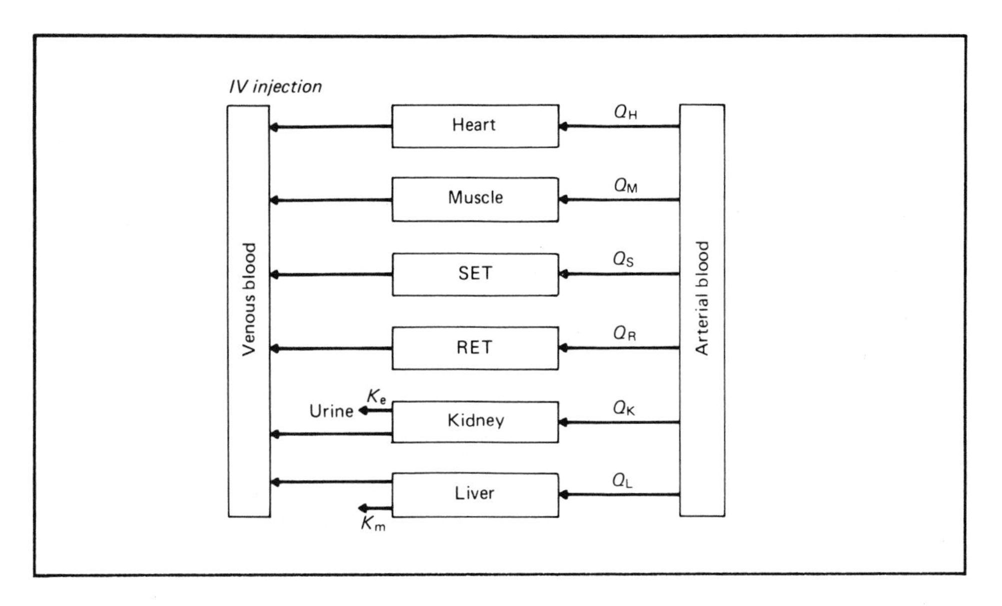

Figure 3-7. Pharmacokinetic model of drug perfusion. The *K*'s represent kinetic constants: K_0 is the first-order rate constant for urinary drug excretion and K_m is the rate constant for hepatic elimination. Each "box" represents a tissue compartment. Organs of major importance in drug absorption are considered separately, while other tissues are grouped as RET (rapidly equilibrating tissue) and SET (slowly equilibrating tissue). The size or mass of each tissue compartment is determined physiologically rather than by mathematical estimation. The concentration of drug in the tissue is determined by the ability of the tissue to accumulate drug as well as by the rate of blood perfusion to the tissue, represented by *Q*.

central nervous system are often excluded, since most drugs have little penetration into these organs. To describe each organ separately with a differential equation would make the model very complex and mathematically difficult. A simpler but equally good approach is to group all the tissues with similar blood perfusion properties into a single compartment. A perfusion model has been successfully used to describe the distribution of lidocaine in blood and various organs.[1] In this case organs such as lung, liver, brain, and muscle were individually described by differential equations, whereas other tissues were grouped as RET (rapidly equilibrating tissue) and SET (slowly equilibrating tissue), as shown in Figure 3-7.

The systems of differential equations which describe drug distribution are usually solved by numerical integration. With the model as a base, the entire time course of drug levels in various tissue organs can be predicted.

The real significance of the physiologically based model is the potential application of this model in the prediction of human pharmacokinetics from animal data. The mass of various body organs or tissues, the extent of protein binding, the drug metabolism capacity, and the blood flow in man and other species are often known or can be determined. Thus, physiologic and anatomic parameters can be used to predict the effects of drugs on man from the effects on animals in cases where human experimentation is difficult or restricted.

QUESTIONS

1. What is the significance of the plasma level–time curve? How does the plasma level–time curve relate to the pharmacologic activity of a drug?
2. What is the purpose of pharmacokinetic models?
3. Draw a diagram describing a three-compartment model with first-order absorption and drug elimination from compartment 1.
4. The pharmacokinetic model presented in Figure 3-8 represents a drug that is eliminated by renal excretion, biliary excretion, and drug metabolism. The metabolite distribution is described by a one-compartment open model. The following questions pertain to Figure 3-8.
   a. How many parameters are needed to describe the model if the drug is injected intravenously (i.e., the rate of drug absorption may be neglected)?

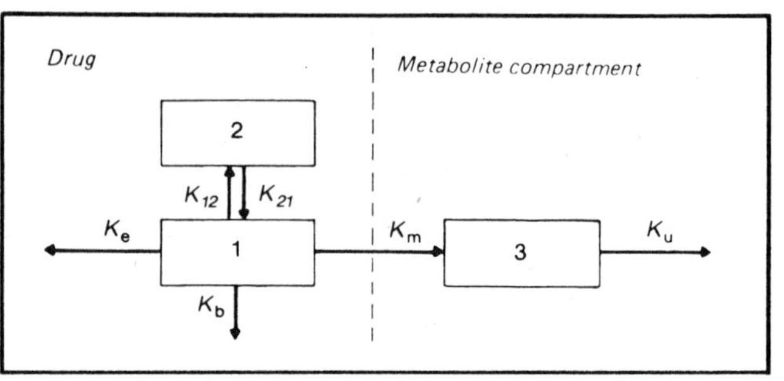

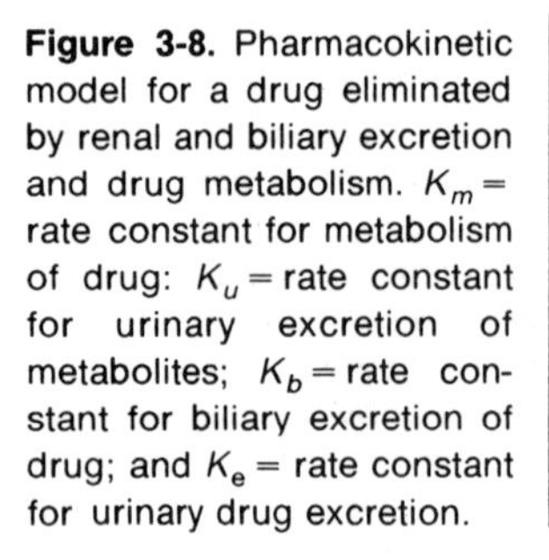

Figure 3-8. Pharmacokinetic model for a drug eliminated by renal and biliary excretion and drug metabolism. K_m = rate constant for metabolism of drug: K_u = rate constant for urinary excretion of metabolites; K_b = rate constant for biliary excretion of drug; and K_e = rate constant for urinary drug excretion.

b. Which compartment(s) can be sampled?
c. What would be the overall elimination rate constant for excretion of drug from compartment 1?
d. Write an expression describing the rate of change of drug concentration in compartment 1 (dC_1/dt).

REFERENCES

1. Benowitz N, Forsyth R, Melmon K, Rowland M: Lidocaine disposition kinetics in monkey and man. Clin Pharmacol Ther 15:87–98. 1974

BIBLIOGRAPHY

Benet LZ: General treatment of linear mammillary models with elimination from any compartment as used in pharmacokinetics. J Pharm Sci 61:536–41, 1972

Bischoff K, Brown R: Drug distribution in mammals. Chem Eng Med 62:33–45, 1966

Bischoff K, Dedrick R, Zaharko D, Longstreth T: Methotrexate pharmacokinetics. J Pharm Sci 60:1128–33, 1971

Chiou W: Quantitation of hepatic and pulmonary first-pass effect and its implications in pharmacokinetic study, I: Pharmacokinetics of chloroform in man. J Pharm Biopharm 3:193–201, 1975

Cowles A, Borgstedt H, Gilles A: Tissue weights and rates of blood flow in man for the prediction of anesthetic uptake and distribution. Anesthesiology 35:523–26, 1971

Dedrick R, Forrester D, Cannon T, et al.: Pharmacokinetics of 1-B-D-arabinofurinosulcytosine (ARA-C) deamination in several species. Biochem Pharmacol 22:2405–17, 1972

Gerlowski LE., Jain RK: Physiologically based pharmacokinetic modeling: Principles and applications. J Pharm Sci 72:1103–27, 1983

Gibaldi M: Estimation of the pharmacokinetic parameters of the two-compartment open model from post-infusion plasma concentration data. J Pharm Sci 58: 1133–35, 1969

Himmelstein KJ, Lutz RJ: A review of the applications of physiologically based pharmacokinetic modeling. J Pharm Biopharm 7:127–45, 1979

Lutz R, Dedrick R, Straw J, et al.: The kinetics of methotrexate distribution in spontaneous canine lymphosarcoma. J Pharm Biopharm 3:77–97, 1975

Montandon B., Roberts R, Fischer L: Computer simulation of sulfobromophthalein kinetics in the rat using flow-limited models with extrapolation to man. J Pharm Biopharm 3:277–90, 1975

Rowland M, Thomson P, Guichard A, Melmon K: Disposition kinetics of lidocaine in normal subjects. Ann NY Acad Sci 179:383–98, 1971

Segre G: Pharmacokinetics: Compartmental representation. Pharm. Ther 17:111–27, 1982

Tozer TN: Pharmacokinetic principles relevant to bioavailability studies. In Blanchard J, Sawchuk RJ, Brodie BB, (eds). Principles and Perspectives in Drug Bioavailability. New York, S. Karger, 1979, pp. 120–55

CHAPTER FOUR

One-Compartment Open Model

INTRAVENOUS ROUTE OF ADMINISTRATION OF DRUG

When a drug is given in the form of a rapid intravenous injection (IV bolus), the entire dose of drug enters the body immediately. Therefore, the rate of absorption is neglected in calculations. In most cases the drug distributes via the circulatory system to all the tissues in the body and equilibrates rapidly in the body. The most simple pharmacokinetic model for describing the dissolution of the drug in an apparent volume within the body is given in Figure 4-1.

The one-compartment open model assumes that any changes that occur in the plasma levels of a drug reflect proportional changes in tissue drug levels. However, this model does not assume that drug concentrations in each tissue are the same at any given point in time. Furthermore, the drug in the body (D_B) cannot be determined directly. Only the accessible body fluids (such as the blood) can be sampled to determine drug concentrations. The term *apparent volume of distribution*, V_d, is the apparent volume in the body in which the drug is dissolved.

ELIMINATION RATE CONSTANT

The rate of elimination for most drugs is a first-order process. The elimination rate constant, K, is a first-order elimination rate constant with units of time^{-1} (e.g., hr^{-1}). In general, only the parent or active drug is measured in the vascular compartment. Total removal or elimination of drug from this compartment is effected by metabolism (biotransformation) and excretion. The elimination rate constant represents the sum of each of these processes:

$$K = K_m + K_e \tag{4.1}$$

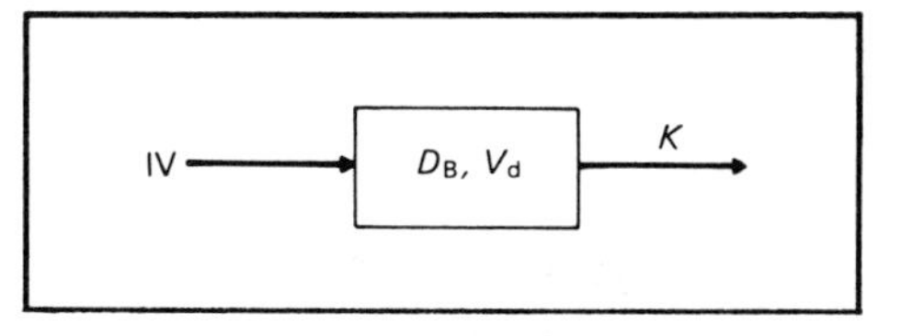

Figure 4-1. Pharmacokinetic model for a drug administered by rapid intravenous injection D_B = drug in body; V_d = apparent volume of distribution; k = elimination rate constant.

where K_m = first-order rate process of metabolism and K_e = first-order rate process of excretion. There may be several routes of elimination of drug by metabolism or excretion. In such a case each of the processes has its own first-order rate constant.

A rate expression for Figure 4-1 is

$$\frac{dD_B}{dt} = -KD_B \tag{4.2}$$

This expression shows that the rate of elimination of drug in the body is a first-order process, depending on the elimination rate constant, K, and the amount of drug, D_B, remaining. Integration of Equation 4.2 gives the following expression:

$$\log D_B = \frac{-Kt}{2.3} + \log D_B^0 \tag{4.3}$$

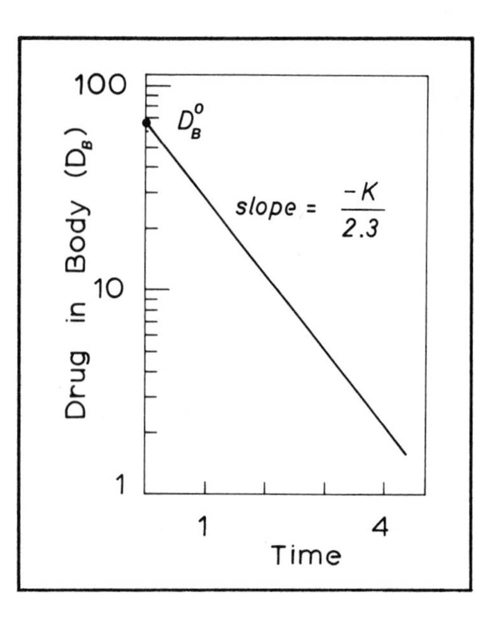

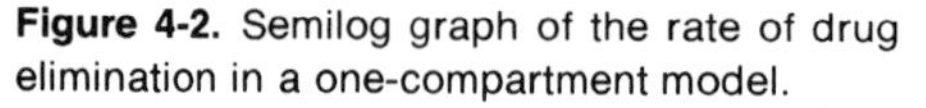
Figure 4-2. Semilog graph of the rate of drug elimination in a one-compartment model.

where D_B = drug in body at time t and D_B^0 = drug in body at $t = 0$. When $\log D_B$ is plotted against t for this equation, a straight line is obtained (Fig. 4-2). In practice, instead of transforming values of D_B to their corresponding logarithms, each value of D_B is placed at logarithmic intervals on semilog paper.

Equation 4.3 can also be expressed as

$$D_B = D_B^0 e^{-Kt} \qquad (4.4)$$

APPARENT VOLUME OF DISTRIBUTION

The volume of distribution represents a factor that must be taken into account in estimating the amount of drug in the body from the concentration of drug found in the sampling compartment. The volume of distribution can also be considered as the apparent volume (V_d) in which the drug is dissolved (Eq. 4.5).

It is usually assumed that the drug equilibrates rapidly in the body, which is true for most drugs. However, each individual tissue may contain a different concentration of drug due to differences in drug affinity for that tissue. Since the value of the volume of distribution does not have a true physiologic meaning in terms of an anatomic space, the term *apparent volume of distribution* is used.

The amount of drug in the body is not determined directly. Instead, a blood sample is removed at periodic intervals and analyzed for its concentration of drug. The V_d is useful for relating the concentration of drug in plasma (C_p) and the amount of drug in the body (D_B), as in the following equation:

$$D_B = V_d C_p \qquad (4.5)$$

By substituting Equation 4.5 into Equation 4.3, a similar expression based on drug concentration in plasma is obtained for the first-order decline of drug plasma levels.

$$\log C_p = \frac{-Kt}{2.3} + \log C_p^0 \qquad (4.6)$$

where C_p = concentration of drug in plasma at time t and C_p^0 = concentration of drug in plasma at $t = 0$. Equation 4.6 can also be expressed as

$$C_p = C_p^0 e^{-Kt} \qquad (4.7)$$

The relationship between apparent volume, drug concentration, and total amount of drug may be better understood by the following example.

EXAMPLE

Exactly 1 g of a drug is dissolved in an unknown volume of water. Upon assay, the concentration of this solution is 1 mg/ml. What is the original volume of this solution?

The original volume of the solution may be obtained by the following proportion and remembering that 1 g = 1000 mg.

$$\frac{1000 \text{ mg}}{x \text{ ml}} = \frac{1 \text{ mg}}{\text{ml}} \qquad x = 1000 \text{ ml}$$

Therefore, the original volume was 1000 ml or 1 L.

If in the above example the volume of the solution is known to be 1 L, and the concentration of the solution is 1 mg/ml, then to calculate the total amount of drug present,

$$\frac{x \text{ mg}}{1000 \text{ ml}} = \frac{1 \text{ mg}}{\text{ml}} \qquad x = 1000 \text{ mg}$$

Therefore, the total amount of drug in the solution is 1000 mg, or 1 g.

From the preceding example it should be reasoned that if the volume of solution in which the drug is dissolved and the concentration of the solution are known, then the total amount of drug present in the solution may be calculated. This relationship between drug concentration, volume in which the drug is dissolved, and total amount of drug present is given in the following equation.

$$D = VC \tag{4.5a}$$

where D = total drug; V = total volume; C = drug concentration. From Equation 4.5a, which is similar to Equation 4.5, if any two parameters are known, then the third term may be calculated.

The body may be considered as a constant-volume system. Therefore, the apparent volume of distribution for a given drug is generally a constant. If both the concentration of drug in the plasma and the apparent volume of distribution for the drug are known, then the total amount of drug in the body (at the time in which the plasma sample was obtained) may be calculated from Equation 4.5.

Calculation of Volume of Distribution

In a one-compartment model (IV administration), the V_d is calculated with the following equation:

$$V_d = \frac{\text{dose}}{C_p^0} = \frac{D_B^0}{C_p^0} \tag{4.8}$$

with a rapid IV injection, the dose is identical to D_B^0. The term C_p^0 is the initial plasma concentration of drug at $t = 0$; its value can be obtained by extrapolation of the regression line to the y axis (Fig. 4-3).

When determined by extrapolation, C_p^0 represents the instantaneous drug concentration (concentration of drug at $t = 0$) after drug has time for equilibration in the body. The dose of drug given by IV bolus (rapid IV injection) represents the amount of drug in the body, D_B^0, at $t = 0$. Since both D_B^0 and C_p^0 are know at $t = 0$, then the apparent volume of distribution, V_d, may be calculated from Equation 4.8.

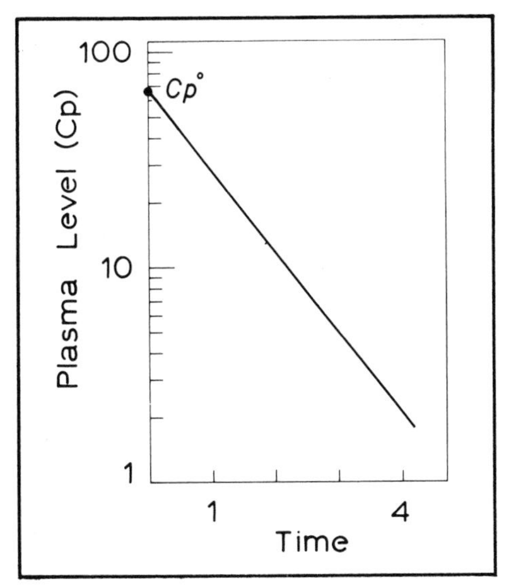

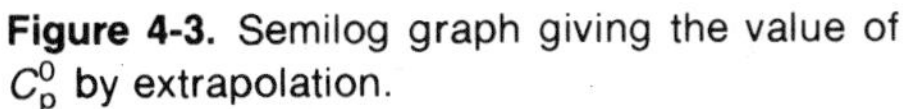

Figure 4-3. Semilog graph giving the value of C_p^0 by extrapolation.

The apparent V_d may also be calculated from knowledge of the dose, elimination rate constant, and AUC from $t = 0$ to $t = \infty$.

From Equation 4.2 (repeated here), the rate of drug elimination is

$$\frac{dD_B}{dt} = -KD_B$$

By substitution of Equation 4.5, $D_B = V_d C_p$, into Equation 4.2, the following expression is obtained:

$$\frac{dD_B}{dt} = -KV_d C_p \tag{4.9}$$

Rearrangement of Equation 4.9 gives

$$dD_B = -KV_d C_p \, dt \tag{4.10}$$

Since both K and V_d are constants, Equation 4.9 may be integrated as follows:

$$\int_0^\infty dD_B = -KV_d \int_0^\infty C_p \, dt \tag{4.11}$$

Equation 4.11 shows that a small change in time (dt) results in a small change in the amount of drug in the body, D_B.

The integral $\int C_p \, dt$ represents summation of the area under the curve from $t = 0$ to $t = \infty$ of AUC_0 and may be estimated by using the trapezoidal rule (Chapter 1). After integration, Equation 4.11 above becomes

$$\text{dose} = KV_d \text{ AUC}$$

TABLE 4-1. FLUID COMPARTMENT IN THE BODY

Water Compartment	Percent of Body Weight	Percent of Total Body Water
Plasma	4.5	7.5
Total extracellular water	27.0	45.0
Total intracellular water	33.0	55.0
Total body water	60.0	100.0

which upon rearrangement yields the following equation:

$$V_d = \frac{D_0}{K[\mathrm{AUC}]_0^\infty} \tag{4.12}$$

The calculation of the apparent V_d by means of Equation 4.12 is a model-independent method. No pharmacokinetic model is considered. The AUC may be determined directly by using the trapezoidal rule.

Significance of the Apparent Volume of Distribution

The apparent volume of distribution bears no physiologic meaning. Most drugs have an apparent volume of distribution smaller than or equal to the body mass. For some drugs the volume of distribution may be several times the body mass. Equation 4.8 shows that the apparent V_d is dependent on C_p^0. For example, a small C_p^0 will result in a large V_d since the given dose is constant. A very small C_p^0 often occurs in the body due to concentration of the drug in peripheral tissues and organs.

Drugs with a large apparent V_d are more concentrated in extravascular tissues and less concentrated intravascularly. If a drug is highly bound to plasma proteins or remains in the vascular region, then C_p^0 will be higher, resulting in a smaller apparent V_d. Consequently, binding of a drug to peripheral tissues or plasma proteins will significantly affect V_d.

The apparent V_d can be expressed as a simple volume or in terms of percent of body weight. For example, if V_d is found to be 3500 ml for a subject weighing 70 kg, V_d expressed as percent of body weight would be

$$\frac{3.5 \text{ kg}}{70 \text{ kg}} \times 100 = 5\% \text{ of body weight}$$

If V_d is found to be a very large number—i.e., $\geq 100\%$ of body weight—then it may be assumed that the drug is concentrated in certain tissue compartments. Thus the apparent V_d is a useful parameter in considering the relative amount of drug outside the central compartment or in the tissues.

Pharmacologists often attempt to visualize the apparent V_d as a true physiologic or anatomic fluid compartment. By expressing the V_d in terms of percent of body weight, values for the V_d may be found which correspond to true anatomic volumes (Table 4-1). However, it may be only fortuitous that the value for the apparent V_d of a drug has the same value as a real anatomic volume. If a drug is to be considered to be distributed in a true volume, then an investigation to test this hypothesis is required.

Given the apparent V_d for a particular drug, the total amount of drug in the body at any time after administration of the drug may be determined by the measurement of the drug concentration in the blood (Eq. 4.5). Since the magnitude of the apparent V_d is a useful indicator for the amount of drug outside the sampling compartment (usually the blood), the larger the apparent V_d, the greater the amount of drug in the extravascular compartment or tissues.

For each drug the apparent V_d is a constant. In certain pathologic cases the apparent V_d for the drug may be altered if the distribution of the drug is changed. For example, in edematous conditions the total body water and total extracellular water increase; this is reflected in a larger apparent V_d value for a drug that is highly water soluble. Similarly, changes in total body weight and lean body mass (which normally occur with age) may also affect the apparent V_d.

CALCULATION OF *K* FROM URINARY EXCRETION DATA

The elimination of rate constant K may be calculated from urinary excretion data. In this calculation the excretion rate of the drug is assumed to be first order. The term K_e is the renal excretion rate constant, and D_u is the amount of drug excreted in the urine.

$$\frac{dD_u}{dt} = K_e D_B \tag{4.13}$$

From Equation 4.4, D_B can be substituted for $D_B^0 e^{-Kt}$:

$$\frac{dD_u}{dt} = K_e D_B^0 e^{-Kt} \tag{4.14}$$

Taking the natural logarithm of both sides and then transforming to common logarithms, the following expression is obtained:

$$\log \frac{dD_u}{dt} = \frac{-Kt}{2.3} + \log K_e D_B^0 \tag{4.15}$$

A straight line can be obtained from this equation by plotting $\log dD_u/dt$ against time (Fig. 4-4). The slope of this curve is equal to $-K/2.3$ and the y intercept is equal to $\log K_e D_B^0$. For rapid intravenous administration, D_B^0 is equal to the dose D_0. Therefore, if D_B^0 is known, the renal excretion rate constant (K_e) can be obtained. Since both K_e and K can be determined by this method, the rate constant (K_{nr}) for any route of elimination other than renal excretion can be found as follows:

$$K - K_e = K_{nr} \tag{4.16}$$

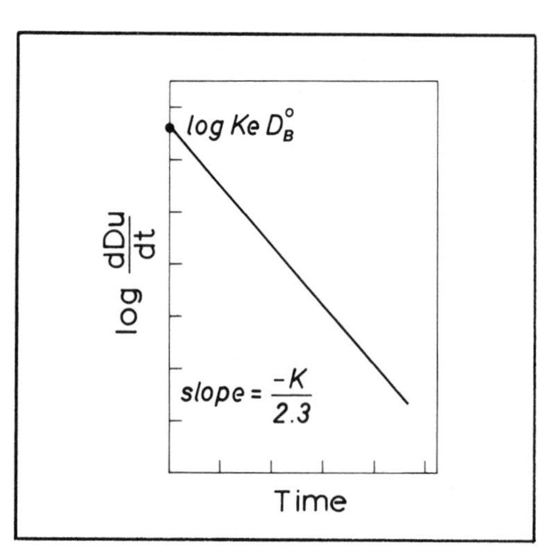

Figure 4-4. Semilog graph of Equation 4.15.

However, since elimination of a drug is usually effected by renal excretion and metabolism (biotransformation) of the drug,

$$K_{nr} \approx K_m \tag{4.17}$$

Substitution of K_m for K_{nr} in Equation 4.17 gives Equation 4.1. Since the major routes of elimination for most drugs are renal excretion and metabolism (biotransformation), then K_{nr} is approximately equal to K_m.

The drug urinary excretion rate (dD_u/dt) cannot be determined experimentally for any given instant. In practice, urine is collected over a specified time interval and the urine specimen is analyzed for drug. An average urinary excretion rate is then calculated for that collection period. The average value of dD_u/dt is plotted on a semilogarithmic scale against the time which corresponds to the midpoint of the collection period.

PRACTICE PROBLEMS

1. A single IV dose of a new antibiotic was given to a 50-kg woman at a dose level of 20 mg/kg. Urine and blood samples were removed periodically and examined for parent drug. The following data were obtained:

Time (hr)	C_p *(μg/ml)*	D_u *(mg)*
0.25	4.2	160
0.50	3.5	140
1.0	2.5	200
2.0	1.25	250
4.0	0.31	188
6.0	0.08	46

Solution

Set up the following table:

Time (hr)	D_u *(mg)*	D_u/t	*mg/hr*	t^**(hr)*
0.25	160	160/0.25	640	0.125
0.50	140	140/0.25	560	0.375
1.0	200	200/0.5	400	0.750
2.0	250	250/1	250	1.50
4.0	188	188/2	94	3.0
6.0	46	46/2	23	5.0

t^* = midpoint of collection period; t = time interval for collection of urine sample.

Construct a graph on a semilogarithmic scale of D_u/t versus t^*. The slope of this line should equal $-K/2.3$. It is usually easier to determine the elimination $t_{1/2}$ directly from the curve and then calculate K from

$$K = \frac{0.693}{t_{1/2}}$$

In this problem the $t_{1/2} = 1.0$ hr and $K = 0.693\ \text{hr}^{-1}$. A similar graph of the C_p values versus t should yield a curve with a slope of the same value as that derived from the previous curve. Note that the slope of the log excretion rate constant is a function of elimination rate constant K and not of the urinary excretion rate constant K_e.

An alternative method for the calculation of the elimination rate constant K from urinary excretion data is the *sigma-minus* method. The sigma-minus method is sometimes preferred over the previous method because fluctuations in the rate of elimination are minimized.

The amount of unchanged drug in the urine can be expressed as a function of time through the following equation:

$$D_u = \frac{K_e D_0}{K}(1 - e^{-Kt}) \tag{4.18}$$

where D_u is the cumulative amount of unchanged drug excreted in the urine.

The amount of unchanged drug that is ultimately excreted in the urine, D_u^∞, can be determined by making time t equal to infinity. Thus, the term e^{-Kt} becomes negligible and the following expression is obtained:

$$D_u^\infty = \frac{K_e D_0}{K} \tag{4.19}$$

Substitution of D_u^∞ for $K_e D_0/K$ in Equation 4.18 and rearrangement yields

$$D_u^\infty - D_u = D_u^\infty e^{-Kt} \tag{4.20}$$

Equation 4.20 can be written in logarithmic form to obtain a linear equation:

$$\log(D_u^\infty - D_u) = \frac{-Kt}{2.3} + \log D_u^\infty \tag{4.21}$$

A linear curve is obtained by graphing the logarithm of the amount of unchanged drug yet to be eliminated ($\log D_u^\infty - D_u$) versus time. The slope of this curve is $-K/2.3$ and the y intercept is $\log D_u^\infty$.

2. Using the data in the preceding problem, determine the elimination constant.

Solution

Construct the following table:

Time (hr)	D_u *(mg)*	*Cumulative* D_u	$D_u^\infty - D_u$
0.25	160	160	824
0.50	140	300	684
1.0	200	500	484
2.0	250	750	234
4.0	188	938	46
6.0	46	984	0

Plot $\log(D_u^\infty - D_u)$ versus time. Use a semilogarithmic scale for $(D_u^\infty - D)$. Evaluate K from slope or $t_{1/2}$.

Problems in Obtaining Valid Urinary Excretion Data

Certain factors can make it difficult to obtain valid urinary excretion data. Some of these factors are as follows:

1. A significant fraction of the unchanged drug must be excreted in the urine.
2. The assay technique must be specific for the unchanged drug and must not have interference due to drug metabolites which have similar chemical structures.

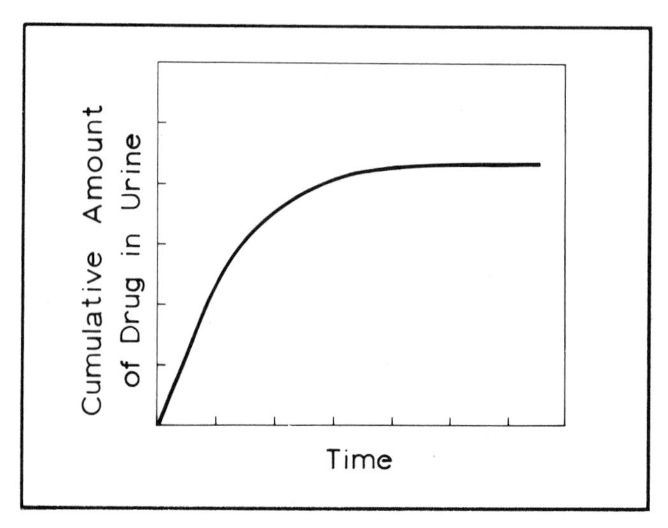

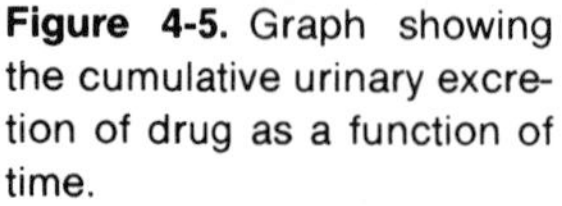

Figure 4-5. Graph showing the cumulative urinary excretion of drug as a function of time.

3. Frequent sampling is necessary for a good curve description.
4. Urine samples should be collected periodically until almost all of the drug is excreted. A graph of the cumulative drug excreted versus time will yield a curve that approaches an asymptote at "infinite" time (Fig. 4-5). In practice, approximately seven elimination half-lives are needed for 99% of the drug to be eliminated.
5. Variations in urinary pH and volume may cause significant variation in urinary excretion rates.
6. Subjects should be carefully instructed as to the necessity of giving a complete urine specimen (i.e., completely emptying the bladder).

QUESTIONS

1. A 70-kg volunteer is given an intravenous dose of an antibiotic and serum concentrations were determined at 2 and 5 hr after administration. The concentrations were 1.2 and 0.3 μg/ml, respectively. What is the biologic half-life for this drug, assuming first-order elimination kinetics?
2. A 50-kg woman was given a single IV dose of an antibacterial drug at a dose level of 6 mg/kg. Blood samples were taken at various time intervals. The concentration of the drug (C_p) was determined in the plasma fraction of each blood sample and the following data were obtained:

t (hr)	C_p (μg/ml)
0.25	8.21
0.50	7.87
1.0	7.23
3.0	5.15
6.0	3.09
12.0	1.11
18.0	0.40

   a. What are the values for V_d, K, and $t_{1/2}$ for this drug?
   b. This antibacterial agent is not effective at a plasma concentration of less than 2 μg/ml. What is the duration of activity for this drug?
   c. How long would it take for 99.9% of this drug to be eliminated?
   d. If the dose of the antibiotic were doubled exactly, what would be the increase in duration of activity?
3. A new drug was given in a single intravenous dose of 200 mg to an 80-kg male. After 6 hr, the blood concentration of drug was found to be 1.5 mg/100 ml of blood. Assuming that the apparent V_d is 10% of body weight, compute the total amount of drug in the body fluids after 6 hr. What is the half-life of this drug?
4. A new antibiotic drug was given in a single intravenous bolus of 4 mg/kg to five healthy male adults ranging in age from 23 to 38 years (average

weight 75 kg). The plasma level–time curve for this drug fits a one-compartment model. The equation of the curve that best fits the data is

$$C_p = 78e^{-0.46t}$$

Determine the following (assume units of micrograms per milliliter for C_p and hours for t):

a. What is the $t_{1/2}$?
b. What is the V_d?
c. What is the plasma level of the drug after 4 hr?
d. How much drug is left in the body after 4 hr?
e. Predict what body water compartment this drug might occupy and explain why you made this prediction.
f. Assuming the drug is no longer effective when levels decline to less than 2 μg/ml, when would you administer the next dose?

5. Define the term *apparent volume of distribution*. What criteria are necessary for the measurement of the apparent volume of distribution to be useful in pharmacokinetic calculations?

6. A drug has an elimination $t_{1/2}$ of 6 hr and follows first-order kinetics. If a single 200-mg dose is given to an adult male patient (68 kg) by IV bolus injection, what percent of the dose is lost in 24 hr?

7. A rather intoxicated young man (75 kg, age 21) was admitted to a rehabilitation center. His blood alcohol content was found to be 210 mg%. Assuming the average elimination rate of alcohol is 10 ml ethanol per hour, how long would it take for his blood alcohol concentration to decline to less than the legal blood alcohol concentration of 100 mg%? (*Hint*: Alcohol is eliminated by *zero*-order kinetics.) The specific gravity of alcohol is 0.8. The apparent volume of distribution for alcohol is 60% of body weight.

8. A single intravenous bolus injection containing 500 mg of cefamandole nafate (Mandol, Lilly) is given to an adult female patient (63 years, 55 kg) for a septicemic infection. The apparent volume of distribution is 0.1 L/kg and the elimination half-life is 0.75 hr. Assuming the drug is eliminated by first-order kinetics and may be described by a one-compartment model, calculate the following:

a. The C_p^0
b. The amount of drug in the body at 4 hr after the dose is given.
c. The time for the drug to decline to 0.5 μg/ml, the minimum inhibitory concentration for streptococci.

9. If the amount of drug in the body declines from 100% of the dose (IV bolus injection) to 25% of the dose in 8 hr, what is the elimination half-life for this drug? (Assume first order-kinetics.)

10. A drug has an elimination half-life of 8 hr and follows first-order elimination kinetics. If a single 600-mg dose is given to an adult female patient (62 kg) by rapid IV injection, what *percent* of the dose is eliminated (lost) in 24 hr assuming the apparent V_d is 400 ml/kg. What is the expected plasma drug concentration (C_p) at 24 hr postdose?

11. For drugs that follow the kinetics of a one-compartment open model must the tissues and plasma have the same drug concentration? Why?
12. An adult male patient (age 35 years, weight 72 kg) with a urinary tract infection was given a single intravenous bolus of an antibiotic (dose = 300 mg). The patient was instructed to empty his bladder prior to being medicated and to save his urine specimens for analysis. The specimens were analyzed for both drug content and sterility (lack of bacteriuria). The drug assays gave the following results:

t (*hr*)	*Amount of Drug in Urine (mg)*
0	0
4	100
8	26

Assuming first-order elimination, calculate the elimination half-life for the antibiotic in this patient.

BIBLIOGRAPHY

Gibaldi M, Nagashima R, Levy G: Relationship between drug concentration in plasma or serum and amount of drug in the body. J Pharm Sci 58:193–97, 1969

Riegelman S, Loo JCK, Rowland M: Shortcomings in pharmacokinetic analysis by conceiving the body to exhibit properties of a single compartment. J Pharm Sci 57:117–23, 1968

Riegelman S, Loo J, Rowland M: Concepts of volume of distribution and possible errors in evaluation of this parameter. Science 57:128–33, 1968

Wagner JG, Northam JI: Estimation of volume of distribution and half-life of a compound after rapid intravenous injection. J Pharm Sci 58:529–31, 1975

CHAPTER FIVE

Multicompartment Models

Multicompartment models are needed to explain the observation that after a rapid IV injection the plasma level–time curve does not decline linearly as a single first-order rate process. In a multicompartment model the drug distributes at various rates into different tissue groups. Those tissues which have the highest blood flow may equilibrate with the plasma compartments. These highly perfused tissues and blood make up the central compartment. While this initial drug distribution is taking place, the drug is delivered to one or more peripheral compartments composed of groups of tissues with lower but similar blood flow and affinity for the drug. These differences account for the appearance of a nonlinear log plasma drug concentration versus time curve. After equilibration of the drug within these peripheral tissues, the plasma level–time curve reflects first-order elimination of the drug from the body.

A drug will concentrate in a tissue in accordance with the affinity of the drug for that particular tissue. For example, lipid-soluble drugs tend to accumulate in fat tissues. Drugs which bind proteins may be more concentrated in the plasma, since protein-bound drugs do not diffuse into the tissues. Drugs may also bind with tissue proteins and other macromolecules, such as DNA and melanin.

In order to apply kinetic analysis of a multicompartment model, one must assume that all rate processes for the passage of drug into or out of individual compartments are first-order processes. On the basis of this assumption, the plasma level–time curve for a drug which follows a multicompartment model is best described by the summation of several first-order rate processes.

Because of the aforementioned distribution factors, drugs will generally concentrate unevenly in the tissues, and different groups of tissues will accumulate the drug at different rates. A summary of the approximate blood flow to major human tissues is presented in Table 5-1.

TABLE 5-1. BLOOD FLOW TO HUMAN TISSUES

Tissue	Percent Body Weight	Percent Cardiac Output	Blood Flow (ml / 100 g tissue / min)
Adrenals	0.02	1	550
Kidneys	0.4	24	450
Thyroid	0.04	2	400
Liver			
Hepatic	2.0	5	20
Portal		20	75
Portal-drained viscera	2.0	20	75
Heart (basal)	0.4	4	70
Brain	2.0	15	55
Skin	7.0	5	5
Muscle (basal)	40.0	15	3
Connective tissue	7.0	1	1
Fat	15.0	2	1

After Butler TC,[1] 1972, with permission.

TWO-COMPARTMENT OPEN MODEL

Many drugs given in a single intravenous dose demonstrate a plasma level–time curve which can be described by assuming first-order transfer of drugs between compartments (Fig. 5-1).

In the case of a two-compartment model it is assumed that the drug distributes into two compartments. One compartment, known as the central compartment, represents the blood, extracellular water, and highly perfused tissues; this compart-

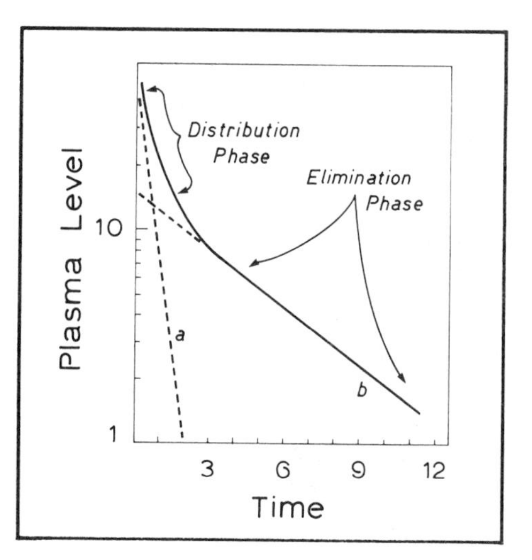

Figure 5-1. Plasma level–time curve for the two-compartment open model (single IV dose) described in Figure 5-2.

ment is rapidly diffused with drug (Fig. 5-2). A second compartment, known as the tissue compartment, contains tissues which equilibrate more slowly with the drug. This model assumes that the drug is eliminated from the central compartment.

After an intravenous injection drug concentrations in plasma and the highly perfused tissues constituting the central compartment decline rapidly due to distribution of the drug into other, more slowly perfused tissues. This initial rapid decline of drug concentration in the central compartment is known as the distribution phase of the curve (Fig. 5-1, line *a*). In time the drug attains a state of equilibrium between the central compartment and the more poorly perfused tissue compartment. After this equilibrium is established, the loss of the drug from the central compartment appears to be a single first-order process due to the overall processes of elimination of the drug from the body. This second, slower rate process is known as the elimination phase (Fig. 5-1, line *b*).

The two-compartment model assumes that at $t = 0$ there is no drug in the tissue compartment. After an intravenous dose drug is rapidly transferred into the tissue compartment while the blood level of drug declines rapidly due to both elimination of the drug and transfer of the drug out of the central compartment into various tissues. A typical tissue drug level curve after a single intravenous dose of drug is shown in Figure 5-3. The tissue drug level will eventually peak and then start to decline as the concentration gradient between the two compartments narrows.

The drug level in the theoretical tissue compartment can be calculated once the parameters for the model are determined. However, the drug concentration in the tissue compartment represents the average drug concentration in a group of tissues rather than any real anatomic tissue drug concentration. Real tissue drug concentration can sometimes be calculated by the addition of compartments to the model until a compartment which mimics the experimental tissue concentrations is found.

In spite of the hypothetical nature of the tissue compartment, the theoretical tissue level is still a valuable piece of information for clinicians. The theoretical tissue concentration, together with the blood concentration, gives an accurate method of calculating the total amount of drug remaining in the body at any time. This information would not be available without using pharmacokinetic models.

In practice, samples of blood are removed from the central compartment and analyzed for the presence of drug. The drug plasma level–time curve represents a phase of initial rapid equilibration with the central compartment (the distribution phase) followed by an elimination phase after the tissue compartment has also been diffused with drug. The distribution phase may take minutes or hours and may be missed entirely if the blood is sampled too late after administration of the drug.

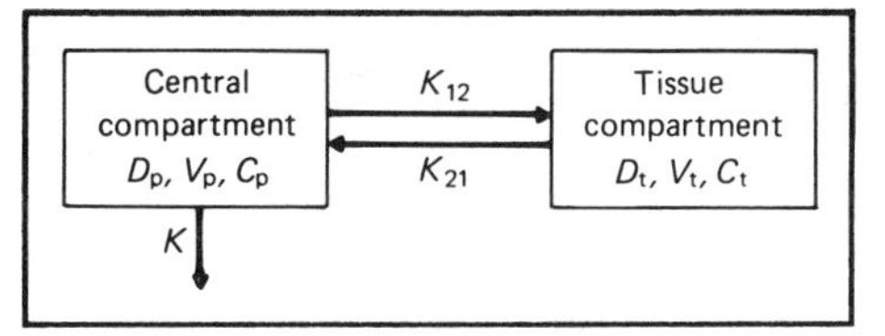

Figure 5-2. Two-compartment open model, intravenous injection.

In the model depicted above K_{12} and K_{21} are first-order rate constants. Similarly, the rate of drug change in the tissues is

$$\frac{dC_t}{dt} = K_{12}C_p - K_{21}C_t \tag{5.1}$$

The relationship between the amount of drug in each compartment and the concentration of drug in each compartment is shown by Equations 5.2 and 5.3:

$$C_p = \frac{D_p}{V_p} \tag{5.2}$$

$$C_t = \frac{D_t}{V_t} \tag{5.3}$$

where D_p = amount of drug in the central compartment; D_t = amount of drug in the tissue compartment; V_p = volume of drug in the central compartment; and V_t = volume of drug in the tissue compartment.

$$\frac{dC_p}{dt} = K_{21}\frac{D_t}{V_t} - K_{12}\frac{D_p}{V_p} - K\frac{D_p}{V_p} \tag{5.4}$$

$$\frac{dC_t}{dt} = K_{12}\frac{D_p}{V_p} - K_{21}\frac{D_t}{V_t} \tag{5.5}$$

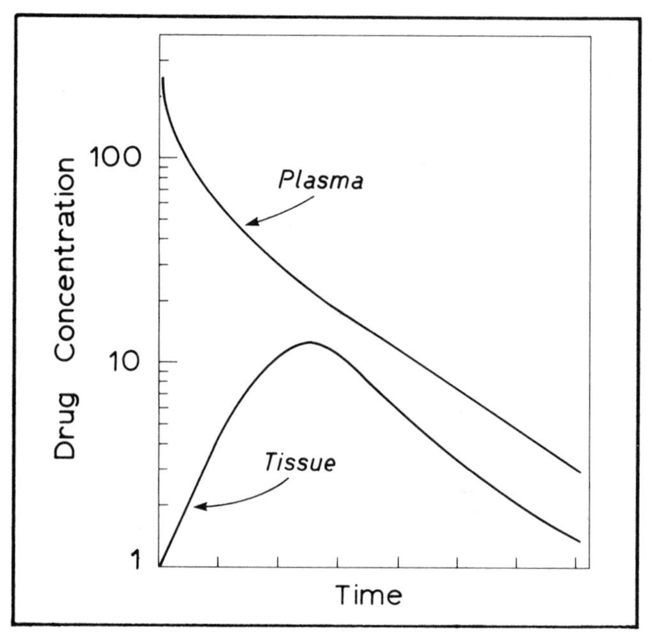

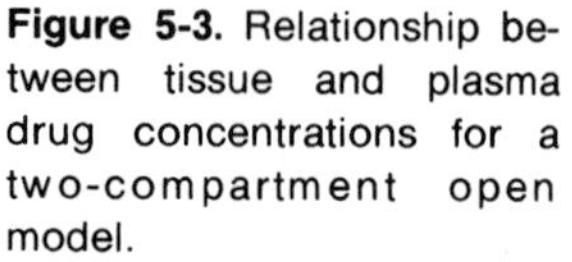
Figure 5-3. Relationship between tissue and plasma drug concentrations for a two-compartment open model.

Solving Equations 5.4 and 5.5 will give Equations 5.6 and 5.7, which describe the change in drug concentration in the blood and in the tissue with respect to time:

$$C_p = \frac{D_p^0}{V_p}\left[\frac{K_{21} - a}{b - a}\right]e^{-at} + \left[\frac{K_{21} - b}{a - b}\right]e^{-bt} \tag{5.6}$$

$$C_t = \frac{D_p^0}{V_t}\left[\frac{K_{12}}{b - a}\right]e^{-at} + \left[\frac{K_{12}}{a - b}\right]e^{-bt} \tag{5.7}$$

where D_p^0 = dose given intravenously; t = time after administration of dose; and a and b are constants that depend solely on K_{12}, K_{21}, and K.

The rate constants for the transfer of drug between compartments are referred to as *microconstants* or *transfer constants* and relate the amount of drug being transferred per unit time from one compartment to the other. The values for these microconstants cannot be determined by direct measurement since the drug concentration in each compartment cannot be sampled directly.

$$a + b = K_{12} + K_{21} + K \tag{5.8}$$

$$ab = K_{21}K \tag{5.9}$$

The constants a and b are hybrid first-order rate constants for the distribution phase and elimination phase, respectively. The mathematical relationship of a and b to the rate constants are given by Equations 5.8 and 5.9, which are derived after integration of Equations 5.4 and 5.5. Equation 5.6 can be transformed into the following expression:

$$C_p = Ae^{-at} + Be^{-bt} \tag{5.10}$$

The constants a and b are rate constants for the distribution phase and elimination phase, respectively. The constants A and B are intercepts on the y axis for each exponential segment of the curve in Equation 5.10. These values may be obtained graphically by the method of residuals or by computer. Intercepts A and B are actually hybrid constants, as shown in Equations 5.11 and 5.12.

$$A = \frac{D_0(a - K_{21})}{V_p(a - b)} \tag{5.11}$$

$$B = \frac{D_0(K_{21} - b)}{V_p(a - b)} \tag{5.12}$$

Method of Residuals

The method of residuals (also known as *feathering* or *peeling*) is a useful procedure for fitting a curve to the experimental data of a drug, which demonstrates the necessity of a multicompartment model. For example, 100 mg of a drug was administered by rapid IV injection to a 70-kg healthy adult male. Blood samples were taken periodically after the administration of drug and the plasma fraction of each sample was assayed for drug. The following data were obtained:

Time (hr)	*Plasma Concentration (μg/ml)*	*Time (hr)*	*Plasma Concentration (μg/ml)*
0.25	43	4.0	6.5
0.5	32	8.0	2.8
1.0	20	12.0	1.2
1.5	14	16.0	0.52
2.0	11		

When these data are plotted on semilogarithmic graph paper, a curved line is observed (Fig. 5-4). The curved-line relationship between the logarithm of the plasma concentration and time indicates that the drug is distributed in more than one compartment. From these data a biexponential equation, Equation 5.10, may be derived, either by computer or by the method of residuals.

From the biexponential curve in Figure 5-4 one can see that the initial distribution rate is more rapid than the elimination rate. This means that rate constant a will be larger than rate constant b. Therefore, at some later time the term Ae^{-at} will approach zero while B will still have a value. At this time Equation 5.10 will reduce to

$$C_p = Be^{-bt} \tag{5.13}$$

which in common logarithms is

$$\log C_p = \frac{-bt}{2.3} + \log B \tag{5.14}$$

From Equation 5.14 the rate constant b can be obtained from the slope $(-b/2.3)$ of a straight line representing the terminal exponential phase (Fig. 5-3). The $t_{1/2}$ for the elimination phase can be derived from the following relationship:

$$t_{1/2} = \frac{0.693}{b} \tag{5.15}$$

In the sample case considered here, b was found to be 0.21 hr^{-1}. From this information the regression line for the terminal exponential or b phase is extrapolated to the y axis; the y intercept is equal to B, or 15 μg/ml. Values from the extrapolated line are then subtracted from the original experimental data points (Table 5-2) and a straight line is obtained. This line represents the rapidly distributed a phase (Fig. 5-4).

The new line obtained by graphing the logarithm of the residual plasma concentration $(C_p - C_{p'})$ against time represents the a phase. The value for a is 1.8 hr^{-1} and the y intercept is 45 μg/ml. The elimination $t_{1/2}$ is computed from b by use of Equation 5.15 and has the value of 3.3 hr.

A number of pharmacokinetic parameters may be derived by proper substitu-

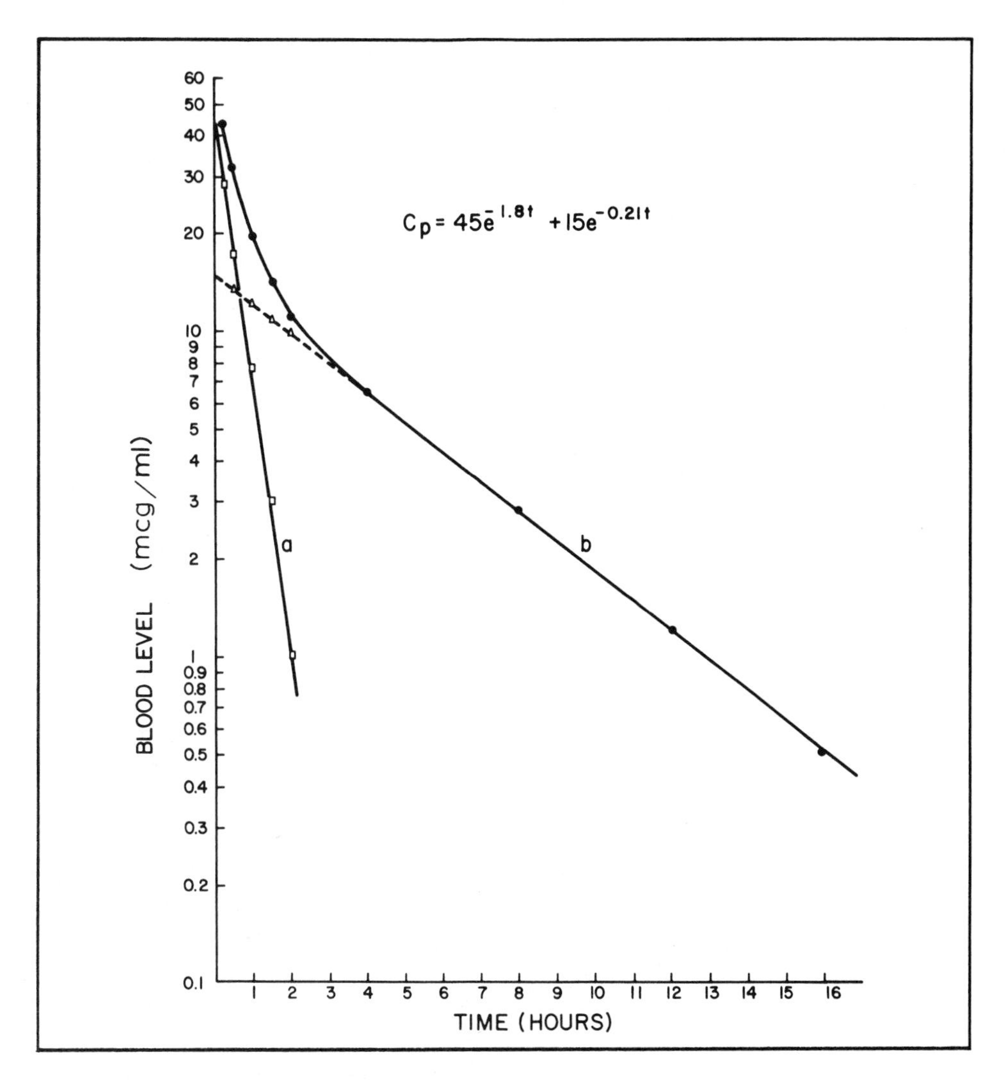

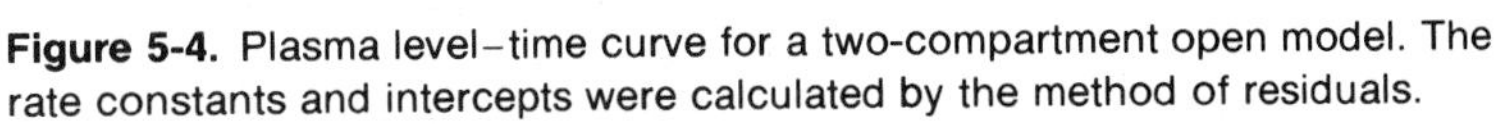

Figure 5-4. Plasma level–time curve for a two-compartment open model. The rate constants and intercepts were calculated by the method of residuals.

tion of rate constants a and b and y intercepts A and B into the following equations:

$$K = \frac{ab(A + B)}{Ab + Ba} \tag{5.16}$$

$$K_{12} = \frac{AB(b - a)^2}{(A + B)(Ab + Ba)} \tag{5.17}$$

$$K_{21} = \frac{Ab + Ba}{A + B} \tag{5.18}$$

TABLE 5-2. APPLICATION OF THE METHOD OF RESIDUALS

Time (hr)	C_p, Observed Plasma Level	C'_p Extrapolated Plasma Concentration	$C_p - C_{p'}$, Residual Plasma Concentration
0.25	43.0	14.5	28.5
0.5	32.0	13.5	18.5
1.0	20.0	12.3	7.7
1.5	14.0	11.0	3.0
2.0	11.0	10.0	1.0
4.0	6.5		
8.0	2.8		
12.0	1.2		
16.0	0.52		

Apparent Volumes of Distribution

As discussed in Chapter 4, the apparent V_d is a useful parameter that relates plasma concentration to the amount of drug in the body. In multiple-compartment kinetics we may consider mathematically hypothetical volumes, such as the volume of the central compartment and the volume of the peripheral or tissue compartment. There are several volumes of distribution that may be considered for a drug that assumes a two-compartment open model. The calculations for each of these volumes are shown below.

Volume of the Central Compartment. The volume of the central compartment, V_p, is useful for describing changes in drug concentration, since the central compartment is usually the sampling compartment. V_p is useful in the determination of drug clearance. In addition, the magnitude of V_p gives an indication of the distribution of the drug in body water. As in the case of the one-compartment model, V_p may be determined from the dose and the instantaneous plasma drug concentration C_p^0.

$$V_p = \frac{D_0}{C_p^0} \tag{5.19}$$

At zero time ($t = 0$) all of the drug in the body is in the central compartment. C_p^0 can be shown to be equal to $A + B$ by the following equations.

$$C_p = Ae^{-at} + Be^{-bt} \tag{5.20}$$

At $t = 0$, $e^0 = 1$. Therefore,

$$C_p^0 = A + B$$

V_p is determined from Equation 5.21 by measuring A and B after feathering the curve, as discussed previously:

$$V_p = \frac{D_0}{A + B} \tag{5.21}$$

Alternatively, the volume of the central compartment may be calculated from the $[AUC]_0^\infty$ in a manner similar to the calculation for the apparent V_d in the one-compartment model. For a one-compartment model

$$[AUC]_0^\infty = \frac{D_0}{KV_d} \quad (5.22)$$

In contrast, $[AUC]_0^\infty$ for the two-compartment model is

$$[AUC]_0^\infty = \frac{D_0}{KV_p} \quad (5.23)$$

Rearrangement of this equation yields

$$V_p = \frac{D_0}{K[AUC]_0^\infty} \quad (5.24)$$

Apparent Volume of Distribution at Steady State. At steady-state conditions the rate of drug entry into the tissue compartment from the central compartment is equal to the rate of drug exit from the tissue compartment into the central compartment. These rates of drug transfer are described by the following expressions:

$$D_t K_{21} = D_p K_{12} \quad (5.25)$$

$$D_t = \frac{K_{12} D_p}{K_{21}} \quad (5.26)$$

Since the amount of drug in the central compartment D_p is equal to $V_p C_p$, then by substitution in the above equation,

$$D_t = \frac{K_{12} C_p V_p}{K_{21}} \quad (5.27)$$

The total amount of drug in the body at steady state is equal to the sum of the amount of drug in the tissue compartment, D_t, and the amount of drug in the central compartment, D_p. Therefore, the apparent volume of drug at steady state $(V_d)_{ss}$ may be calculated by dividing the total amount of drug in the body by the concentration of drug in the central compartment at steady state:

$$(V_d)_{ss} = \frac{D_p + D_t}{C_p} \quad (5.28)$$

By substitution of Equation 5.27 into Equation 5.25, and by expressing D_p as $V_p C_p$, a more useful equation for the calculation of $(V_d)_{ss}$ is obtained:

$$(V_d)_{ss} = \frac{C_p V_p + K_{12} V_p C_p / K_{21}}{C_p} \quad (5.29)$$

which reduces to

$$(V_d)_{ss} = V_p + \frac{K_{12}}{K_{21}} V_p \quad (5.30)$$

In practice, Equation 5.30 is used to calculate $(V_d)_{ss}$. The $(V_d)_{ss}$ is a function of the transfer constants, K_{12} and K_{21}, which represent the rate constants of drug into and out of the tissue compartment, respectively.

Extrapolated Volume of Distribution. The extrapolated volume of distribution $(V_d)_{exp}$ is calculated by the following equation:

$$(V_d)_{exp} = \frac{D_0}{B} \tag{5.31}$$

where B is the y intercept obtained by extrapolation of the b phase of the plasma level curve to the y axis (Fig. 5-1). Since the y intercept is a hybrid constant, as shown by Equation 5.12, $(V_d)_{exp}$ may also be calculated by the following expression:

$$(V_d)_{exp} = V_p \frac{a - b}{K_{21} - b} \tag{5.32}$$

This equation shows that a change in the distribution of a drug, which is observed by a change in the value for V_p, will be reflected in a change in $(V_d)_{exp}$.

Volume of Distribution by Area. The volume of distribution by area $(V_d)_{area}$, also known as $(V_d)_\beta$, is obtained through calculations similar to those used to find V_p, except that the rate constant b is used instead of the overall elimination rate constant K.

$$(V_d)_\beta = (V_d)_{area} = \frac{D_0}{b[\mathrm{AUC}]_0^\infty} \tag{5.33}$$

Since total body clearance is equal to $D_0/[\mathrm{AUC}]_0^\infty$, $(V_d)_\beta$ may be expressed in terms of clearance and the rate constant b:

$$(V_d)_\beta = \frac{\text{clearance}}{b} \tag{5.34}$$

By substitution of KV_p for clearance in Equation 5.34, one obtains

$$(V_d)_\beta = \frac{KV_p}{b} \tag{5.35}$$

Significance of the Volumes of Distribution

From Equations 5.34 and 5.35 we can observe that $(V_d)_\beta$ is affected by changes in the overall elimination rate (i.e., changes in K) and by change in total body clearance of the drug. After the drug is distributed, the total amount of drug in the body during the elimination of b phase is calculated by using $(V_d)_\beta$.

In contrast, $(V_d)_{ss}$ is not affected by changes in drug elimination. $(V_d)_{ss}$ reflects the true distributional volume changes and not changes due to renal function. As mentioned previously, V_p represents the apparent volume of the central compartment and is useful in the calculation of drug clearance. The magnitude of the various apparent volumes of distribution have the following relationship to each other:

$$(V_d)_{exp} > (V_d)_\beta > V_p$$

In a study involving a cardiotonic drug given intravenously to a group of normal and congestive heart failure (CHF) patients, it was found that the average AUC for CHF was 40% higher than the normal subjects, and that the b elimination constant was 40% less in CHF patients whereas the average $(V_d)_\beta$ remained essentially the same. In spite of the edematous conditions of these patients, the volume of distribution apparently remained constant. No change was found in the V_p or $(V_d)_\beta$. In this case the volume of distribution was estimated by using Equation 5.33. In this study a 40% increase in AUC in the CHF subjects was offset by a 40% smaller b elimination constant estimated by using computer methods. Since the dose was the same, the $(V_d)_\beta$ would not change unless the increase in AUC is not accompanied by a change in b elimination constant.

From Equation 5.34 the clearance of the drug in CHF patients was reduced by 40% as a result of decrease in the b elimination constant, possibly due to a reduction in renal blood flow as a result of reduced cardiac output in CHF patients.

In dealing with drugs that follow two-compartment model kinetics, changes in disease states may not result in different pharmacokinetic parameters. Conversely, changes in pharmacokinetic parameters should not be attributed to physiologic changes without careful consideration of method of curve fitting and intersubject differences. Equation 5.35 shows that unlike a simple one-compartment open model, $(V_d)_\beta$ may be estimated from K, b, and V_p. Error in fitting is easily carried over to the others even if they are estimated by computer method. The terms K_{12} and K_{21} often fluctuate due to minor fitting and experimental difference and may affect calculation of other parameters.

Drug in the Tissue Compartment

The apparent volume of the tissue compartment (V_t) is a conceptual volume only and does not represent true anatomic volumes. The V_t may be calculated from knowledge of the transfer rate constants and V_p.

$$V_t = \frac{V_p K_{12}}{K_{21}} \tag{5.36}$$

The calculation of the amount of drug in the tissue compartment does not entail the use of V_t. Calculation of the drug concentration in the tissue compartment is useful, since the pharmacologic activity may correlate better with the tissue drug level–time curve. To calculate the amount of drug in the tissue compartment D_t, the following expression is used:

$$D_t = \frac{K_{12} D_0}{a - b}(e^{-bt} - e^{-at}) \tag{5.37}$$

The amount of drug in the tissue compartment is also related to the amount of drug in the central compartment and the transfer constants, as shown in Equation 5.37.

Elimination Rate Constant

In the two-compartment model (IV administration) the elimination rate constant K represents the elimination of drug from the central compartment, whereas b represents drug elimination from the entire body after the diffusable drug has established an equilibrium. Therefore, b is useful in calculating $t_{1/2}$ and multiple-dosage regimens.

THREE-COMPARTMENT OPEN MODEL

The three-compartment model is an extension of the two-compartment model, with an additional deep tissue compartment. A drug which demonstrates the necessity of a three-compartment open model is distributed most rapidly to a highly perfused central compartment, less rapidly to the second or tissue compartment, and very slowly to the third or deep tissue compartment, containing such poorly perfused tissue as bone and fat. The deep tissue compartment may also represent tightly bound drug in the tissues. The three-compartment open model is shown in Figure 5-5.

A solution of the differential equation describing the rates of flow of drug into and out of the central compartment gives the following equation:

$$C_p = Ae^{-at} + Be^{-bt} + Ce^{-ct} \tag{5.38}$$

where A, B, and C are the y intercepts of extrapolated lines for the central, tissue, and deep tissue compartments, respectively, and a, b, and c are first-order rate constants for the central, tissue, and deep tissue compartments, respectively.

The parameters in Equation 5.23 may be solved graphically by the method of residuals (Fig. 5-6) or by computer. The equations for the elimination rate constant

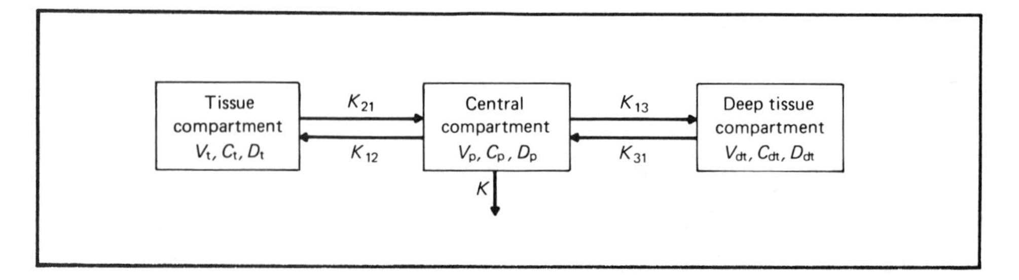

Figure 5-5. Three-compartment open model. This model, as with the previous two-compartment models, assumes that all drug elimination occurs via the central compartment.

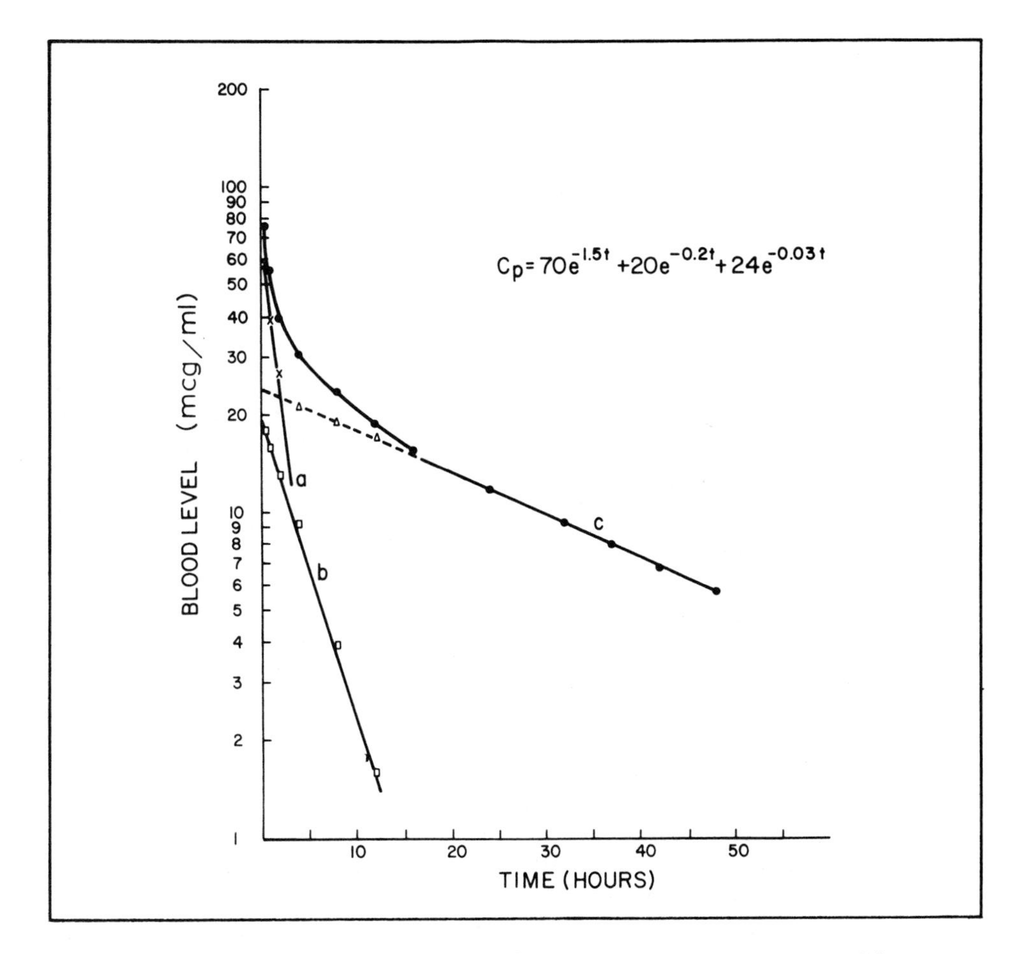

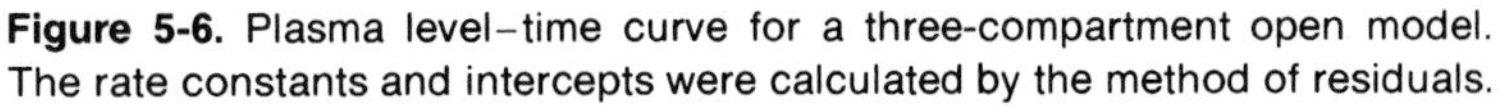

Figure 5-6. Plasma level–time curve for a three-compartment open model. The rate constants and intercepts were calculated by the method of residuals.

K, volume of the central compartment, and area are shown in the following equations:

$$K = \frac{(A + B + C)abc}{Abc + Bac + Cab} \tag{5.39}$$

$$V_p = \frac{D_0}{A + B + C} \tag{5.40}$$

$$[\text{AUC}] = \frac{A}{a} + \frac{B}{b} + \frac{C}{c} \tag{5.41}$$

DETERMINATION OF COMPARTMENT MODELS

Models based on compartmental analysis always use the fewest number of compartments necessary to adequately describe the experimental data. Once an empirical equation is derived from the experimental observations, it becomes necessary to

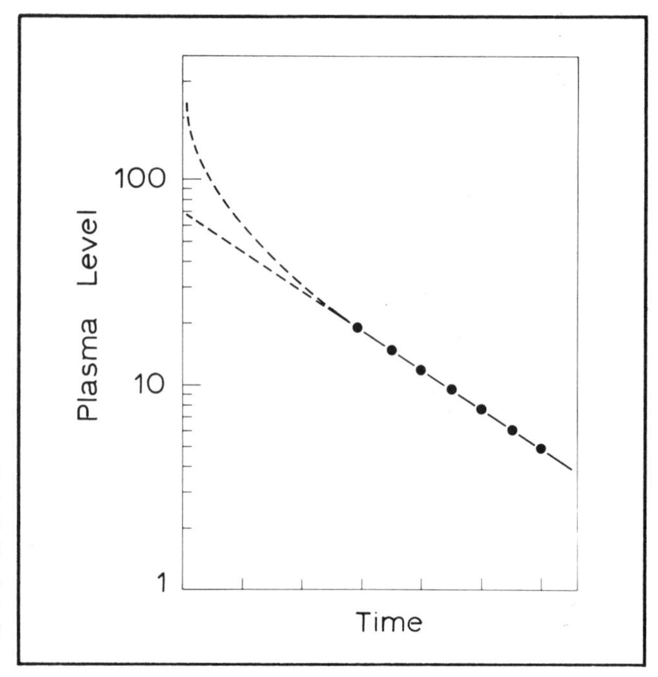

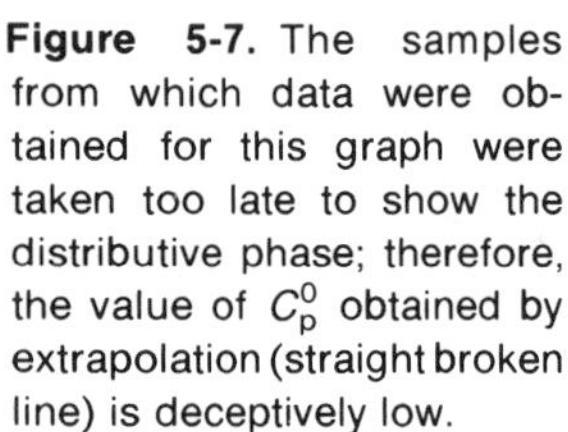

Figure 5-7. The samples from which data were obtained for this graph were taken too late to show the distributive phase; therefore, the value of C_p^0 obtained by extrapolation (straight broken line) is deceptively low.

examine how well the theoretical values calculated from the derived equation fit the experimental data.

Depending on the sampling intervals, it is also possible to miss a compartment, since samples may be taken too late after administration of the dose to observe a possible distributive phase. For example, the data plotted in Figure 5-7 could easily be mistaken for those of a one-compartment model, since the distributive phase has been missed and extrapolation of the data to C_p^0 will give a lower value than was actually the case.

In describing compartments, each new compartment requires an additional first-order plot. Compartment models having more than three compartments are rarely of pharmacologic significance. In certain cases it is possible to "lump" a few compartments together to get a smaller number of compartments which together will describe the data adequately.

An adequate description of several tissue compartments can be difficult. When addition of a compartment to the model seems necessary, it is important to realize that the drug may be retained or slowly concentrated in a deep tissue compartment.

QUESTIONS

1. A drug was administered by rapid IV injection into an 70-kg adult male. Blood samples were withdrawn over a 7-hr period and assayed for intact drug. The results are tabulated below. Calculate the values for intercepts A

and B and slopes a, b, K, K_{12}, and K_{21}.

Time (hr)	C_p *(μg/ml)*	*Time (hr)*	C_p *(μg/ml)*
0.00	70.0	2.5	14.3
0.25	53.8	3.0	12.6
0.50	43.3	4.0	10.5
0.75	35.0	5.0	9.0
1.00	29.1	6.0	8.0
1.50	21.2	7.0	7.0
2.00	17.0		

2. A 70-kg male subject was given 150 mg of a drug by IV injection. Blood samples were removed and assayed for intact drug. Calculate the slopes and intercepts of the three phases of the plasma level versus time plot from the results tabulated below. Give the equation for the curve.

Time (hr)	C_p *(μg/ml)*	*Time (hr)*	C_p *(μg/ml)*
0.17	36.2	3.0	13.9
0.33	34.0	4.0	12.0
0.50	27.0	6.0	8.7
0.67	23.0	7.7	7.7
1.0	20.8	18.0	3.2
1.5	17.8	23.0	2.4
2.0	16.5		

3. Mitenko and Ogilvie[2] demonstrated that theophylline followed a two-compartment pharmacokinetic model in human subjects. After administering a single intravenous dose (5.6 mg/kg) in nine normal volunteers, these investigators demonstrated that the equation best describing theophylline kinetics in humans was

$$C_p = 12e^{-5.8t} + 18e^{-0.16t}$$

What is the plasma level of the drug 3 hr after the IV dose?

4. A drug has a distribution that can be described by a two-compartment open model. If the drug is given by IV bolus, then what is the cause of the initial or rapid decline in blood levels (a phase)? What is the cause of the slower decline in blood levels (b phase)?

5. What does it mean when a drug demonstrates a plasma level–time curve that indicates a three-compartment open model? Can this curve be described by a two-compartment model?

6. A drug that follows a multicompartment pharmacokinetic model is given to a patient by rapid intravenous injection. Would the drug concentration in each tissue be the same after the drug equilibrates with the plasma and all the tissues in the body? Explain.

7. Polk et al.[3] studied the pharmacokinetics of amrinone after a single IV bolus injection (75 mg) in 14 healthy adult male volunteers. The pharmacokinetics of this drug followed a two-compartment open model and fitted the following equation:

$$C_p = Ae^{-at} + Be^{-bt}$$

where

$$A = 4.62 \pm 12.0\ \mu g/ml$$
$$B = 0.64 \pm 0.17\ \mu g/ml$$
$$a = 8.94 \pm 13\ hr^{-1}$$
$$b = 0.19 \pm 0.06\ hr^{-1}$$

From these data calculate:

a. The volume of the central compartment.
b. The volume of the tissue compartment.
c. The transfer constants K_{12} and K_{21}.
d. The elimination rate constant from the central compartment.
e. The elimination half-life of amrinone after the drug has equilibrated with the tissue compartment.

8. A drug may be described by a three-compartment model involving a central compartment and two peripheral tissue compartments. If you *could* sample the tissue compartments (organs), in which organs would you expect to find a drug level corresponding to the two theoretical peripheral tissue compartments?

REFERENCES

1. Butler TC: The distribution of drugs. In LaDu BN, et al. (eds.), Fundamentals of Drug Metabolism and Disposition. Baltimore, Williams and Wilkins, 1972
2. Mitenko PA, Ogilvie RI: Pharmacokinetics of intravenous theophylline. Clin Pharmacol Ther 14:509, 1973
3. Park GP, Kershner RP, Angellotti J, et al: Oral bioavailability and intravenous pharmacokinetics of amrinone in humans. J Pharm Sci 72:817, 1983

BIBLIOGRAPHY

Dvorchick BH, Vessell ES: Significance of error associated with use of the one-compartment formula to calculate clearance of 38 drugs. Clin Pharmacol Ther 23:617–23, 1978

Jusko WJ, Gibaldo M: Effects of change in elimination on various parameters of the two-compartment open model. J Pharm Sci 61: 1270–73, 1972

Loughman PM, Sitar DS, Olgivie RI, Neims AH: The two-compartment open-system kinetic model: A review of its clinical implications and applications. J Pediatr 88:869–73, 1976

Mayersohn M, Gibaldi M: Mathematical methods in pharmacokinetics, II: Solution of the two-compartment open model. Am J Pharm Ed 35: 19–28, 1971

Riegelman, S, Loo JCK, Rowland M: Concept of a volume of distribution and possible errors in evaluation of this parameter. J Pharm Sci 57:128–33, 1968

Riegelman S, Loo JCK, Rowland M: Shortcomings in pharmacokinetics analysis by conceiving the body to exhibit properties of a single compartment. J Pharm Sci 57:117–23, 1968

CHAPTER SIX

Biopharmaceutic Aspects of Drug Products

Biopharmaceutics is the study of the relationship of the physicochemical properties of a drug formulation to the bioavailability of the drug. Bioavailability refers to the rate and the amount of active drug that reaches the systemic circulation. Because the bioavailability of a drug influences its therapeutic, clinical, and toxic activity, the study of biopharmaceutics is becoming increasingly important. The aim of biopharmaceutics is to adjust the delivery of drug to the systemic circulation in such a way as to provide optimal therapeutic activity for a given clinical situation.

The systemic absorption of a drug from an extravascular site is influenced by the anatomic and physiologic properties of the site and the physicochemical properties of the drug and the drug product. Biopharmaceutics attempts to control these variables by designing a drug product with a specific therapeutic objective. By carefully choosing the route of drug administration and properly designing the drug product, the bioavailability of the active drug can be varied from very rapid and complete absorption to a slow, sustained rate of absorption or even virtually no absorption. Once the drug is systemically absorbed, normal physiologic processes for distribution and elimination occur which usually are not influenced by the specific formulation of the drug. Because of the factors involved in drug bioavailability, particularly in gastrointestinal absorption, drug levels after enteral administration are subject to more variation than are drug levels after parenteral administration.

FACTORS IN DRUG BIOAVAILABILITY

Systemic absorption of most drug products consists of a succession of rate processes (Fig. 6-1). These processes include (1) disintegration of the drug product and subsequent release of the drug; (2) dissolution of the drug in an aqueous environment; and (3) absorption across cell membranes into the systemic circulation. In the process of drug disintegration, dissolution, and absorption, the rate at which drug reaches the circulatory system is determined by the slowest step in the sequence.

The slowest step in a series of kinetic processes is called the *rate-limiting* step. Except for sustained-release or prolonged-action products, disintegration of a solid drug product is usually more rapid than drug dissolution and drug absorption. For drugs that have very poor aqueous solubility, the rate at which the drug dissolves (dissolution) is often the slowest step and therefore exerts a rate-limiting effect on drug bioavailability. In contrast, for a drug which has a high aqueous solubility, the dissolution rate is rapid and the rate at which the drug crosses or permeates cell membranes is the slowest or rate-limiting step.

Physiologic Factors Related to Drug Absorption

Passage of Drug Across Cell Membranes. In order for a drug to reach the site of action in a tissue or organ, it must cross cellular membranes. There are several theories as to the exact structure of cell membranes, including the unit membrane and the fluid (dynamic) mosaic models. In general, cell membranes are considered to be lipoprotein structures which act as semipermeable lipid membranes. Various studies have been carried out with drugs of different structures and physicochemical properties and with various cell membranes, and as a result the mechanisms by which drugs are transported across cellular membranes are to some extent known. One finding is that there appears to be some general physicochemical properties of molecules which influence the rate at which the drug crosses the cell membrane. One major factor is the lipid solubility of the molecule.

Many drugs contain both lipophilic and hydrophilic chemical substituents. Those drugs which are more lipid soluble tend to traverse cell membranes more easily than less lipid-soluble or more water-soluble molecules. For drugs which act as weak electrolytes, such as weak acids and bases, the extent of ionization influences the rate of drug transport. The ionized species of the drug contains a charge and is more water soluble than the nonionized species of the drug, which is more lipid soluble. The extent of ionization of a weak electrolyte will depend on both the pK_a of the drug and the pH of the medium in which the drug is dissolved. Henderson and Hasselbalch used the following expressions pertaining to weak acids and weak bases to describe the relationship between pK_a and pH.

For weak acids:

$$\text{Ratio} = \frac{(\text{salt})}{(\text{acid})} = \frac{(\text{A}^-)}{(\text{HA})} = 10^{(\text{pH} - \text{pK}_a)} \tag{6.1}$$

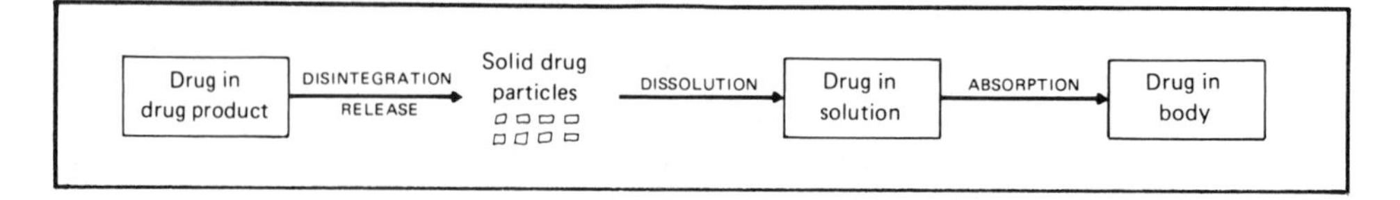

Figure 6-1. Rate processes of drug bioavailability.

For weak bases:

$$\text{Ratio} = \frac{(\text{base})}{(\text{salt})} = \frac{(\text{RNH}_2)}{(\text{RNH}_3^+)} = 10^{(\text{pH}-\text{pK}_\text{a})} \qquad (6.2)$$

With Equations 6.1 and 6.2, the proportion of free acid or free base existing as the nonionized species may be determined at any given pH, assuming the pK_a for the drug is known. For example, at a plasma pH of 7.4, salicylic acid (pK_a 3.0) would exist mostly in its ionized or water-soluble form as shown below:

$$\text{Ratio} = \frac{(\text{salt})}{(\text{acid})} = 10^{(7.4-3.0)}$$

$$\log \frac{(\text{salt})}{(\text{acid})} = 7.4 - 3.0 = 4.4$$

$$\frac{(\text{Salt})}{(\text{Acid})} = 2.51 \times 10^4$$

Another physicochemical property that influences the passage of a drug across a cell membrane is molecular size. Very small molecules (as urea) and small ions (such as Na^+, K^+, and Li^-) move across cell membranes rapidly, as if the membrane contained *pores*. In contrast, very large macromolecules (such as proteins) either do not traverse cell membranes or do so very poorly. Drugs which are tightly bound to proteins act as macromolecules and do not cross cell membranes. This phenomenon occurs very often when drugs bind plasma proteins.

In addition to the physicochemical properties of the drug molecules, there are also a number of physiologic transport phenomena which influence the mechanism by which a drug traverses the cell membrane.

Passive Diffusion. Passive diffusion is the major transmembrane process for most drugs. The driving force for passive diffusion is the difference in drug concentrations on either side of the cell membrane. According to *Fick's law of diffusion*, drug molecules diffuse from a region of high drug concentration to a region of low drug concentration:

$$\frac{dQ}{dt} = \frac{DAK}{h}(C_{\text{GI}} - C_\text{p}) \qquad (6.3)$$

where dQ/dt = rate of diffusion; D = diffusion coefficient; K = partition coefficient; A = surface area of membrane; h = membrane thickness; and $C_{GI} - C_p$ = difference between the concentrations of drug in the gastrointestinal tract and in the plasma.

Since the drug is distributed rapidly into a large volume after entering the blood, the concentration of drug in the blood will be quite low with respect to the concentration at the site of drug administration. For example, drug is usually given in milligram doses, whereas plasma concentrations are often in the microgram per milliliter or nanogram per milliliter range. If the drug is given orally, then $C_{GI} \gg C_p$ and a large concentration gradient is maintained, acting as a "driving force" during absorption.

Given Fick's law of diffusion, several other factors can be seen to influence the rate of passive diffusion of drugs. For example, the degree of lipid solubility of the drug will influence the rate of drug absorption. The partition coefficient, K, represents the oil–water partitioning of a drug. Drugs which are more lipid soluble will have a larger value for K. The surface area of the membrane also influences the rate of absorption. Drugs may be absorbed from most areas of the gastrointestinal tract. However, the duodenal area of the small intestine shows the most rapid drug absorption due to such anatomic features as villi and microvilli, which provide a large surface area. These villi are not found in such numbers in other areas of the gastrointestinal tract.

The thickness of the membrane, h, is a constant for any particular absorption site. Drugs usually diffuse very rapidly through capillary cell membranes in the vascular compartments, in contrast to diffusion through cell membranes of capillaries in the brain. In the brain the capillaries are densely lined with glial cells, so that a drug diffuses slowly into the brain as if a thick lipid membrane existed. The term *blood–brain barrier* is used to describe the poor diffusion of water-soluble molecules across capillary cell membranes into the brain. However, in certain disease states these cell membranes may be disrupted or become more permeable to drug diffusion.

The diffusion coefficient, D, is a constant for each drug and is defined as the number of moles of a drug that diffuses across a membrane of a given unit area per unit time when the concentration gradient is unity. The dimensions of D are area per unit time—e.g., cm^2/sec.

Since D, A, K, and h are constants under usual conditions for absorption, a combined constant P or permeability coefficient may be defined.

$$P = \frac{DAK}{h} \tag{6.4}$$

Furthermore, in Equation 6.3 the drug concentration in the plasma, C_p, is extremely small compared to the drug concentration in the gastrointestinal tract, C_{GI}. If C_p is negligible and P is substituted into Equation 6.3, the following relationship for Fick's law is obtained.

$$\frac{dQ}{dt} = P(C_{GI}) \tag{6.5}$$

Equation 6.5 is an expression for a first-order process. In practice, the extravascular absorption of most drugs tends to be a first-order absorption process. Moreover, due to the large concentration gradient between C_{GI} and C_p, the rate of drug absorption is usually more rapid than the rate of drug elimination.

The concentrations of a drug on either side of a membrane should be the same at equilibrium, assuming Fick's law of diffusion is the only distribution factor involved. For nonelectrolyte drugs, or drugs which do not ionize, the concentrations on both sides of the membrane at distribution equilibrium may be the same. For drugs that ionize, the concentrations on either side of the membrane may not be equal if the pH of the medium differs on respective sides of the membrane. For example, consider the concentration of salicylic acid (pK_a 3.0) in the stomach (pH 1.2) as opposed to the concentration in the plasma (pH 7.4) (Fig. 6-2).

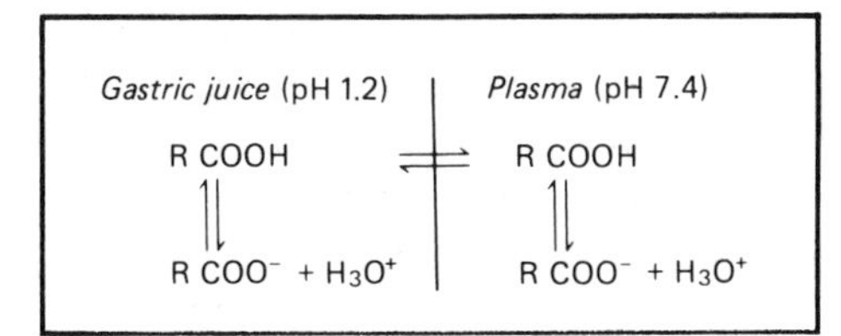

Figure 6-2. Model for the distribution of an orally administered weak electrolyte drug such as salicylic acid.

As shown by the Henderson–Hasselbalch equation (Eq. 6.1) for weak acids, at pH 7.4 and at pH 1.2, salicylic acid would exist in the following ratios.

In the plasma, at pH 7.4:

$$\text{Ratio} = \frac{(\text{R COO}^-)}{(\text{R COOH})} = 2.51 \times 10^4$$

In gastric juice, at pH 1.2:

$$\text{Ratio} = \frac{(\text{R COO}^-)}{(\text{R COOH})} = 10^{(1.2-3.0)} = 1.58 \times 10^{-2}$$

The total drug concentration on either side of the membrane is determined as shown in Table 6-1. Thus it can be seen that the pH affects distribution of salicylic acid (R COOH) and its salt (R COO$^-$) across cell membranes. It is assumed that the acid, R COOH, is freely permeable and the salt, R COO$^-$, is not permeable across the cell membrane. In this example the total concentration of salicylic acid at equilibrium is approximately 25,000 times greater in the plasma than in the stomach (Table 6-1). These calculations can also be applied to weak bases, as well as using Equation 6.2.

According to the *pH–partition hypotheses*, if the pH on one side of a cell membrane differs from the pH on the other side of the membrane, then (1) the drug (weak acid or base) will ionize to different degrees on respective sides of the membrane; (2) the total drug concentrations (ionized plus nonionized drug) on either side of the membrane will be unequal; and (3) the compartment in which the drug is more highly ionized will contain the greater total drug concentration. For these reasons, a weak acid (such as salicylic acid) would be rapidly absorbed from the stomach (pH 1.2), whereas a weak base (such as quinidine) would be poorly absorbed from the stomach.

TABLE 6-1. RELATIVE CONCENTRATIONS OF SALICYLIC ACID AS AFFECTED BY pH

Drug	Gastric Juice (pH 1.2)	Plasma (pH 7.4)
R COOH	1.0000	1
R COO$^-$	0.0158	25100
Total drug concentration	1.0158	25101

Another factor that can influence drug concentrations on either side of a membrane is a particular *affinity* of the drug for a tissue component, which would prevent the drug from freely moving back across the cell membrane. For example, a drug might bind plasma or tissue proteins. This drug–protein binding has been described for dicumarol, certain sulfonamides, and other drugs. Moreover, a drug such as chlordane, a lipid-soluble insecticide, might dissolve in the adipose (fat) tissue. In addition, a drug such as tetracycline might form a complex with calcium in the bones and teeth. Finally, a drug may concentrate in a tissue due to a specific uptake or active transport process. Such processes have been demonstrated for iodide in thyroid tissue, potassium in the intracellular water, and certain catecholamines in adrenergic storage sites.

Active Transport. *Active transport* is a carrier-mediated transmembrane process which plays an important role in the renal and biliary secretion of many drugs and metabolites. A few lipid-insoluble drugs which resemble natural physiologic metabolites (such as 5-fluorouracil) are absorbed from the gastrointestinal tract by this process. Active transport is characterized by the fact that the drug is transported against a concentration gradient—i.e., from regions of low drug concentrations to regions of high concentrations. Therefore, this is an energy-consuming system. In addition, active transport is a specialized process requiring a carrier that binds the drug to form a carrier–drug complex which shuttles the drug across the membrane and then dissociates the drug on the other side of the membrane (Fig. 6-3).

The carrier molecule may be highly selective for the drug molecule. If the drug structurally resembles a natural substrate that is actively transported, then it is likely to be actively transported by the same carrier mechanism. Therefore, drugs of similar structure may compete for sites of adsorption on the carrier. Furthermore, since only a certain amount of carrier is available, all the adsorption sites on the carrier may become saturated if the drug concentration gets very high. A comparison between the rate of drug absorption and the concentration of drug at the absorption site is shown in Figure 6-4. Notice that for a drug absorbed by passive diffusion, the rate of absorption increases in a linear relationship to drug concentration. In contrast, when a drug is absorbed by a carrier-mediated process, the rate of drug absorption increases with drug concentration until the carrier molecules are completely saturated. At higher drug concentrations the rate of drug absorption remains constant.

Facilitated Diffusion. Facilitated diffusion is also a carrier-mediated transport system, differing from active transport in that the drug moves along a concentration

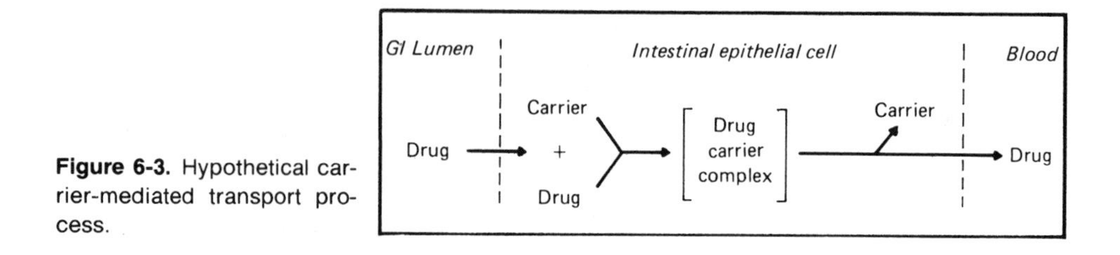

Figure 6-3. Hypothetical carrier-mediated transport process.

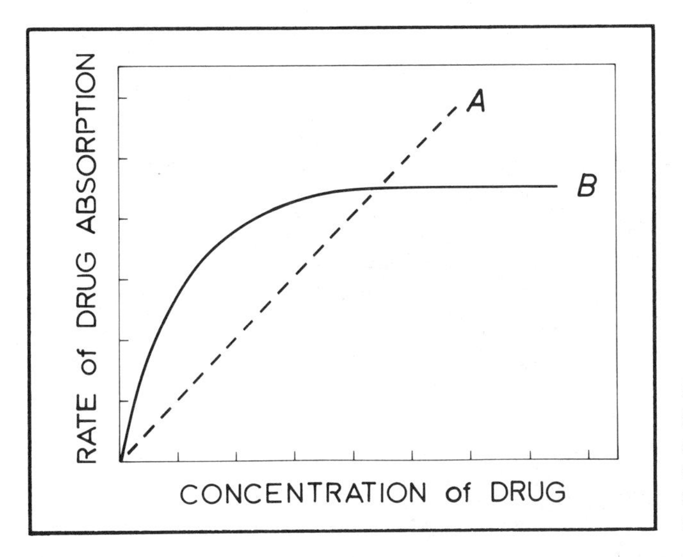

Figure 6-4. Comparison of the rates of drug absorption of a drug absorbed by passive diffusion (line *A*) and a drug absorbed by a carrier mediated system (line *B*).

gradient (i.e., moves from a region of high drug concentration to a region of low drug concentration). Therefore, this system does not require energy input. However, since this system is carrier mediated, it is saturable and structurally selective for the drug and shows competition kinetics for drugs of similar structure. In terms of drug absorption, facilitated diffusion seems to play a very minor role.

Pinocytosis (Vesicular Transport). *Pinocytosis* is the process of the engulfment of large macromolecules. This is a process of phagocytosis by which the cell membrane invaginates to surround macromolecular material and then engulfs the material into the cell. The macromolecule remains within the cell as a vesicle or vacuole. Pinocytosis is the proposed process for the absorption of the orally administered sabin polio vaccine and various large protein molecules.

Pore (Convective) Transport. Very small molecules (such as urea, water, and sugars) are able to rapidly cross cell membranes as if the membrane contained channels or pores. Although such pores have never been directly observed by microscopy, the model of drug permeation through aqueous pores is used to explain renal excretion of drugs and uptake of drugs into the liver.

Transit Time of Drug in the Gastrointestinal Tract. The small intestine, and particularly the duodenal mucosa, provides a large surface area for drug absorption. To ensure rapid absorption of a drug after oral administration, the drug should reach the duodenal area quickly.

Anatomically, the swallowed drug first reaches the stomach. Eventually, the stomach empties its contents into the small intestine, which has the best capacity for drug absorption. Therefore, any factor which affects gastrointestinal motility can affect the rate of drug absorption.

A delay in *gastric emptying* of drug into the duodenum will slow the rate of drug absorption and thereby delay the onset of the therapeutic effect. A number of factors have been shown to affect the gastric emptying time. Some factors which tend to delay gastric emptying include consumption of meals high in fat, cold beverages, and anticholinergic drugs. Many of these factors were described by Gibaldi (1977). In addition, drugs which are unstable at acid pH, such as penicillin, may decompose if stomach emptying is delayed.

Normal peristaltic movements of the duodenum are helpful to absorption, since these movements bring the drug particles into intimate contact with the intestinal mucosa cells. For optimum absorption, a drug must have a certain *residence time* in the duodenum. When there is a high motility of the duodenum, as in diarrhea, the drug has a very brief residence time in the duodenum and very little opportunity to be absorbed.

Blood Perfusion of the Gastrointestinal Tract. The blood flow to the gastrointestinal tract is important in carrying the drug to the systemic circulation and thence to the site of action. The intestinal area is perfused by the mesenteric blood vessels. The drug is delivered into the liver via the hepatic portal vein and then to the general or systemic circulation. Any decrease in the mesenteric blood flow, as in congestive heart failure, will decrease the rate of removal of drug from the intestinal tract and thereby reduce the rate of drug bioavailability.

Pharmaceutic Factors Affecting Drug Bioavailability

In order to design a drug product that will deliver the active drug in the most bioavailable form, the pharmacist must consider (1) the type of drug product (e.g., solution, suspension, suppository); (2) the nature of the excipients in the drug product; and (3) the physicochemical properties of the drug itself.

As discussed previously, the bioavailability of the active drug in a solid dosage form is dependent on several factors, including (1) disintegration of the drug product and release of the active drug particles; (2) dissolution of the drug; and (3) absorption or permeation of the drug across the cell membranes (Fig. 6-1).

Disintegration. It was generally recognized some years ago that a solid drug product had to disintegrate into small particles and release the drug before absorption could take place. For the purpose of monitoring uniform tablet disintegration, the United States Pharmacopeia (USP) established an official disintegration test. Solid drug products exempted from disintegration tests include troches, tablets which are intended to be chewed, and drug products intended for sustained release or prolonged or repeat action. The process of disintegration does not imply complete dissolution of the tablet and/or the drug. Complete disintegration is defined by the USPXX as "that state in which any residue of the tablet, except fragments of insoluble coating, remaining on the screen of the test apparatus in the soft mass have no palpably firm core." The official apparatus for the disintegration test and procedure is described in the USPXX. Separate specifications are given for uncoated tablets, plain coated tablets, enteric tablets, buccal tablets, and sublingual tablets.

Although disintegration tests allow for precise measurement of the formation of fragments, granules, or aggregates from solid dosage forms, no information is obtained from these tests on the rate of dissolution of the active drug. However, the disintegration tests do serve as a component in the overall quality control of tablet manufacture.

Dissolution. *Dissolution* is the process by which a chemical or drug becomes dissolved in a solvent. In biologic systems drug dissolution in an aqueous medium is an important prior condition of systemic absorption. The rate at which drugs with poor aqueous solubility dissolve from an intact or disintegrated solid dosage form in the gastrointestinal tract often controls the rate of systemic absorption of the drug.

Noyes and Whitney and other investigators studied the rate of dissolution of solid drugs. According to their observations, the steps in dissolution include the process of drug dissolution at the surface of the solid particle, thus forming a saturated solution around the particle. The dissolved drug in the saturated solution known as the "stagnant layer" diffuses to the bulk of the solvent from regions of high drug concentration to regions of low drug concentrations. (Fig. 6-5).

The overall rate of drug dissolution may be described by the *Noyes–Whitney equation*, which resembles Fick's law of diffusion (Eq. 6.3):

$$\frac{dc}{dt} = \frac{DAK}{h}(C_S - C) \tag{6.6}$$

where dc/dt = rate of drug dissolution; D = diffusion rate constant; A = surface area of the particle; C_S = concentration of drug in the stagnant layer; C = concentration of drug in the bulk solvent; K = oil/water partition coefficient; and h = thickness of the stagnant layer.

The rate of dissolution, $(dc/dt) \cdot (1/A)$, is the amount of drug dissolved per unit area per time (e.g., g/cm^2 min).

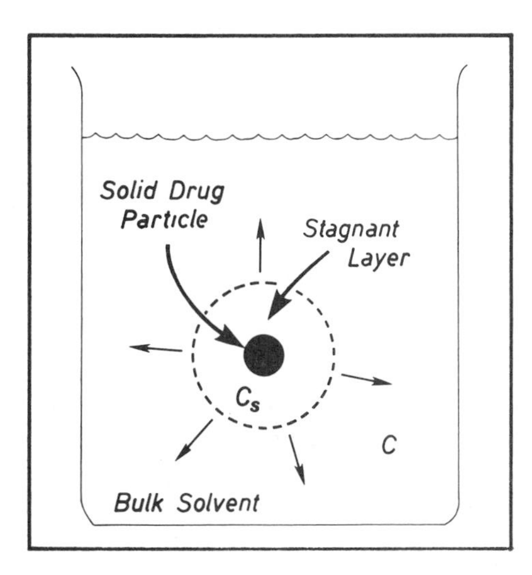

Figure 6-5. Dissolution of a solid drug particle in a solvent. C_S = concentration of drug in the stagnant layer, and C = concentration of drug in the bulk solvent.

It can be seen from the Noyes–Whitney equation (Eq. 6.6) that dissolution kinetics may be influenced by the physicochemical characteristics of the drug, the formulation, and the solvent. Drug in the body, particularly in the gastrointestinal tract, is considered to be dissolving in an aqueous environment.

In addition to these factors, the temperature of the medium and the agitation rate also affect the rate of drug dissolution. In vivo, the temperature is maintained at a constant 37°C, and the agitation (primarily peristaltic movements in the gastrointestinal tract) is reasonably constant. In contrast, in vitro study of dissolution kinetics requires maintenance of constant temperature and agitation. Temperature is generally kept at 37°C, and the agitation or stirring rate is held to a specified constant. An increase in temperature will increase the kinetic energy of the molecules and increase the diffusion constant, D. On the other hand, an increase in agitation of the solvent medium will reduce the thickness, h, of the stagnant layer, allowing for more rapid drug dissolution.

Physicochemical Nature of the Drug. The nature of the physical and chemical properties of the solid drug particles has a great effect on dissolution kinetics. The effective surface area of the drug may be enlarged enormously by a reduction in the particle size. Since dissolution is thought to take place at the surface of the solute, the greater the surface area, the more rapid the rate of drug dissolution. The geometric shape of the particle also affects the surface area, and during dissolution the surface is constantly changing. In calculation, it is usually assumed that the solute particle has retained its geometric shape.

The degree of aqueous solubility of the drug also affects the rate of dissolution. Generally, the ionizable salt of the drug is more water soluble than the free acid or free base. By chemical manipulation, the pharmacist can synthesize various salts of the drug, providing a range of solubility from very water soluble to practically water insoluble. Moreover, if the drug is in the anhydrous state, the rate of dissolution is usually faster than with the hydrous salt.

The drug may also exist in more than one of the crystalline forms known as polymorphs. These polymorphs, which have identical chemical structures, demonstrate different dissolution kinetics. In general, crystalline structures are more rigid and thermodynamically more stable than the amorphous forms of the drug. Thus the amorphous forms of the drug demonstrate faster dissolution rates than the crystalline forms of the drug.

Formulation Factors Affecting Drug Dissolution. The various excipients in the drug product may also affect dissolution kinetics of the drug by either altering the medium in which the drug is dissolving or by reacting with the drug itself. For example, excipients such as suspending agents increase the viscosity of the drug vehicle and thereby diminish the rate of drug dissolution of suspensions. Tablet lubricants such as magnesium stearate may repel water and reduce dissolution when used in large quantities. Surfactants may, however, affect drug dissolution in an unpredictable fashion. Low concentrations of surfactants lower the surface tension and increase the rate of drug dissolution, whereas higher concentrations of surfactants tend to form micelles with the drug and thus decrease the dissolution rate.

Some excipients, such as sodium bicarbonate, may change the pH of the medium. With a solid acid drug, such as aspirin, an alkaline medium adjacent to the acid drug will cause the drug to form a water-soluble salt in which the drug rapidly dissolves. This type of process is called dissolution in a reactive medium. The solid drug may dissolve rapidly in the reactive solvent surrounding the solid particle. However, as the dissolved drug molecules diffuse outward into the bulk solvent, the drug may precipitate out of solution with a very fine particle size. These small particles have enormous collective surface area and disperse easily, coming into contact with the intestinal membrane and redissolving readily for more rapid absorption.

In addition, the excipients in a formulation may interact directly with the drug to form a water-soluble or water-insoluble complex. For example, if tetracycline is formulated with calcium carbonate, an insoluble complex of calcium tetracycline is formed, demonstrating a slow rate of dissolution and poor absorption.

In Vitro Dissolution Testing. Dissolution tests in vitro measure the rate and extent of dissolution of the drug in an aqueous medium in the presence of one or more excipients contained in the drug products. There are a number of factors that must be considered when performing a dissolution test.

For one thing, the size and shape of the container may affect the rate and extent of dissolution. For example, the container may range in size from several milliliters to several liters. The shape of the container may be round-bottomed or flat, so that the tablet might be in a different position in different experiments. Drugs that are not very water soluble may require use of a very-large-capacity container to observe significant dissolution.

A second consideration is the amount of agitation and the nature of the stirrer. Stirring rates must be controlled, and specifications differ between drug products.

The temperature of the dissolution medium must also be controlled and variations in temperature must be avoided. Most dissolution tests are performed at 37°C.

The nature of the dissolution medium will also affect the dissolution test. The solubility of the drug must be considered as well as the amount of drug in the dosage form. The dissolution medium should not be saturated by the drug. Usually, a volume of medium larger than the amount of solvent needed to completely dissolve the drug is used in such tests. Which medium is best is a matter of considerable controversy. Various investigators have used diluted gastric juice, 0.1 N HCl, phosphate buffer, simulated gastric juice, water, and simulated intestinal juice, depending on the nature of the drug product and the location in the gastrointestinal tract where it is predicted the drug will dissolve.

The design of the dissolution apparatus, along with the factors described above, has a marked effect on the outcome of the dissolution test. No single apparatus and test can be used for all drug products. Each drug product must be tested individually with the dissolution test which best correlates to in vivo bioavailability.

Usually, the report on the dissolution test will state that a certain percentage of the labeled amount of drug in the drug product must dissolve within a specified period of time. In practice, the absolute amount of drug in the drug product may vary from tablet to tablet. Therefore, a number of tablets from each lot are usually tested to get a representative dissolution rate for the product.

COMPENDIAL METHODS OF DISSOLUTION

The USP-XXI/NF-XVI provides several official methods for carrying out dissolution tests of tablets and capsules. The selection of a particular method for a drug is usually specified in the monograph for a particular drug product.

The Rotating Basket Method (Apparatus 1)

The rotating basket method consists of a cylindrical basket held by a motor shaft. The basket holds the sample and rotates in a round flask containing the dissolution medium. The entire flask is immersed in a constant temperature bath set at 37°C. The rotating speed and the position of the basket must meet specific requirements set forth in the current USP. Dissolution calibration standards are available to make sure that these mechanical and operating requirements are met. Calibration tablets containing prednisone are made specially for dissolution tests requiring disintegrating tablets whereas salicylic acid calibration tablets are used as a standard requiring nondisintegrating tablets.

The Paddle Method (Apparatus 2)

The paddle method or apparatus 2 consists of a special coated paddle that minimizes turbulence due to stirring (Fig. 6-6). The paddle is vertically attached to a variable-speed motor which rotates at a controlled speed. The tablet or capsule is placed into the round bottom dissolution flask which also minimizes turbulence of the dissolution medium. The apparatus is housed in a constant-temperature water bath maintained at 37°C similar to that of the rotating basket method. The position and alignment of the paddle are specified in the USP. The paddle method is very sensitive to tilting. Improper alignment may drastically affect the dissolution results with some drug products. The same set of dissolution calibration standards are used to check the equipment before tests are run.

The Modified Disintegration Method (Apparatus 3)

This method essentially adopts the USP disintegration "basket-and-rack" assembly for the dissolution test. The disks are omitted when this apparatus is used for dissolution. The basket screen is also changed so that particles will not fall through the screen during dissolution. This method is used infrequently and is included in the USP for an older drug formulation.

The amount of agitation and vibration makes this method less suitable for precise dissolution testing.

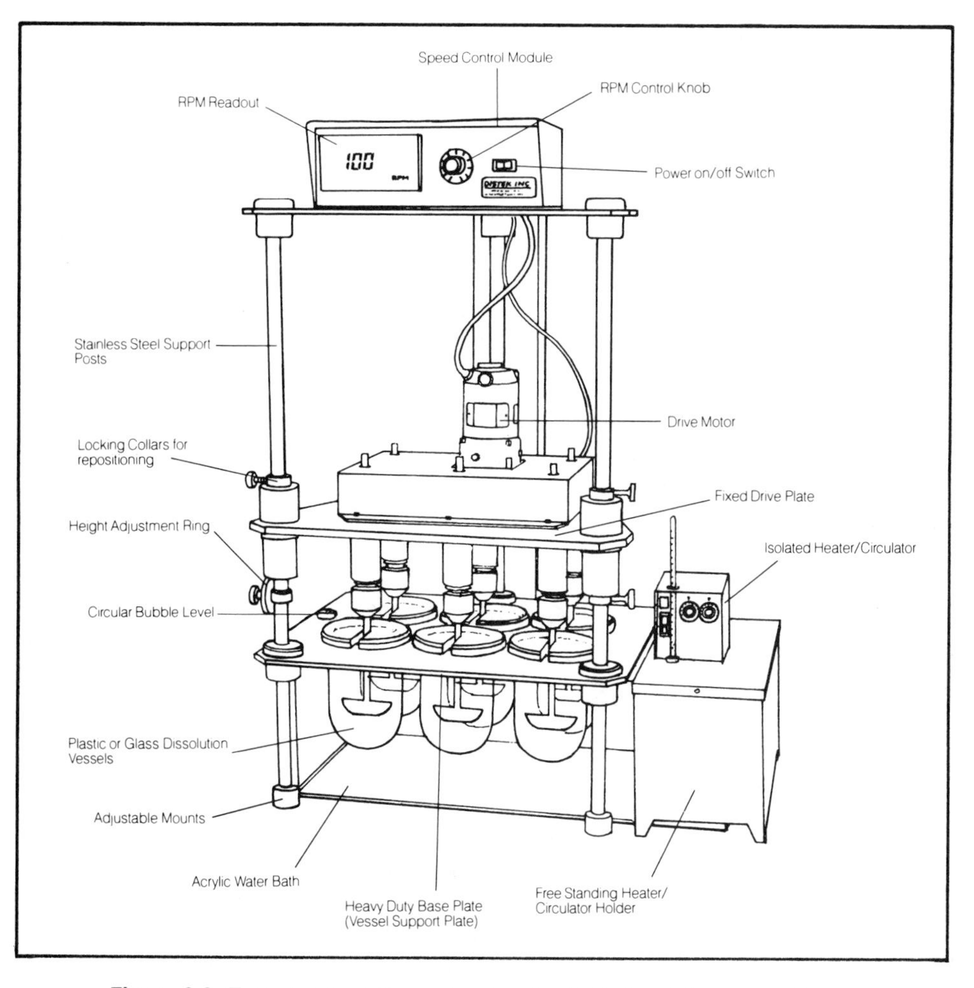

Figure 6-6. Typical set up for performing the USP dissolution test with the Distek 2000. The system is equipped with a height adjustment ring for easy adjustment of paddle height. (*Drawing courtesy of Distek Inc., Somerset, N.J.*)

MEETING DISSOLUTION REQUIREMENTS

The USP–NF sets dissolution requirements for many products (see Table 6-2). The requirements apply to both the basket and the paddle methods. Amount of drug dissolved within a given time period, Q, is expressed as a percentage of label content. The Q is generally specified in the monograph for a drug product to pass the dissolution test. For each dissolution run, six tablets or capsules are tested, and the dissolution test continues until the criteria is met or the stages are exhausted.

For many products the passing of Q is set at 75% in 45 min, and this standard has been proposed for all products. For a new drug product setting the dissolution specification requires a thorough consideration of the physical and chemical proper-

TABLE 6-2. DISSOLUTION ACCEPTANCE

Stage	Number Tested	Acceptance Criteria
S_1	6	Each unit is not less than $Q + 5\%$
S_2	6	Average of 12 units ($S_1 + S_2$) is equal to or greater than Q, and no unit is less than $Q - 15\%$
S_3	12	Average of 24 units ($S_1 + S_2 + S_3$) is equal to or greater than Q, and not more than 2 units are less than $Q - 15\%$

Adapted from United States Pharmacopeia, 1980[1].

ties of the drug. In addition to the consideration that the dissolution test must ensure consistent bioavailability of the product, the test must provide for variation in manufacturing and testing variables so that a product may not be improperly rejected.

UNOFFICIAL METHODS OF DISSOLUTION TESTING

The Rotating Bottle Method

This method was suggested in NF XIII and has become less popular. The rotating bottle method was used mainly for controlled release beads. For this purpose the dissolution media may be easily changed, such as from artificial gastric juice to artificial intestinal juice. The equipment consists of a rotating rack that holds the sample drug products in bottles. The bottles are capped tightly and rotated in a 37°C temperature bath. At various times the samples are removed from the bottle, decanted through a 40-mesh screen, and the residues are assayed. To the remaining drug residues within the bottles are added an equal volume of fresh medium and the dissolution test is continued. A dissolution test with pH 1.2 medium for 1 hr, pH 2.5 medium for the next 1 hr, followed by pH 4.5 medium for 1.5 hr, pH 7.0 medium for 1.5 hr, and pH 7.5 medium for 2 hr was recommended to simulate condition of the gastrointestinal tract. The main disadvantage is that this procedure is manual and tedious. Moreover, it is not known if the rotating bottle procedure results in a better in vitro–in vivo correlation for drugs.

Flow-Through Dissolution Method

There are many variations of this method. Essentially, the sample is held in a fixed position while the dissolution medium is pumped through the sample holder dissolving the drug. Laminar flow of the medium is achieved by using a pulseless pump. Peristaltic or centrifugal pumps are not recommended. The flow rate is usually maintained between 10 and 100 ml/min. The dissolution medium may be fresh or recirculated. In the case of fresh medium the dissolution rate at any moment may be obtained, whereas in the official paddle or basket methods cumulative dissolution rates are monitored. A major advantage of the flow-through method is the easy maintenance of a sink condition for dissolution. A large volume of dissolution medium may be used also, and the mode of operation is easily adapted to automated equipment.

Intrinsic Dissolution Method

Most methods for dissolution deal with a finished drug product. Sometimes a new drug or substance may be tested for dissolution without the effect of excipients or the fabrication effect of processing. The dissolution of a drug powder by maintaining a constant surface area is called *intrinsic dissolution*. Intrinsic dissolution is usually expressed as mg/cm^2 min. In one method the basket method is adapted to test dissolution of powder by placing the powder in a disk attached with clipper to the bottom of the basket.

The Peristalsis Method

This method attempts to simulate the hydrodynamic conditions of the gastrointestinal tract in an in vitro dissolution device. The apparatus consists of a rigid plastic cylindrical tubing fitted with a septum and rubber stoppers at both ends. The dissolution chamber consists of a space between the septum and the lower stopper. The apparatus is placed in a beaker containing the dissolution medium. The dissolution medium is pumped with peristaltic action through the dosage form.

PROBLEMS OF VARIABLE CONTROL IN DISSOLUTION TESTING

There are a number of equipment and operating variables associated with dissolution testing. Depending on the particular dosage form involved, the variables may or may not exert a pronounced effect on the rate of dissolution of the drug or drug product. Variations of 25% or more may occur with the same type of equipment and procedure. The centering and alignment of the paddle is critical in the paddle method. Turbulence can create increased agitation resulting in a higher dissolution rate. Wobbling and tilting due to worn equipment should be avoided. The basket method is less sensitive to the tilting effect. However, the basket method is more sensitive to clogging due to gummy materials. Pieces of small particles can also clog up the basket screen and create a local nonsink condition for dissolution. Furthermore, dissolved gas in the medium may form air bubbles on the surface of the dosage form unit and can affect dissolution in both the basket and paddle methods.

The interpretation of dissolution data is probably the most difficult job for the pharmacist. In the absence of in vivo data, it is generally impossible to make valid conclusions about bioavailability from the dissolution data alone. The use of various testing methods makes it even more difficult to interpret dissolution results since there is no simple correlation among dissolution results obtained with various methods. For many drug products the dissolution rates are higher with the paddle method. Dissolution results at 50 rpm with the paddle method may be equivalent to the dissolution at 100 rpm with the basket method. In the study of sustained theophylline tablets compressed at various hardness, McGinity[10] found that at 50 rpm dissolution with the paddle method was faster than that of the basket method for tablets of 4.0 kg hardness. However, with tablets of 6.8 kg hardness, similar dissolution profiles were obtained at 125 rpm for the basket and paddle methods over a period of 6 hrs. With both methods increased dissolution rates were observed as the rates were increased. Apparently, the composition of the formulation as well as the process variables in manufacturing may be both important. No simple correlation can be made for dissolution results obtained with different methods.

In a comparison of the paddle and basket methods in evaluating sustained-release pseudoephedrine–guaifenesin preparation, Masih et al.[11] found that the paddle method was more discriminating in demonstrating dissolution differences among drug products. At 100 rpm the basket method failed to pick up formulation differences detected by the paddle method.

In the absence of in vivo data, the selection of the dissolution method is based on the type drug product to be tested. For example, a low-density preparation may be poorly wetted in the basket method. A gummy preparation may clog up the basket screen, and therefore the paddle method is preferred. For many drugs a satisfactory dissolution test may be obtained with more than one method by optimizing testing conditions.

IN VITRO–IN VIVO CORRELATION OF DISSOLUTION

The various methods of dissolution provide a convenient means of testing a drug product. When a proper dissolution method is chosen, the rate of dissolution of the product may be correlated to the rate of absorption of the drug into the body.

This dissolution test then becomes a part of the standard quality control procedure for the drug product. For example, the USP-XX/NF-XV has separate and distinct dissolution test requirements for the two different phenytoin sodium capsules. Regarding the Extended Phenytoin Sodium Capsules, USP states that "not more than 35%, between 30% and 70% and not less than 85% of the labeled amount of $C_{15}H_{11}N_2NaO_2$ in the Extended Capsules dissolves in 30 minutes, 60 minutes and 120 minutes, respectively, under the specified dissolution conditions." In contrast, the tolerances for the Prompt Phenytoin Sodium Capsules USP states that "not less than 85% of the labeled amount of $C_{15}H_{11}N_2NaO_2$ in the Prompt Capsules dissolves in 30 minutes." There are several ways of checking for in vitro–in vivo correlation.

Dissolution Rate Versus Absorption Rate

If dissolution of the drug is rate limiting, a faster dissolution rate may result in a faster rate of appearance of the drug in the plasma. It may be possible to establish a correlation between rate of dissolution and rate of absorption of the drug.

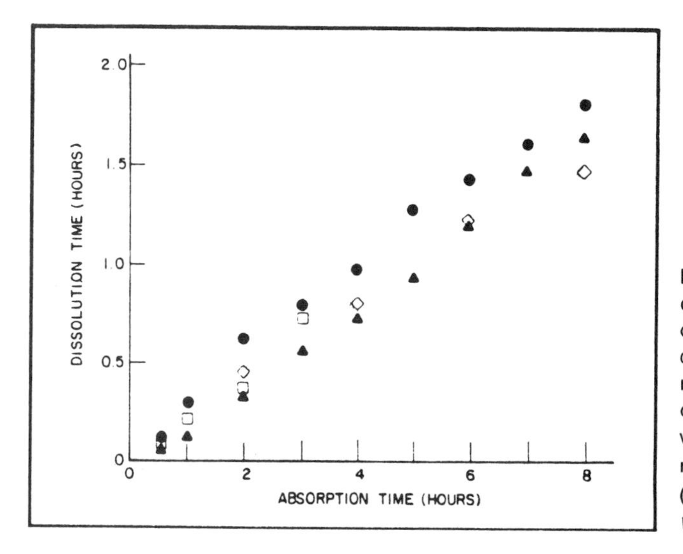

Figure 6-7. An example of correlation between time required for a given amount of drug to be absorbed and time required for the same amount of drug to be dissolved in vitro for three sustained-release aspirin products. *(From Wood JH, 1966, with permission.[2])*

The absorption rate is usually more difficult to determine than absorption time. Therefore, the absorption time may be used in correlating dissolution data to absorption data. In the analysis of in vitro–in vivo drug correlation, rapid drug absorption may be distinguished from the slower drug absorption by observation of the absorption time for the preparation. The absorption time refers to the time for a constant amount of drug to be absorbed. In one study involving three sustained-release aspirin products, the dissolution time for the preparations were linearly correlated to the absorption times for various amounts of aspirin absorbed (Fig. 6-7). The results from this study demonstrated that aspirin was rapidly absorbed and was very much dependent on the dissolution rate for absorption.

Percent of Drug Dissolved Versus Percent of Drug Absorbed

If a drug is absorbed completely after dissolution, a linear correlation may be obtained by comparing the percent of drug absorbed to the percent of drug dissolved. In choosing the dissolution method, one must consider the appropriate dissolution medium and use a slow dissolution stirring rate so that in vivo dissolution is approximated.

Figure 6-8 shows the percent of aspirin absorbed and the percent of aspirin dissolved of three aspirin products.

Aspirin is absorbed rapidly and a slight change in formulation may be reflected in a change in the amount and rate of drug absorption during the period of observation. If the drug is slow absorbing, which occurs when the absorption is the rate-limiting step, a difference in dissolution rate of the product may not be observed. In this case the drug would have been absorbed very slowly independent of the dissolution rate.

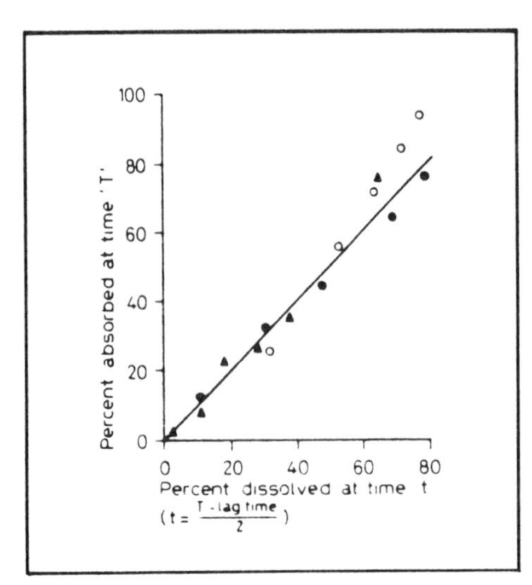

Figure 6-8. An example of continuous in vivo–in vitro correlation of aspirin. (*From Levy G, et al, 1965, with permission.*[3])

Maximum Plasma Concentrations Versus Percent of Drug Dissolved In Vitro

When different drug formulations are tested for dissolution, a poorly formulated drug will not be completely dissolved and released, resulting in lower plasma drug concentrations. The percent of drug released at any time interval will be greater for the more available drug product. When such drug products are tested in vivo, the peak drug serum concentration will be higher for the drug product which shows the highest percent of drug dissolved. An example of in vitro–in vivo correlation for 100 mg phenytoin sodium capsules is shown in Figure 6-9. Several products were tested. A linear correlation was observed between the maximum drug concentration in the body and the percent of the drug dissolved in vitro.

The dissolution study on the phenytoin sodium products showed that the fastest dissolution rate was product *C*, for which about 100% of the labeled contents dissolved in the test (Fig. 6-10). Interestingly, these products also show the shortest time for peak concentration (T_{max}). The T_{max} is dependent on the absorption rate constant. In this case the fastest absorption would also result in the shortest T_{max} (see Chapter 7, Eq. 7.12).

Serum Drug Concentration Versus Percent of Drug Dissolved

In a study on aspirin absorption the serum concentration of aspirin was correlated to the percent of drug dissolved using an in vitro dissolution method. The dissolution medium was simulated gastric juice. Since aspirin is rapidly absorbed from the stomach, the dissolution of the drug is the rate-limiting step and various formulations with different dissolution rates would cause differences in the serum concentration of aspirin by minutes (Fig. 6-11).

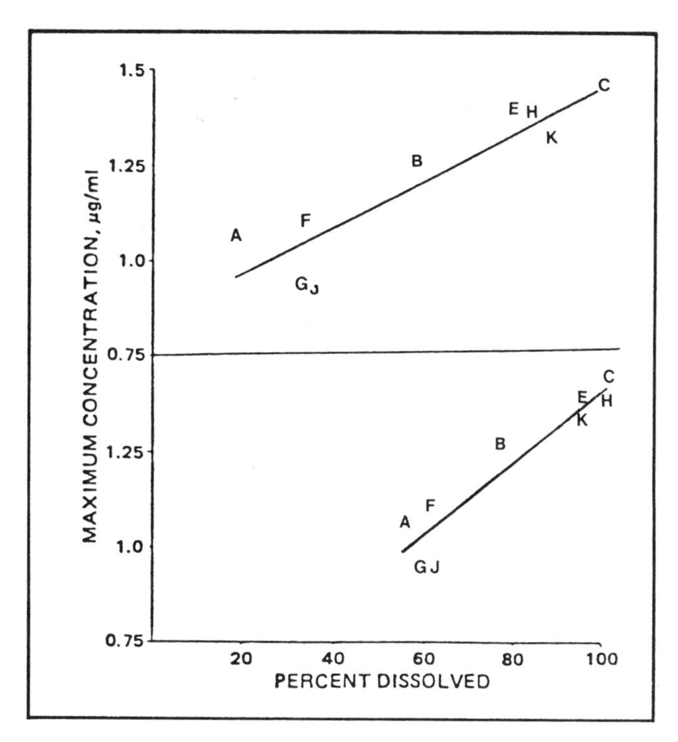

Figure 6-9. In vitro–in vivo correlation between C_{max} and percent drug dissolved in 30 min (slope = 0.06, r = 0.902, $p < 0.001$) (A); 60 min (slope = 0.10, r = 0.940, $p < 0.001$) (B). Letters on graph indicate different products. *(From Shah VP, et al, 1983, with permission.[4])*

Failure of Correlation of In Vitro Dissolution to In Vivo Absorption

Although there are many published examples of drugs with dissolution data that correlate well with drug absorption in the body, there are also many examples indicating poor correlation of dissolution to drug absorption. There are also instances where a drug has failed the dissolution test and yet is well absorbed. The problem of no correlation between bioavailability and dissolution may be due to the complexity of drug absorption and the weakness of the dissolution design. For example, a product which involves fatty components may be subjected to longer retention in the gastrointestinal tract. The effect of digestive enzymes may also play an important role in the dissolution of the drug in vivo. These factors may not be adequately simulated with a simple dissolution medium. An excellent example showing the importance of dissolution design is shown in Figure 6-12. Dissolution tests using four different dissolution media were performed for two quinidine gluconate sustained-release tablets. Brand BE was known to be bioavailable whereas product BO-1 was known to be incompletely absorbed. It is interesting to see that using acid media as well as acid followed by pH 7.4 buffer did not distinguish the two products well, whereas using water or pH 5.4 buffer as dissolution media clearly distinguishes the "good" product from the one that is not completely available. In this case the use of an acid medium is consistent with the physiologic condition in the stomach, but this procedure would be misleading as a quality control tool. It is

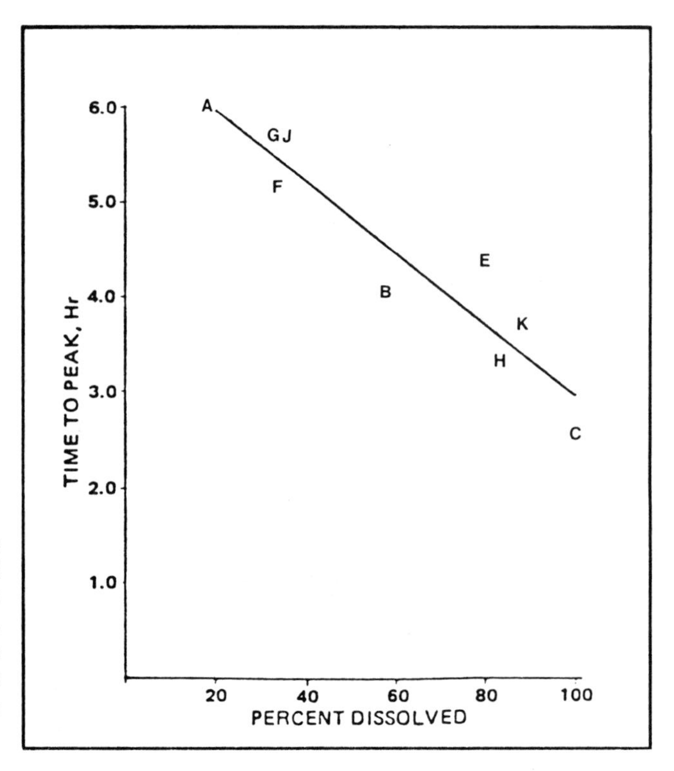

Figure 6-10. In vitro–in vivo correlation between T_{max} and percent drug dissolved in 30 minutes by Basket Method. Letters on graph indicate different products. (*From Shah VP, et al, 1983, with permission.*[4])

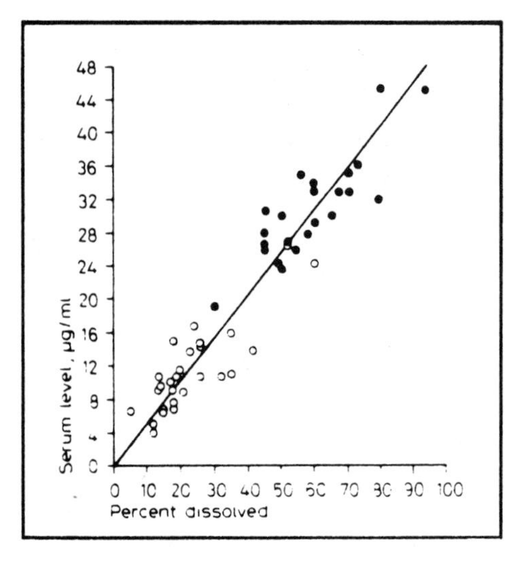

Figure 6-11. Example of in vivo–in vitro two-point correlation between 10-min serum level and percent dissolved at 1.2 min (○) and the 20-min serum level and percent dissolved at 4.2 min (●). (*From Wood J, 1967, with permission.*[2])

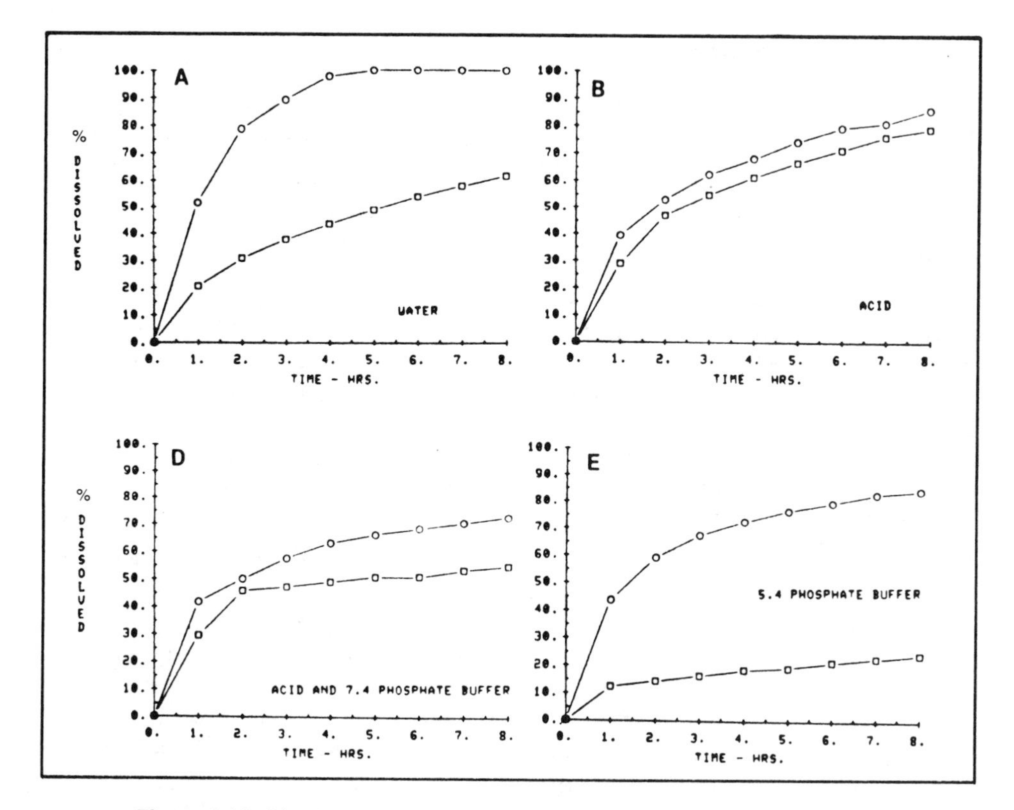

Figure 6-12. Dissolution profile of two quinidine gluconate sustained release products in different dissolution media. Each data point is the mean of 12 tablets. Key: ○ = product BE; □ = product BO-1. (*From Prasad V, Shah VP, et al, 1983)*

important that any new dissolution test be carefully researched before being adopted as a method for predicting drug absorption.

CONSIDERATIONS IN DOSAGE FORM DESIGN

The most important considerations in designing a dosage form are safety and efficacy. The active and inactive ingredients must be safe when used as intended. The drug must be effectively delivered to the target so that the intended therapeutic effect can be achieved. The dosage form must not add any additional side effect or discomfort to the drug. In preparing the drug product, the pharmacist tries to consider the needs of the physician, the patient, and the cost of manufacturing. These considerations are then balanced out by the physical, chemical, and biologic limitations of the drug.

Patient Consideration

The dosage form must be acceptable for the patient. A bitter drug should be encapsulated or coated if taken as tablet. The size of the tablet or capsule should be small enough for easy swallowing. Dosing frequency should be kept to a minimum.

Dose Consideration

The dosage form must be designed with dose consideration. Some drugs have wide individual dose variation, and a number of dosing strengths must be available so that a convenient dose can be taken from the available dosage forms. With certain drugs, dosing of drug is based on body surface or body weight, and the dosage may be readjusted by monitoring the concentration of the drug in the body.

Dosing Frequency Consideration

The dose frequency of a drug is related to the elimination half-life of the drug as well as the therapeutic concentration of the drug. For a drug with a short half-life, considerations are often given to sustain the duration of action of the drug. The risk of dose dumping and the potential for reduced bioavailability of the drug must be considered if a larger dose is formulated to achieve a longer duration of action. On the other hand, the sustained product must not reduce the total amount of drug absorbed. A reduced absorption usually leaves an increased amount of residual drug in the gastrointestinal tract, which may cause local irritation or side effects.

Therapeutic Consideration

Knowledge of the therapeutic indication of the drug is important to the formulator. A drug that is used for an immediate and acute condition should be formulated so that it reaches the target rapidly. A drug that is used for longer-term therapy may reach the target more slowly. For example, a pain-relieving drug should be rapidly absorbed so that quick relief can be obtained, whereas a drug designed to prevent asthmatic episodes may be absorbed slowly so that the protective effect of the drug lasts over a long period of time. The rate of drug absorption may affect the intensity of a drug response, and the drug product must be designed to optimize the absorption rate which gives the best therapeutic response. For example, formulation of the antidiabetic drug tolbutamide as a fast absorbing product consisting of the soluble salt may result in abrupt fall in sugar level in the patient causing temporary hypoglycemic shock. In contrast, the more slowly absorbed tolbutamide as the base may bring about a gradual and controlled drop in sugar level without any undesirable hypoglycemic effect. The formulation of any sympathomimetic bronchiodilating agent requires careful consideration of drug absorption rate, since rapid absorption of the drug may cause an exaggerated increase in heart rate (tachycardia); a more gradual absorption of the drug may deliver the antiasthmatic effect without causing any tachycardia side effect. The separation of side effect from therapeutic effect requires a systematic screening of a series of formulations with different absorption rates. For many of the sympathomimetic agents, it is best to avoid a "burst" type of sudden absorption since this is usually translated to a "burst" type of response that is not well tolerated by the patient.

Gastrointestinal Side Effect

Many orally administered drugs are irritating to the stomach. These drugs may cause nausea or stomach pain when taken on an empty stomach. In some cases food or antacids may be given together with the drug to reduce stomach irritation. Alternatively, the drug may be enteric coated to reduce gastric irritation. A common drug that causes irritation is aspirin. Buffered aspirin tablets, enteric coated tablets, and granules are available. However, enteric coating may sometimes delay or reduce the amount of drug absorbed. Furthermore, enteric coating may not abolish gastric irritation completely since the drug may be regurgitated back to the stomach occasionally after the coating dissolves in the intestine.

Enteric coated tablets may be greatly affected by the presence of food in the stomach. Drug may not be released from the stomach for several hours when stomach emptying is delayed by food.

The use of buffering material or antacid ingredients with aspirin has been used to reduce stomach irritation. When a large amount of antacid or buffering material is included in the formulation, dissolution of aspirin may occur quickly leading to reduced irritation to the stomach. However, many buffered aspirin formulations do not contain sufficient buffering material to make a difference in dissolution in the stomach.

Certain drugs have been formulated into soft gelatin capsules to improve drug bioavailability and reduce gastrointestinal side effects. If the drug is formulated in the soft gelatin capsule as a solution, the drug may disperse and dissolve more rapidly leaving less residual drug in the gut and causing irritation. This approach may be useful for a drug that causes local irritation but would be ineffective if the drug is inherently ulcerogenic. Indomethacin, for example, may cause ulceration even when administered parenterally to animals.

There are many options available to the formulator to improve the tolerance of the drug and minimize gastric irritation. The nature of excipients and the physical state of the drug are important and must be carefully assessed before a drug product is formulated. Some excipients may improve the solubility of the drug and facilitate absorption, whereas others may physically adsorb the drug to reduce irritation. Often, a great number of formulations must be tested before an acceptable one is chosen.

ROUTE OF ADMINISTRATION CONSIDERATIONS

A drug may be administered in various routes and still result in equivalent activity; however, the duration and onset of action may be very different because of pharmacokinetic changes due to the route of administration. Before a product is made for a certain route of administration, it is important to consider the physiologic and physicochemical changes that may be brought about by the dosage form change.

PARENTERAL PRODUCTS

In general, intravenous administration provides the most rapid onset of action. Drugs injected intravenously go directly into the blood and circulate to all parts of the body within a few minutes. A drug injected intramuscularly involves an absorption delay in which the drug travels from the injection site to the blood stream. Figure 6-13 shows a drug administered by three different routes. Plasma drug input of both the oral and intramuscular administration involve an absorption phase in which the drug concentration rises slowly to a peak and then declines according to the elimination half-life of the drug. (Notice the elimination phases for all products are the same because changing the formulation only changes the absorption, not the elimination.) In the case of intravenous administration, plasma level peaks instantaneously so that a peak is usually not visible. After 3 hr, however, the plasma level of the drug after intravenous administration has declined to a lower level than that of the oral and intramuscular administration. It should be pointed out that in this case the area under the plasma curves are all equal, indicating that the oral and intramuscular preparations are both well formulated and are 100% available. Frequently, because of absorption or metabolism, oral preparations may have lower area under the curve.

The intramuscular injection shown has a faster absorption than that of the oral preparation; however, it is possible that an intramuscular preparation may release drug relatively slowly. Intramuscular preparations are generally injected into a muscle mass. Drug absorption occurs as the drug diffuses from the muscle to the surrounding tissue fluid and then the blood. Intramuscular injections may be formulated to have a fast or slow release by changing the vehicle of the injection preparation. Solutions generally distribute rapidly from the injection site whereas a viscous, oily, or suspension vehicle may result in a slow and sustained blood level. Viscous vehicles generally slow down drug diffusion and distribution. Preparations in oily vehicles may first partition into aqueous phase before distribution. A drug that is very soluble in the oil and relatively insoluble in water may have a relatively long and sustained release because of slow partitioning.

A major advantage of the intramuscular injection over intravenous injection is the flexibility of formulation. A drug that is not water soluble cannot be easily administered by intravenous route. There are a few nonaqueous injections for intravenous use; however, they must be administered very slowly to avoid any drug precipitation. Propylene glycol in combination with other solvents has been used in intravenous preparations.

BUCCAL TABLET

A drug that diffuses and penetrates rapidly may be administered and absorbed in the oral cavity. A tablet designed for drug absorption in the oral cavity is called a *buccal tablet*. Nitroglycerin sublingual tablet, for example, is dissolved under the tongue

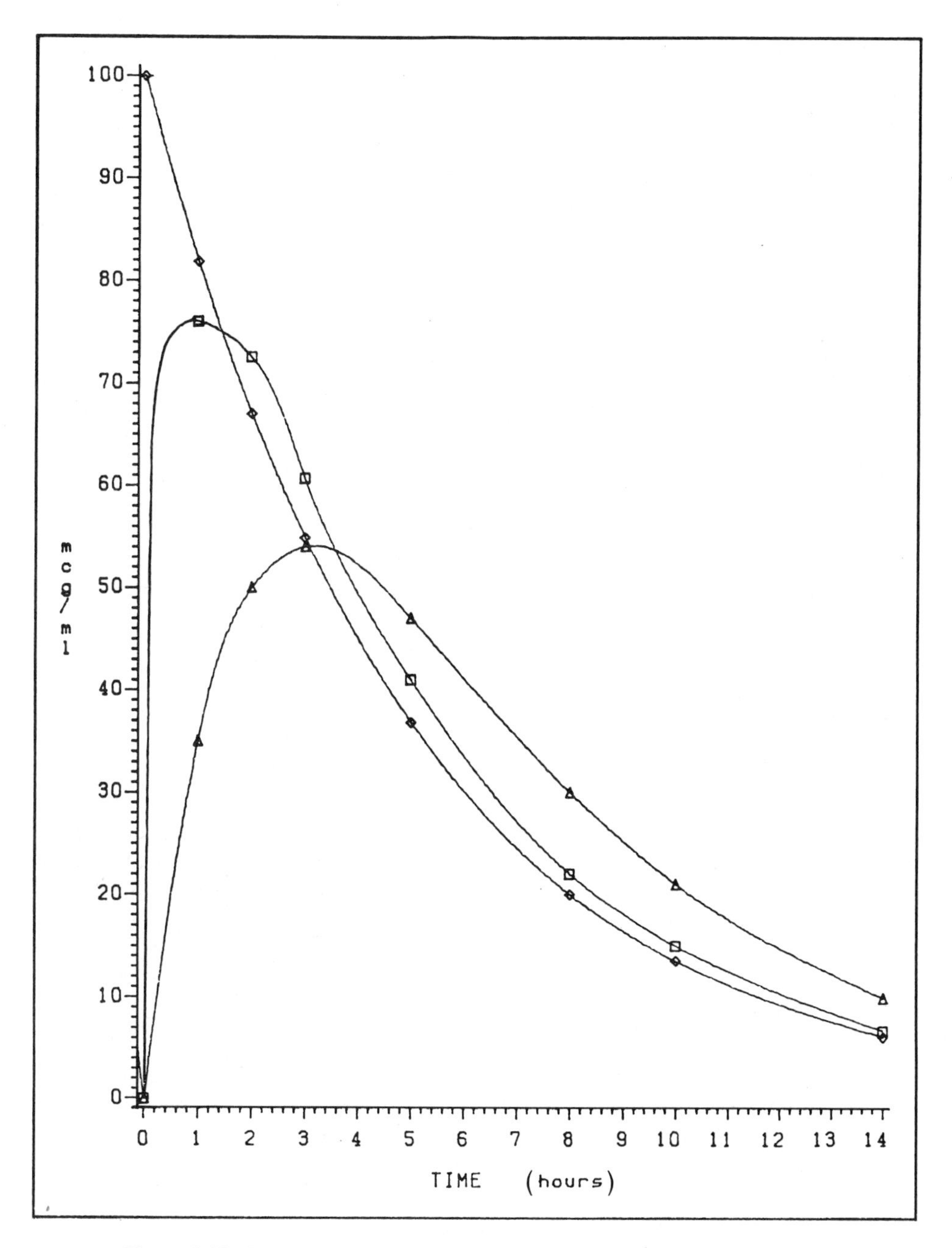

Figure 6-13. Plasma concentration of a drug after the same dose is administered by three different routes. Key: ◇ = Intravenous, □ = Intramuscular, and △ = Oral.

and absorbed through the oral mucosa. Buccal tablets generally contain a fast dissolving excipient such as lactose so that the drug is released rapidly. The onset of nitroglycerin sublingually is rapid, much faster than that taken orally or absorbed through the skin. The duration of action, however, is shorter than that of the other two routes. Drug absorbed through the oral mucosa will not pass through the liver before general distribution. Consequently, for a drug with significant first-pass effect, buccal absorption may provide better bioavailability over oral administration.

AEROSOL

Drugs administered into the respiratory system, such as antiasthmatics, may be formulated into an aerosol or inhalation solution. An aerosol preparation with suitable propellant can administer drug rapidly into the bronchial region. The particle size of the suspension (or in the case of a solution the size of the mist particles) is important in determining the extent of penetration. For coarse particles the inertia carries the drug for a short distance up the nasal cavity. Drugs with small particles move by sedimentation or Brownian movements deeper into the bronchioles. Isoetharine and isoproterenol have been formulated for administration by this route. These drugs provide rapid relief and are not as effective by oral administration due to first-pass effects or metabolism prior to systemic absorption.

TRANSDERMAL PREPARATIONS

Transdermal administration refers to the delivery of a drug to the body system through the skin. An example of a drug delivered transdermally is Transderm-V. Transderm-V delivers scopolamine through the ear skin for motion sickness. This route of administration may release the drug over an extended period of several hours without the discomforts of gastrointestinal side effects. A drug administered transdermally is not affected by first-pass effects.

ORAL PREPARATIONS

The major advantages of oral preparations are the convenience of administration and the elimination of discomforts involved with injections. Also, the hazards of rapid intravenous administration causing toxic high concentration of drug in the blood is avoided. The main disadvantages of oral preparations are the potential problems of reduced and erratic bioavailability due to either incomplete absorption or drug interaction. Nausea or stomach discomfort may occur with some drugs that cause local gastrointestinal irritation. Poor bioavailability or reduced absorption may be due to antacids or food interaction. Many drugs are adsorbed to antacids or food substances. These drugs would not diffuse effectively across the gastrointestinal tract to be absorbed. Drug molecules do not get absorbed easily when ionized. The ganglion-blocking drugs, hexamethonium, pentolinium, and bretylium, become ionized at intestinal pH. Therefore, they are not absorbed orally to be effective. Neomycin, gentamycin, and cefamandole are not well absorbed orally. In the case of neomycin, after oral administration the drug will concentrate on the gastrointestinal tract to exert its local antibacterial effect.

In general, drugs with large molecular weights may not be well absorbed when administered orally. There is some evidence that large drug molecules may be absorbed through the lymphatic system when formulated with a "carrier." The mechanism is not known. Some large molecules are absorbed when administered in solution with a surface-active agent. For example, the drug cyclosporin has been administered orally with good absorption when formulated with a surfactant in oil. A possible role of the oil is to stimulate the flow of lymph as well as delay the retention of the drug. Oily vehicles have been used to lengthen the gastrointestinal transit time of oral preparations.

RECTAL PREPARATIONS

Rectal preparations may be administered either in solid or liquid form. Rectal administration is preferred with drugs that cause nausea or in situations where it is not possible to give the drug orally. A sustained-release preparation may be prepared for rectal administration. The rate of release of the drug from this preparation is dependent on the nature of the base composition and the solubility of the drug involved.

Rectal drug absorption may bypass first pass effects due to enzymes in the liver. In general, the drug absorbed in the lower rectal region does not pass through the liver, whereas a drug absorbed through the upper rectal region passes through the hepatic portal vein and may be inactivated by the liver.

Although drug responses are quite similar with different routes of administration, there are examples where severe differences in response may occur. For example, with the drug isoproterenol a difference in activity of a thousand-fold has been found attributing to different routes of administration. Figure 6-14 shows the

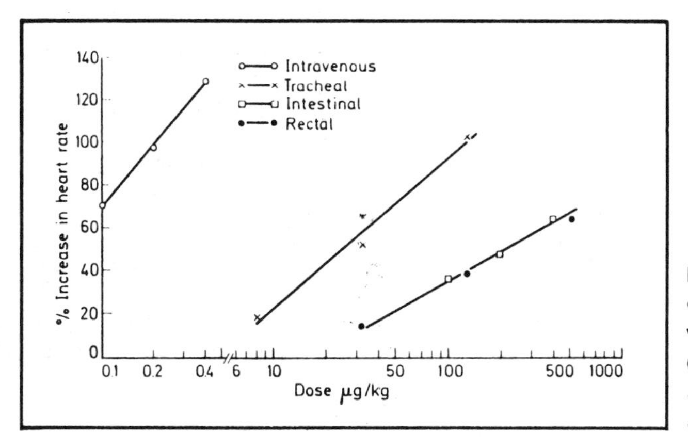

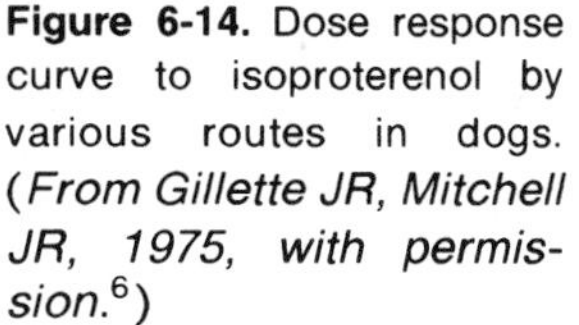
Figure 6-14. Dose response curve to isoproterenol by various routes in dogs. *(From Gillette JR, Mitchell JR, 1975, with permission.*[6]*)*

change in heart rate due to isoproterenol with different routes of administration.[6] Studies have shown that isoproterenol is metabolized in the gut and during the passage through the liver. The rate and types of metabolite formed are found to be different depending on the routes of administration.

Physicochemical Considerations

The physicochemical profile of a drug is a very important consideration in designing the dosage form. For example, a drug with poor water solubility is very difficult to formulate as an intravenous dosage form; however, an intramuscular dosage form would be much easier to formulate. Some of the important physicochemical factors considered in formulation are given in Table 6-3.

Solubility, pH, and Drug Absorption

The solubility–pH profile is a plot of solubility of the drug at various physiologic pH. This information is used in formulation design because the natural pH environment of the gastrointestinal tract varies from acidic in the stomach to slightly alkaline in the small intestine. A basic drug would be soluble in the acidic medium because of the formation of soluble salts. Conversely, an acid drug would be more soluble in the intestine forming a soluble salt at the more alkaline pH. The solubility–pH profile gives a rough estimation of the completeness of dissolution for a dose of a drug in the stomach. Solubility may be improved with the addition of an acidic or basic excipient. Solubilization of aspirin, for example, may be increased by the addition of an alkaline buffer. In the formulation of controlled-release drugs, buffering agents may be added to slow or modify the release rate of a fast dissolving

TABLE 6-3. PHYSICOCHEMICAL PROPERTIES FOR CONSIDERATION IN DRUG PRODUCT DESIGN

pK_a and pH profile	Necessary for optimum stability and solubility of the final product.
Particle size	May affect the solubility of the drug and therefore the dissolution rate of the product.
Polymorphism	The ability of a drug to exist in various crystal forms may change the solubility of the drug. Also, the stability of each form is important since polymorphs may convert from one form to another.
Hygroscopicity	Moisture absorption may affect the physical structure as well as stability of the product.
Partition coefficient	May give some indication of the relative affinity of the drug for oil and water. A drug that has high affinity for oil may have poor release and dissolution from the formulation.
Excipient interaction	The compatibility of the excipients with the drug and sometimes trace elements in excipients may affect the stability of the product. It is important to have specifications of all raw materials.
pH stability profile	The stability of solutions are often affected by the pH of the vehicle; furthermore, since the pH in the stomach and gut are different, knowledge of the stability profile would help to avoid or prevent degradation of the product during storage or after administration.

drug. To be effective, however, the controlled-release drug product must be a nondisintegrating dosage form. The buffering agent is released slowly rather than rapidly so that the drug does not dissolve immediately in the surrounding gastrointestinal fluid.

Stability, pH, and Drug Absorption

The pH–stability profile is a plot of reaction rate constant versus pH for the drug. If drug decomposition occurs by either acid or base catalysis, some prediction for degradation of the drug in the gastrointestinal tract may be made. For example, the drug erythromycin has a pH-dependent stability profile. In an acidic medium, such as in the stomach, decomposition occurs rapidly, whereas at neutral or alkaline pH the drug is relatively stable. Consequently, erythromycin tablets are enteric coated to protect against acid degradation in the stomach. This information also leads subsequently to the preparation of a less soluble salt which is stable in the stomach.

Particle Size and Drug Absorption

Particle size and particle size distribution studies are important for drugs that have low water solubility. Many hydrophobic drugs are very active intravenously but are not very effective when given orally due to poor absorption. Griseofulvin, nitrofurantoin, and many steroids are drugs with low solubility; reduction of the particle size may increase the amount of drug absorbed. Milling of these drugs to micronized form has improved their absorption significantly. Smaller particle size results in an increase in the total surface area of the particles, enhances water penetration into the particles, and increases the dissolution rates. With poorly soluble drugs a disintegrant may be added to the formulation to ensure rapid disintegration of the tablet and release of the particles. Addition of surface-active agents may increase wetting as well as solubility of these drugs.

Polymorphic Crystals, Solvates, and Drug Absorption

Polymorphism refers to the arrangement of a drug in various crystal forms or polymorphs. Polymorphs have the same chemical structure but different physical properties, such as solubility, density, hardness, and compression characteristics. Some polymorphic crystals may have much lower aqueous solubility than the amorphous forms, causing a product to be incompletely absorbed. Choramphenicol, for example, has several crystal forms, and when given orally as a suspension, the drug concentration in the body was found to be dependent on the percent of β polymorph in the suspension. The β form is more soluble and better absorbed (Fig. 6-15). In general, the crystal form with the lowest free energy is the most stable polymorph. The other polymorphs are metastable and may convert to the more stable form over time. A change in crystal form may cause problems in manufacturing the product; for example, a change in crystal structure of the drug may cause cracking in a tablet or even inability for a granulation to be compressed to form a tablet. Reformulation of a product is often necessary if a new crystal form of a drug

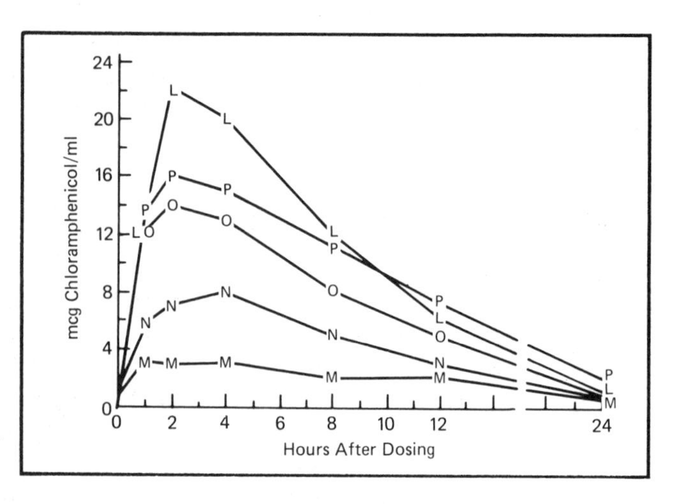

Figure 6-15. Comparison of mean blood serum levels obtained with chloramphenicol palmitate suspensions containing varying ratios of A and B polymorphs, following single oral dose equivalent to 1.5 g chloramphenicol. Percentage polymorph B in the suspension: M = 0%; N = 25%; O = 50%; P = 75%; L = 100%. (*From Aguiar AJ, et al, 1967 with permssion.*[7])

is used. Some drugs interact with solvent during preparation to form a crystal called *solvate*. Water may form a special crystal with drugs called *hydrates*, which may have quite different solubility compared to the anhydrous form of the drug (Fig. 6-16). Ampicillin trihydrate, for example, was reported to be less absorbed than the anhydrous form of ampicillin due to faster dissolution of the latter.

Formulation Ingredients and Drug Absorption

An apparently inert ingredient in a product may affect drug absorption. Some ingredients may increase the solubility of the drug and therefore increase the rate of drug absorption. Other excipients may increase the retention time of the drug in the

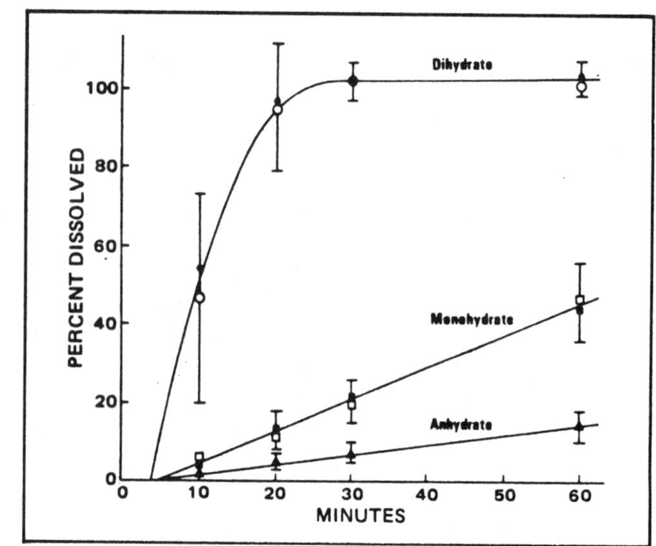

Figure 6-16. Dissolution behaviour of erythromycin dihydrate, monohydrate, and anhydrate in phosphate buffer (pH 7.5) at 37°C. (*From Allen PV, et al, 1978, with permission.*[8])

TABLE 6-4. COMMON EXCIPIENTS USED IN SOLID DOSAGE FORMS

Excipient	Property in Dosage Form
Lactose	Diluent
Dibasic calcium phosphate	Diluent
Starch	Disintegrant, diluent
Microcrystalline cellulose	Disintegrant, diluent
Magnesium stearate	Lubricant
Stearic acid	Lubricant
Hydrogenated vegetable oil	Lubricant
Talc	Lubricant
Sucrose (solution)	Granulating agent
Polyvinyl pyrrolidone (solution)	Granulating agent
Hydroxypropylmethylcellulose	Tablet-coating agent
Titinium dioxide	Combined with dye as colored coating
Methylcellulose	Coating or granulating agent
Cellulose acetate phthalate	Enteric coating agent

gastrointestinal tract and therefore increase the amount of drug to be absorbed. Some ingredients may act as carriers to increase drug diffusion across the intestinal wall. In contrast, many excipients may retard drug dissolution and thus reduce drug absorption. The influence on drug absorption of some common oral tableting ingredients are listed in Tables 6-4 and 6-5. In general, a tablet is formulated with several inactive components: (1) diluent (e.g., lactose); (2) disintegrant (e.g., starch); (3) lubricant (e.g., magnesium stearate); and (4) other components such as binding and stabilizing agents. These ingredients are relatively safe. When improperly used in the formulation, the rate as well as the extent of drug absorption may be affected. For example, Figure 6-17 shows that an excessive quantity of magnesium stearate (a hydrophobic lubricant) in the formulation may retard drug dissolution and cause slower drug absorption. A higher concentration of lubricant may greatly reduce the total amount of drug absorbed in the body (Fig. 6-18). In this case the lubricant level

TABLE 6-5. COMMON EXCIPIENTS USED IN LIQUID DOSAGE FORM

Excipient	Property in Dosage Form
Sodium carboxymethylcellulose	Suspending agent
Tragacanth	Suspending agent
Sodium alginate	Suspending agent
Xanthan gum	Thixotropic suspending agent
Veegum	Thixotropic suspending agent
Sorbitol	Sweetener
Alcohol	Solubilizing agent, preservative
Propylene glycol	Solubilizing agent
Methyl, propylparaben	Preservative
Sucrose	Sweetener
Polysorbates	Surfactant
Sesame oil	For emulsion vehicle
Corn Oil	For emulsion vehicle

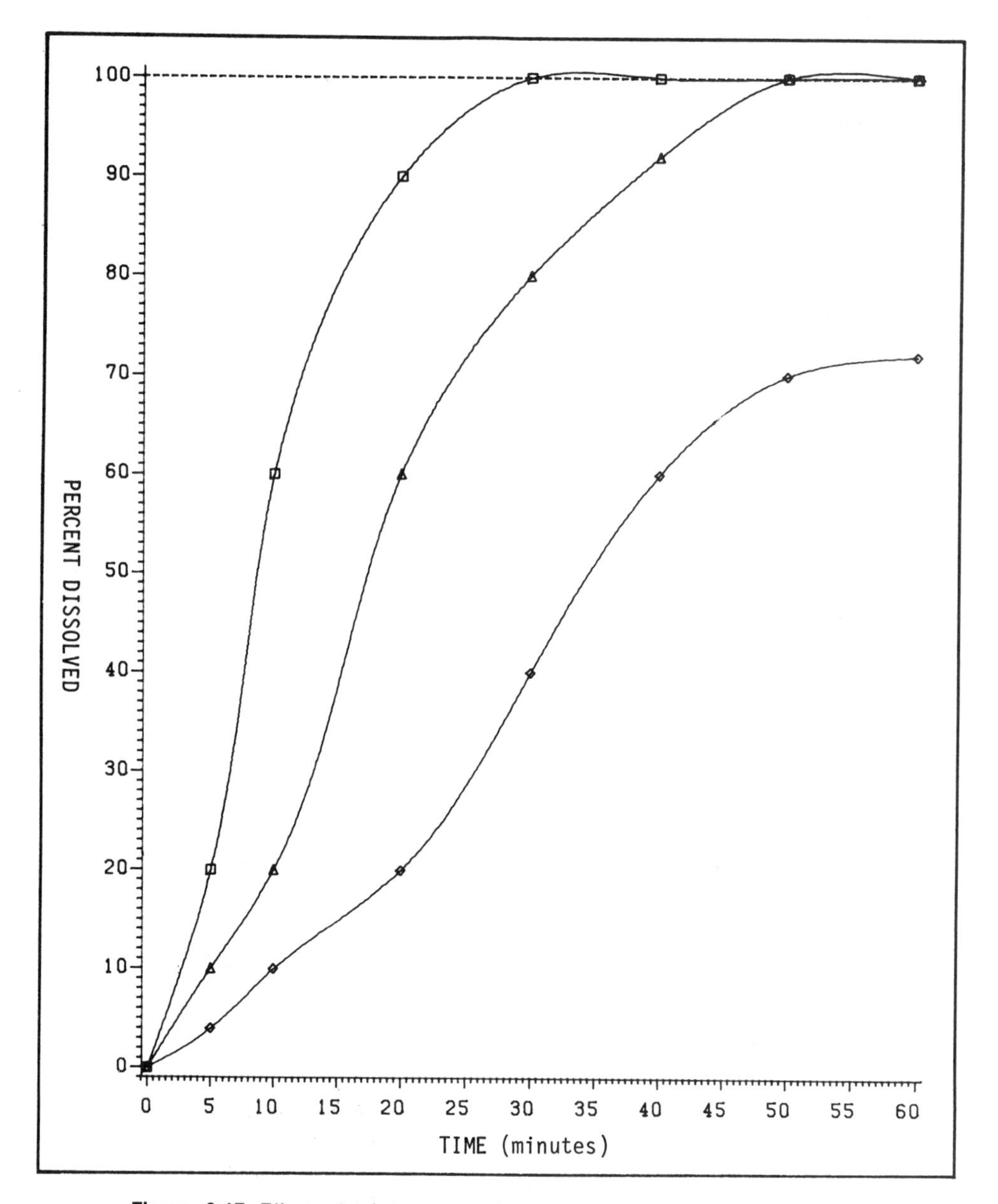

Figure 6-17. Effect of lubricant on drug dissolution. Key (percentage of magnesium stearate in formulation): □ = 0.5%; △ = 1.0%; ◇ = 5.0%.

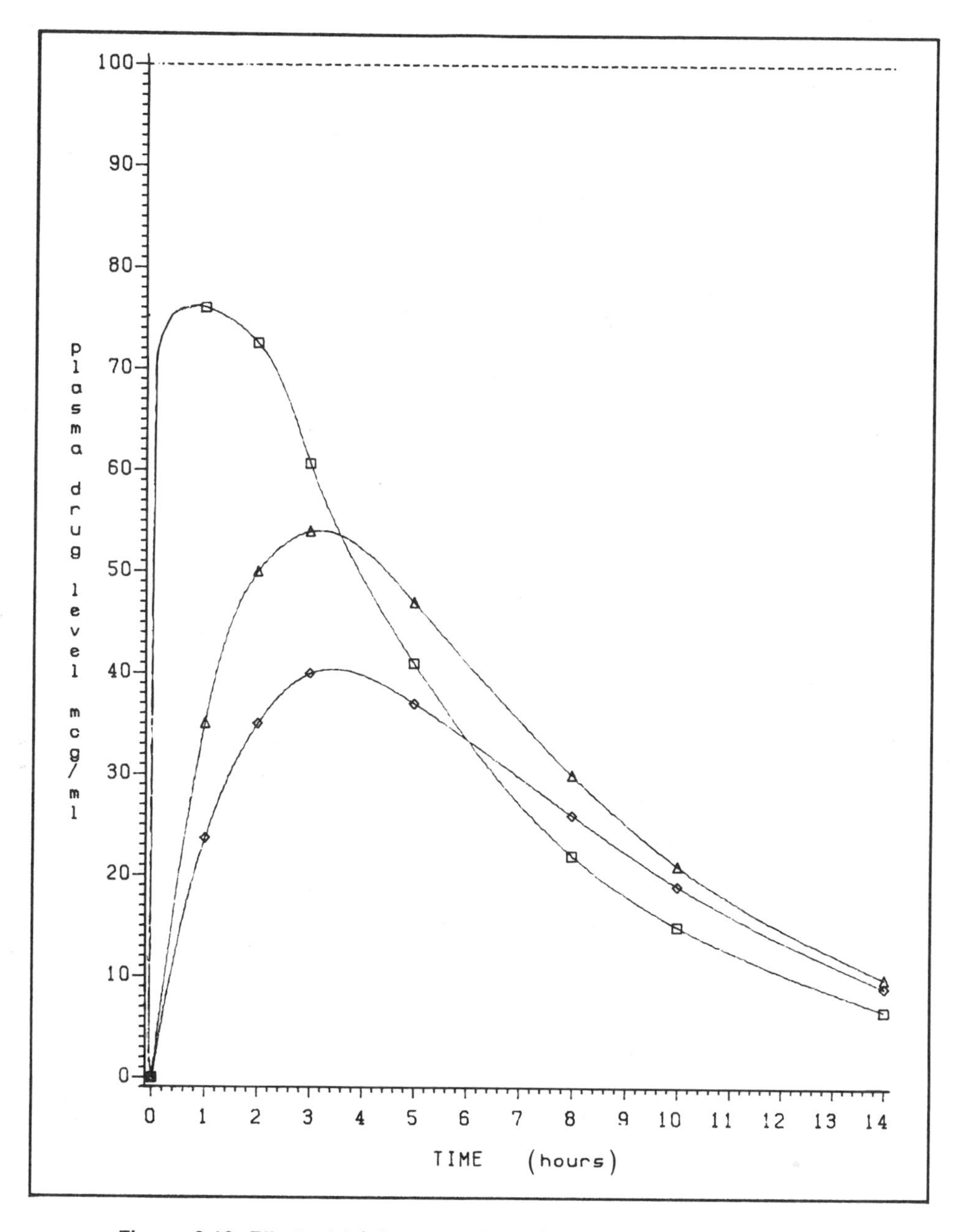

Figure 6-18. Effect of lubricant on drug absorption. Key (percentage of magnesium stearate in formulation): □ = 0.5%; △ = 1.0%; ◇ = 5.0%. Incomplete drug absorption occurs for formulation with 5% magnesium stearate.

TABLE 6-6. EFFECT OF EXCIPIENTS ON THE PHARMACOKINETIC PARAMETERS OF ORAL DRUG PRODUCTS*

Excipients	Example	K_a	T_{max}	AUC
Disintegrants	Avicel, Explotab	↑	↓	↑/—
Lubricants	Talc, hydrogenated vegetable oil	↓	↑	↓/—
Coating agent	Hydroxypropylmethyl cellulose	—	—	—
Enteric coat	Cellulose acetate phthalate	↓	↑	↓/—
Sustained-release agents	Methylcellulose, ethylcellulose	↓	↑	↓/—
Sustained-release agents (waxy agents)	Castorwax, Carbowax	↓	↑	↓/—
Sustained-release agents (gum/viscous)	Veegum, Keltrol	↓	↑	↓/—

*This may be concentration and drug dependent. ↑, Increase; ↓, decrease; —, no effect. K_a, absorption rate constant; T_{max}, time for peak drug concentration in plasma; AUC, area under the plasma drug concentration time curve.

should be decreased or a different lubricant selected. Sometimes, increasing the amount of disintegrant may overcome the retarding effect of lubricants on dissolution. However, with some poorly soluble drugs an increase in disintegrant level has little or no effect on drug dissolution simply because the fine drug particles are not wetted. The influence of some common ingredients on drug absorption parameters are listed in Table 6-6. These are general trends for typical preparations.

The inactive components of a product are commonly referred to as *formulation ingredients* or excipients. The excipients are often needed to produce a drug product with homogeneity and stability. Excipients for both liquid and solid products are listed in Tables 6-4 and 6-5. Some of these ingredients may affect drug release in a product and therefore affect drug absorption.

PRACTICE PROBLEM

Drug formulation of erythromycin including its esters and salts has significant differences in bioavailability. Erythromycin is unstable in acidic medium. Suggest a method for preventing a potential bioavailability problem for this drug.

Solution

A bioavailability problem may be uncovered by a suitable dissolution method. However, the dissolution testing condition reveals that the bioavailability problem differs with each drug formulation. A reasonable approach involves selecting a dissolution method in which the acceptable and unacceptable drug formulation is distinguished by having different dissolution rates. Different agitation rates, different medium (including different pH) and different

TABLE 6-7. DISSOLUTION OF ERYTHROMYCIN STEARATE BULK DRUG AND CORRESPONDING TABLETS

	Percent Dissolution After 1.0 hr:		
Curve No:	Bulk Drug	500-mg Tablet	250-mg Tablet
4	49	44	
6	72	70	
7	75	70	
—	78	—	80
8	82	75	
9	92	85	

From Philip J, Daly RE, 1983, with permission.[9]

dissolution apparatus should be tried. Once differences in dissolution rates are found, the formulation of the drug product may be matched with the dissolution rates to get an empirically acceptable criteria for the product. The composition and supplies of the raw materials may then be examined to reveal the problem. In one example Philip et al.[9] devised a method using pH 6.6 phosphate buffer as the dissolution medium instead of 0.1 N HCl to avoid instability of the drug. Using the testing temperature at 22°C and the USP

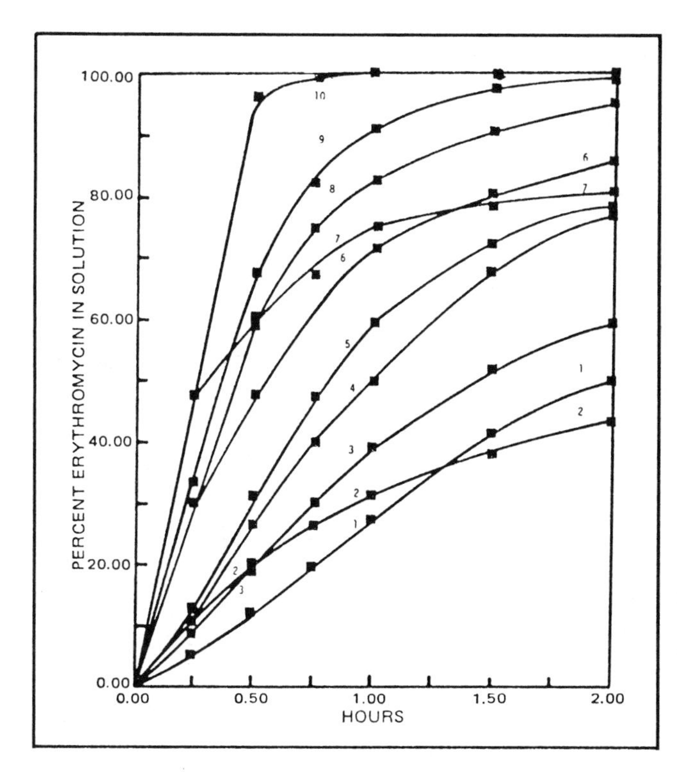

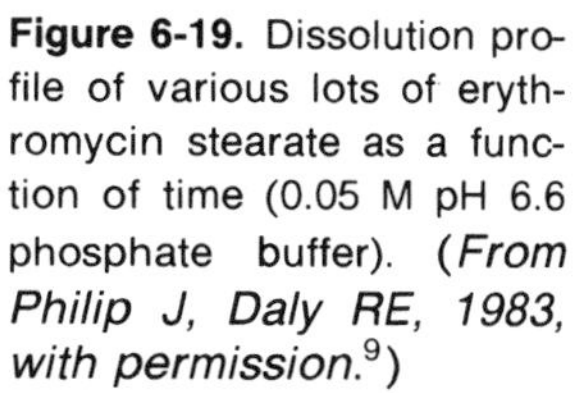
Figure 6-19. Dissolution profile of various lots of erythromycin stearate as a function of time (0.05 M pH 6.6 phosphate buffer). (*From Philip J, Daly RE, 1983, with permission.*[9])

paddle method at 50 rpm, the dissolution of the various erythromycin tablets varied with the source of the bulk drug (as shown in Table 6-7 and Figure 6-19).

The dissolution rate of erythromycin powder varied from 100% dissolved in an hour to less than 40% dissolved in an hour. The slow dissolving raw material also resulted in slow dissolving drug products. Therefore, the dissolution of powdered raw material is a very useful in vitro method for the prediction of a bioavailability problem of the erythromycin product in the body.

QUESTIONS

1. What are the two rate-limiting steps possible in the oral absorption of a solid drug product? Which one would apply to a soluble drug? Which one could be altered by the pharmacist? Give examples.
2. What is the physiologic transport mechanism for the absorption of most drugs from the gastrointestinal tract? What area of the gastrointestinal tract is most favorable for the absorption of drugs? Why?
3. Explain why the absorption rate of a soluble drug tends to be greater than the elimination rate of the drug.
4. What type of oral dosage form generally yields the greatest amount of systemically available drug in the least amount of time? (Assume that the drug can be prepared in any form.) Why?

REFERENCES

1. The United States Pharmacopeia XX/NF-XV. Easton, Mark Publishing Co., 1980, p. 960
2. Wood JH: In vitro evaluation of physiological availability of compressed tablets. Pharm Acta Helv 42:129, 1966
3. Levy G, Leonards J, Procknal JA: Development of in vitro tests which correlate quantitatively with dissolution rate-limited drug absorption in man. J Pharm Sci 54:1719, 1965.
4. Shah VP, Prasad VK, Alston T, Cabana B, Gural RP, Meyer MC: Phenytoin I: In vitro correlation for 100 mg phenytoin sodium capsules. J Pharm Sci 72:306–308, 1983
6. Gillette JR, Mitchell JR: Routes of drug administration and response. In Concept in Biochemical Pharmacology. Berlin, Springer-Verlag, 1975, Chap. 64
7. Aguiar, AJ, Krc J, Kinkel AW, Samyn JC: Effect of polymorphism on the absorption of chloramphenicol from chloramphenical palmitate. J Pharm Sci 56:847–853, 1967
8. Allen PV, Rahn PD, Sarapu AC, Vandewielen AJ: Physical characteristic of erythromycin anhydrate, and dihydrate crystalline solids. J Pharm Sci 67:1087–1093, 1978
9. Philip J, Daly RE: Test for selection of erythromycin stearate bulk drug for tablet preparation. J Pharm Sci 72:979–980, 1983
10. Cameron CG, Cuff GW, McGinity J: Development and Evaluation of Controlled Release Theophylline Tablet Formulations Containing Acrylic Resins; Comparison of Dissolution Test Methodologies A. Ph.A. meeting abstract, April, 1983

11. Masih SZ, Jacob KC, Majuh M, Fatmi A: Comparison of USP Basket and Paddle Method for Evaluation of Sustained Release Formulation Containing Pseudoephedrine and Guaifenesin. P. Ph.A. meeting abstract, April 1983

BIBLIOGRAPHY

Aguiar AJ: Physical properties and pharmaceutical manipulations influencing drug absorption. In Forth IW, Rummel W (eds.), Pharmacology of Intestinal Absorption: Gastrointestinal Absorption of Drugs. New York, Pergamon, 1975, vol. 1, Chap. 6

Barr WH: The use of physical and animal models to assess bioavailability. Pharmacology 8:88–101, 1972

Blanchard J, Sawchuk RJ, Brodie BB: Principles and Perspectives in Drug Bioavailability. New York, Karger, 1979

Cabana BE, O'Neil R: FDA's report on drug dissolution. Pharm Forum 6:71–75, 1980

Cadwalder DE: Biopharmaceutics and Drug Interactions. Nutley, N.J., Roche Laboratories, 1971

Christensen J: The physiology of gastrointestinal transit. Med Clin North Am 58:1165–80, 1974

Dakkuri A, Shah AC: Dissolution methodology: An overview. Pharm Technol 6:28–32, 1982

Gilbaldi M: Biopharmaceutics and Clinical Pharmacokinetics. Philadelphia, Lea and Febiger, 1977

Hansen WA: Handbook of Dissolution Testing. Springfield, OR, Pharmaceutical Technology Publications, 1982

Hardwidge E, Sarapu A, Laughlin W: Comparison of operating characteristics of different dissolution test systems. J Pharm Sci 6:1732–1735, 1978

Jollow DJ, Brodie BB: Mechanisms of drug absorption and drug solution. Pharmacology 8:21–32, 1972

LaDu BN, Mandel HG, Way EL: Fundamentals of Drug Metabolism and Drug Disposition. Baltimore, Williams and Wilkins, 1971

Leeson LJ, Carstensen JT: Industrial pharmaceutical technology. In Dissolution Technology. Washington, D.C., Academy of Pharmaceutical Sciences, 1974

Levine RR: Factors affecting gastrointestinal absorption of drugs. Dig Dis 15:171–88, 1970

Niazi S: Textbook of Biopharmaceutics and Clinical Pharmacokinetics. New York, Appleton, 1979

Notari RE: Biopharmaceutics and Pharmacokinetics: An Introduction. New York, Marcel Dekker, 1975

Parrott EL: Pharmaceutical Technology. Minneapolis, Burgess, 1970

Pernarowski M: Dissolution methodology. In Leeson L, Carstensen JT (eds.), Dissolution Technology. Washington D.C., The Industrial Pharmaceutical Technology Section Of The Academy Of Pharm. Sciences, P. Ph.A., 1975, p. 58

Pharmacopeial Forum: FDA report on drug dissolution. Pharm Forum 6:71–75, 1980

Prasad VK, Shah VP, Hunt J, Purich E, Knight P, Cabana BE: Evaluation of basket and paddle dissolution methods using different performance standards. J Pharm Sci 72:42–44, 1983

Prasad V, Shah V, Knight P, Mallinowski H, Cabana B, Meyer MC: Importance of media selection in establishment of in vitro–in vivo relationship for quinidine gluconate. Int J Pharm 13:1–7, 1983

Robinson JR: Sustained and Controlled Release Drug Delivery Systems. New York, Marcel Dekker, 1978

Robinson JR, Eriken SP: Theoretical formulation of sustained release dosage forms. J Pharm Sci 55:1254, 1966

Shaw JE, Chandrasekaran K: Controlled topical delivery of drugs for system in action. Drug Metab Rev 8:223–33, 1978

Swarbrick J: In vitro models of drug dissolution. In Swarbrick J (ed.), Current Concepts in the Pharmaceutical Sciences: Biopharmaceutics. Philadelphia, Lea and Febiger, 1970

Wagner JG: Biopharmaceutics and Relevant Pharmacokinetics. Hamilton, Ill., Drug Intelligence Publications, 1971

Wurster DE, Taylor PW: Dissolution rates. J Pharm Sci 54:169–75, 1965

York P: Solid state properties of powders in the formulation and processing of solid dosage form. Int J Pharm 14:1–28, 1983

Zaffaroni A: Therapeutic systems: The key to rational drug therapy. Drug Metab Rev 8:191–222, 1978

CHAPTER SEVEN

Pharmacokinetics of Drug Absorption

The systemic absorption of a drug from the gastrointestinal tract or any other extravascular site is dependent on the dosage form of the drug and the anatomy and physiology of the absorption site. Such factors as surface area of the gut, stomach-emptying rate, gastrointestinal mobility, and blood flow to the absorption site all affect the rate and the extent of drug absorption. In spite of these variations, the overall rate of drug absorption may be described mathematically as a first-order or zero-order input process. Most pharmacokinetic models assume first-order absorption unless an assumption of zero-order absorption improves the model significantly or has been verified experimentally.

The rate of change in the amount of drug in the body, dD_B/dt, is dependent on the rates of drug absorption and elimination (Fig. 7-1).

The rate of drug accumulation in the body at any time is equal to the rate of drug absorption less the rate of drug elimination.

$$\frac{dD_B}{dt} = \frac{dD_{GI}}{dt} - \frac{dD_e}{dt} \tag{7.1}$$

A plasma level–time curve describing drug adsorption and elimination rate processes is depicted graphically in Figure 7-2.

During the *absorption phase* of a plasma level–time curve (Fig. 7-2) the rate of drug absorption is greater than the rate of drug elimination:

$$\frac{dD_{GI}}{dt} > \frac{dD_e}{dt} \tag{7.2}$$

At the *time of peak drug concentration* in the plasma, which corresponds to the time of peak absorption in Figure 7-2, the rate of drug absorption just equals the rate of drug elimination, and there is no change in the amount of drug in the body:

$$\frac{dD_{GI}}{dt} = \frac{dD_e}{dt} \tag{7.3}$$

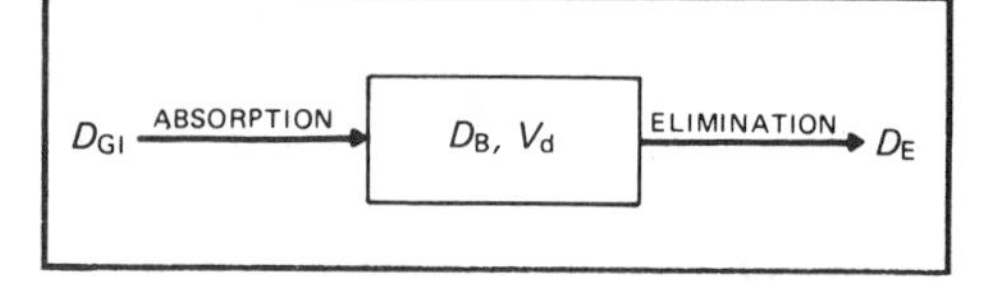

Figure 7-1. Model of drug absorption and elimination.

Immediately after the time of peak drug absorption some drug may still be at the absorption site (i.e., in the gastrointestinal tract). However, the rate of drug elimination is at this time faster than the rate of drug absorption, as represented by the *postabsorption phase* in Figure 7-2.

$$\frac{dD_{\mathrm{GI}}}{dt} < \frac{dD_{\mathrm{e}}}{dt} \tag{7.4}$$

When the drug at the absorption site becomes depleted, the rate of drug absorption approaches zero, or $dD_{\mathrm{GI}}/dt = 0$. The *elimination phase* of the curve then represents only the elimination of drug from the body, usually a first-order process. Therefore, during the elimination phase the rate of change in the amount of drug in the body is described as a first-order process.

$$\frac{dD_{\mathrm{B}}}{dt} = -KD_{\mathrm{B}} \tag{7.5}$$

where K is the first-order elimination rate constant.

ZERO-ORDER ABSORPTION MODEL

In this model drug in the gastrointestinal tract, D_{GI}, is absorbed systemically at a constant rate, K_0. Drug is eliminated from the body by a first-order rate process with a first-order rate constant, K. This model is analogous to that of the adminis-

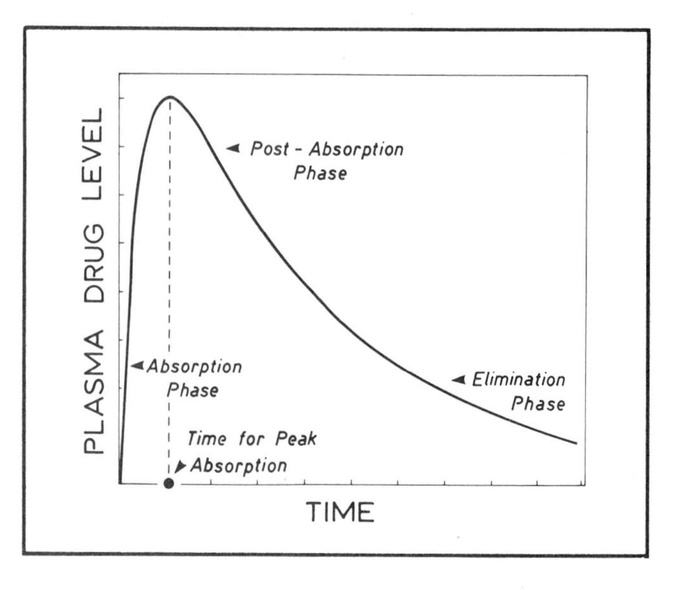

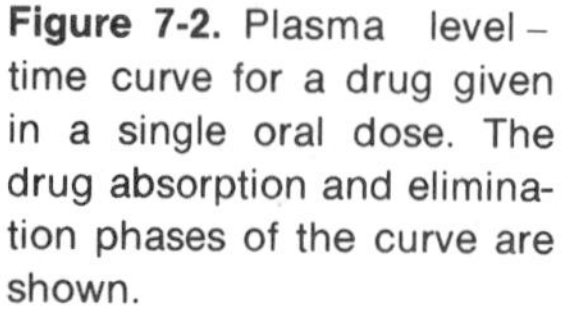

Figure 7-2. Plasma level–time curve for a drug given in a single oral dose. The drug absorption and elimination phases of the curve are shown.

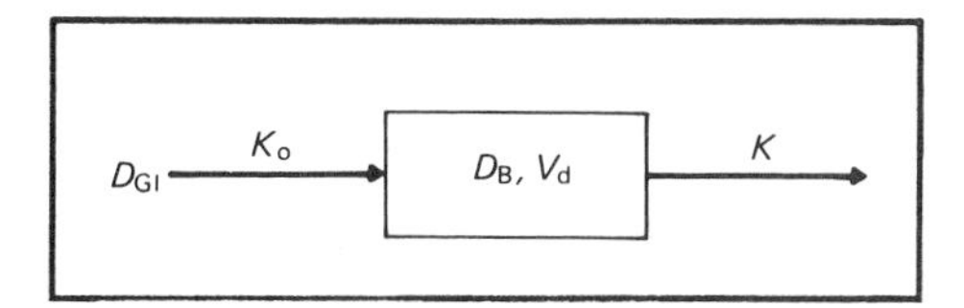

Figure 7-3. One-compartment pharmacokinetic model for zero-order drug absorption and first-order drug elimination.

tration of a drug by intravenous infusion (see Chapter 12). The pharmacokinetic model assuming zero-order absorption is described in Figure 7-3.

The rate of elimination at any time, by first-order process, is equal to $D_B K$. The rate of input is simply K_0. Therefore, the net change per unit time in the body can be expressed as follows:

$$\frac{dD_B}{dt} = K_0 - KD_B \tag{7.6}$$

Integration of this equation with substitution of $V_d C_p$ for D_B produces

$$C_p = \frac{K_0}{V_d K}(1 - e^{-Kt}) \tag{7.7}$$

The rate of drug absorption is constant and continues until the amount of drug in the gut, D_{GI}, is depleted. The time at which drug absorption is continuous is equal to D_{GI}/K_0. After this time the drug is no longer available for absorption from the gut, and Equation 7.7 no longer holds. The drug concentration in the plasma will decline in accordance with a first-order elimination rate process (Fig. 7-2).

FIRST-ORDER ABSORPTION MODEL

This model assumes a first-order input and a first-order elimination (Fig. 7-4). The differential equation that describes the rate of drug change in the body is as follows:

$$\frac{dD_B}{dt} = FK_a D_{GI} - KD_B \tag{7.8}$$

where F is the fraction of drug systemically absorbed. Since the drug in the gastrointestinal tract also follows a first-order decline process (i.e., it is absorbed across the gastrointestinal wall), the amount of drug in the gastrointestinal tract is equal to $D_0 e^{-K_a t}$.

$$\frac{dD_B}{dt} = FK_a D_0 e^{-K_a t} - KD_B \tag{7.9}$$

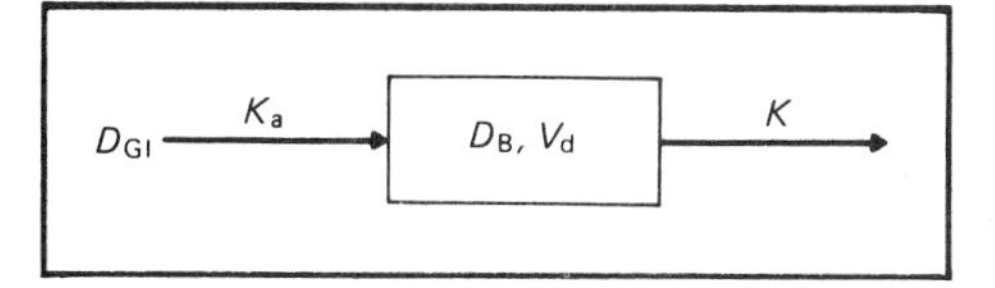

Figure 7-4. One-compartment pharmacokinetic model for first-order drug absorption and first-order elimination.

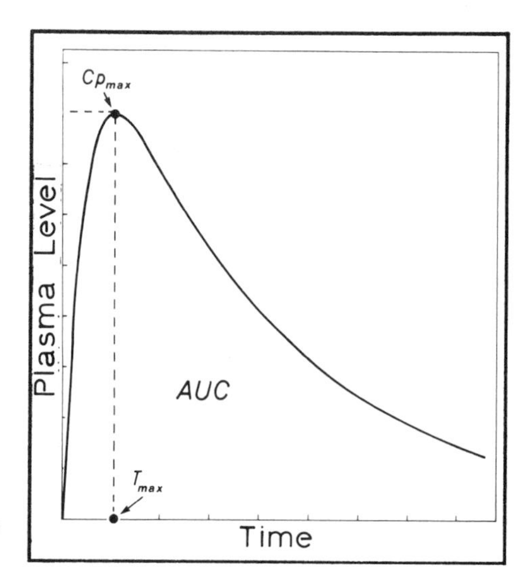

Figure 7-5. Typical plasma level–time curve for a drug given in a single oral dose.

This equation can be integrated to give the general oral absorption equation for calculation of the drug concentration (C_p) in the plasma at any time t:

$$C_p = \frac{FK_a D_0}{V_d(K_a - K)}(e^{-Kt} - e^{-K_a t}) \tag{7.10}$$

A typical plot of the concentration of drug in the body after oral dose is presented in Figure 7-5.

The maximum concentration is $C_{p,\max}$ and the time needed to reach maximum concentration is $t_{\max}$. The time needed to reach maximum concentration is independent of dose and is dependent on the rate constants for absorption (K_a) and elimination (K). At the maximum concentration, sometimes called peak concentration, the rate of drug absorbed is equal to the rate of drug eliminated. Therefore, the rate of concentration change is equal to zero. The rate of concentration change can be obtained by differentiating Equation 7.10:

$$\frac{dC_p}{dt} = \frac{K_a D_0 F}{V_d(K_a - K)}(-Ke^{-Kt} + K_a e^{-K_a t}) = 0 \tag{7.11}$$

This can be simplified as follows:

$$-Ke^{-Kt} + K_a e^{-K_a t} = 0$$

or

$$Ke^{-Kt} = K_a e^{-K_a t}$$

$$\ln K - Kt = \ln K_a - K_a t$$

$$t_{\max} = \frac{\ln K_a - \ln K}{K_a - K} = \frac{\ln(K_a/K)}{K_a - K} = \frac{2.3 \log(K_a/K)}{K_a - K} \tag{7.12}$$

As shown here, the time for maximum drug concentration, t_{max}, is dependent only on the rate constants K_a and K. In order to calculate the peak plasma drug concentration, the value for t_{max} is determined via Equation 7.12 and then substituted into Equation 7.10, solving for $C_{p,max}$. From Equation 7.10 it can be seen that the $C_{p,max}$ is directly proportional to the dose of drug given (D_0) and the fraction of drug absorbed (F). Calculation of t_{max} and $C_{p,max}$ is usually necessary, since direct measurement of drug concentrations may not be possible due to improper timing of the serum samples.

The first-order elimination rate constant may be determined from the elimination phase of the plasma level–time curve (Fig. 7-2). At the later time intervals, when drug absorption has been completed, Equation 7.10 reduces to the following expression:

$$C_p = \frac{FK_a D_0}{V_d(K_a - K)} e^{-Kt} \tag{7.13}$$

Taking the natural logarithm of this expression,

$$\ln C_p = \ln \frac{FK_a D_0}{V_d(K_a - K)} - Kt \tag{7.14}$$

Substitution of common logarithms gives

$$\log C_p = \log \frac{FK_a D_0}{V_d(K_a - K)} - \frac{Kt}{2.3} \tag{7.15}$$

With this equation, a graph constructed by plotting $\log C_p$ versus time will yield a straight line with a slope of $-K/2.3$. With a similar approach, *urinary drug excretion* data may also be used for calculation of the first-order elimination rate constant. The rate of drug excretion after a single oral dose of drug is given by

$$\frac{dD_u}{dt} = \frac{FK_e K_a D_0}{K_a - K}(e^{-Kt} - e^{-K_a t}) \tag{7.16}$$

where dD_u/dt = rate of urinary drug excretion; K_e = first-order renal excretion constant; and F = fraction of dose absorbed.

A graph constructed by plotting dD_u/dt versus time will yield a curve which is identical in appearance to the plasma level–time curve for the drug. After drug absorption is virtually complete, $e^{-K_a t}$ approaches zero, and Equation 7.16 reduces to the following expression:

$$\frac{dD_u}{dt} = \frac{K_e K_a F D_0}{K_a - K} e^{-Kt} \tag{7.17}$$

Taking the natural logarithm of both sides of this expression and substituting in terms of common logarithms, Equation 7.17 becomes

$$\log \frac{dD_u}{dt} = \log \frac{K_e K_a F D_0}{K_a - K} - \frac{Kt}{2.3} \tag{7.18}$$

When $\log(dD_u/dt)$ is plotted against time, a graph of a straight line is obtained with a slope of $-K/2.3$. Since the rate of urinary drug excretion, dD_u/dt, cannot be determined directly, an average rate of urinary drug excretion is obtained, and this value is plotted against the midpoint of the collection period for each urine sample.

To obtain the *cumulative drug excretion* in the urine, Equation 7.16 must be integrated:

$$D_u = \frac{FK_eK_aD_0}{K_a - K}\left(\frac{e^{-K_at}}{K_a} - \frac{e^{-Kt}}{K}\right) + \frac{FK_eD_0}{K} \tag{7.19}$$

A plot of D_u versus time will give the urinary drug excretion curve described in Chapter 8. When all of the drug has been excreted, at $t = \infty$, Equation 7.19 reduces to

$$D_u^\infty = \frac{FK_eD_0}{K} \tag{7.20}$$

where D_u^∞ is the maximum amount of active or parent drug excreted.

Determination of Absorption Rate Constants from Oral Absorption Data

Method of Residuals. Assuming $K_a \gg K$ in Equation 7.10, the value for the second exponential will become insignificantly small with time and can therefore be omitted. When this is the case, drug absorption is virtually complete. Equation 7.10 then reduces to Equation 7.21:

$$C_p = \frac{FK_aD_0}{V_d(K_a - K)}e^{-Kt} \tag{7.21}$$

From this one may also obtain

$$\frac{FK_aD_0}{V_d(K_a - K)} = A$$

where A is a constant. Thus, Equation 7.21 becomes

$$C_p = Ae^{-Kt} \tag{7.22}$$

This equation, which represents first-order drug elimination, will yield a linear plot on semilog paper. The slope is equal to $-K/2.3$. The value for K_a can be obtained by using the method of *residuals* or a *feathering* technique, as described in Chapter 5. The value of K_a is obtained by means of the following procedure.

1. Plot the drug concentration versus time on semilog paper with the concentration values on the logarithmic axis (Fig. 7-6).
2. Obtain the slope of the terminal phase (line BC, Fig. 7-6) by extrapolation.
3. Take any points on the upper part of line BC (e.g., $x_1', x_2', x_3', \ldots$) and drop vertically to obtain corresponding points on the curve (e.g., $x_1, x_2, x_3, \ldots$).
4. Read off the values x_1 and x_1', x_2 and x_2', x_3 and x_3', etc. Plot the values of the differences at the corresponding time points $\Delta_1, \Delta_2, \Delta_3, \ldots$. A straight line will be obtained with a slope of $-K_a/2.3$ (Fig. 7-6).

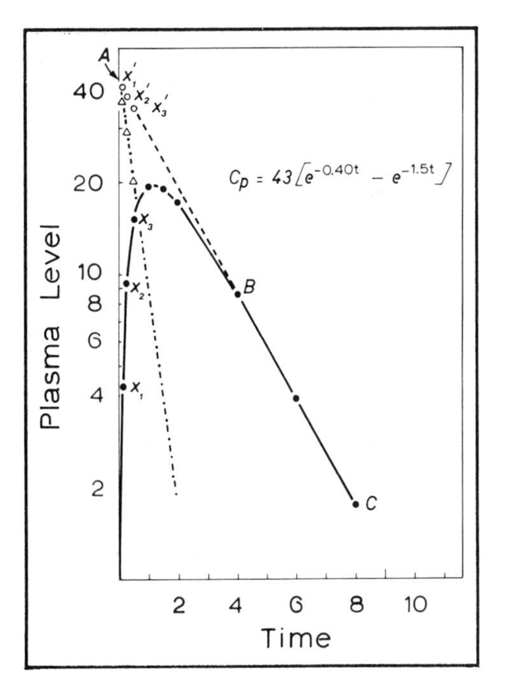

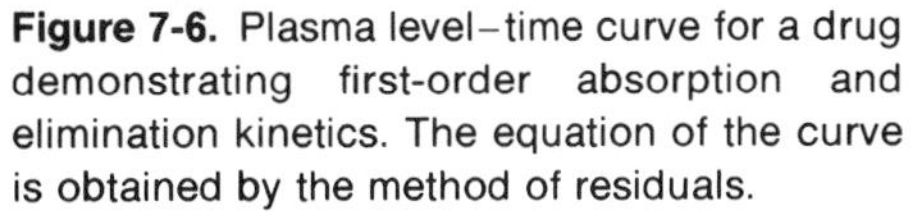

Figure 7-6. Plasma level–time curve for a drug demonstrating first-order absorption and elimination kinetics. The equation of the curve is obtained by the method of residuals.

When using the method of residuals, a minimum of three points should be used to define the straight line. Data points occurring shortly after t_{max} may not be accurate, since drug absorption is still continuing at that time. Since this portion of the curve represents the postabsorption phase, only data points from the elimination phase should be used to define the rate of drug absorption as a first-order process.

If drug absorption begins immediately after oral administration, the residual lines obtained by feathering the plasma level–time curve (as shown in Fig. 7-6) will intersect on the y axis at point A. The value of this y intercept, A, represents a hybrid constant composed of K_a, K, V_d, and FD_0:

$$A = \frac{FK_a D_0}{V_d(K_a - K)}$$

The value for A, as well as the values for K and K_a, may be substituted back into Equation 7.10 to obtain a general theoretical equation that will describe the plasma level–time curve.

Lag Time. In some individuals absorption of drug after a single oral dose does not start immediately, due to such physiologic factors as stomach-emptying time and intestinal mobility. The time delay prior to the commencement of first-order drug absorption is known as *lag time*.

The lag time for a drug may be observed if the two residual lines obtained by feathering the oral absorption plasma level–time curve intersects at a point after $t = 0$ on the x axis. The time at the point of intersection on the x axis is the lag time (Fig. 7-7).

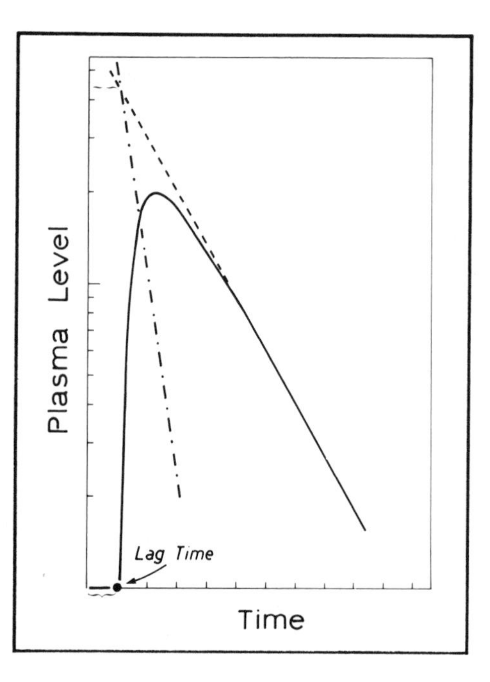

Figure 7-7. The lag time can be determined graphically if the two residual lines obtained by feathering the plasma level–time curve intersect at a point where $t > 0$.

The lag time, t_0, represents the beginning of drug absorption and should not be confused with the pharmacologic term *onset time*, which represents the latency or the time for the drug to just reach the minimum effective concentration.

Two equations can adequately describe the curve in Figure 7-7. In one the lag time t_0 is subtracted from each time point, as shown in Equation 7.23.

$$C_p = \frac{FK_a D_0}{V_d(K_a - K)}\left(e^{-K(t-t_0)} - e^{-K_a(t-t_0)}\right) \tag{7.23}$$

where $FK_a D_0 / V_d(K_a - K)$ is the y value at the point of intersection of the residual lines in Figure 7-7.

The second expression that describes the curve in Figure 7-7 omits the lag time, as follows:

$$C_p = Be^{-Kt} - Ae^{-K_a t} \tag{7.24}$$

where A and B represent the intercepts on the y axis after extrapolation of the residual lines for absorption and elimination, respectively.

Flip-Flop of K_a and K. In using the method of residuals to obtain an estimate of K_a and K, the terminal phase of an oral absorption curve is usually represented by the elimination rate constant and the absorption rate constant is represented by the steeper slope (Fig. 7-6). In a few cases the elimination rate constant K obtained from oral absorption data does not agree with that obtained from intravenous data. For example, the K obtained after an intravenous bolus of a bronchiodilator was

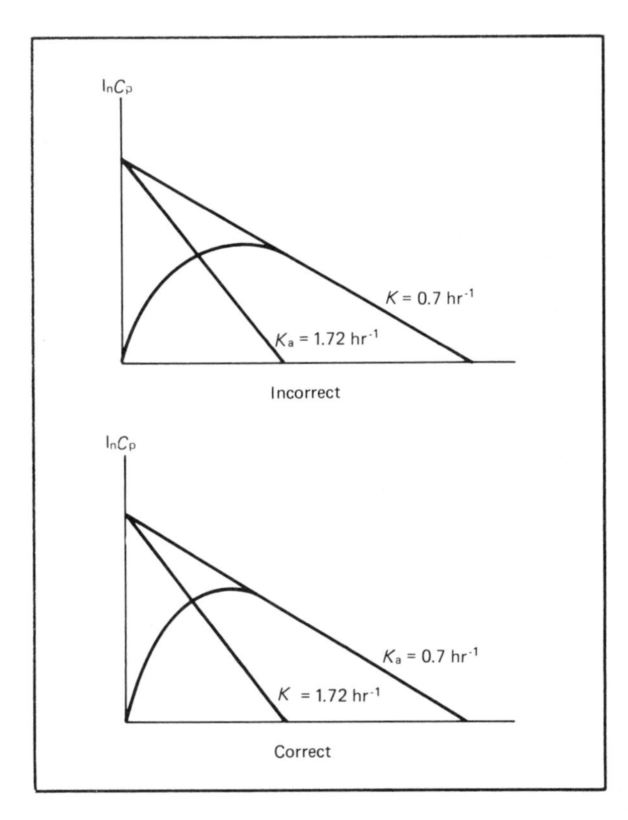

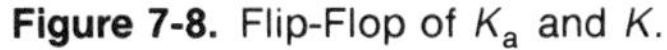

Figure 7-8. Flip-Flop of K_a and K.

1.72 hr^{-1}, whereas the K calculated after oral administration was only 0.7 hr^{-1} (Fig. 7-8). When K_a was obtained by the method of residuals, rather suprisingly, the K_a was 1.72 hr^{-1}.

Apparently, the K_a and K obtained by the method of residuals has been interchanged. This phenomenon is called *flip-flop* of the absorption and elimination rate constants. Flip-flop may occur whenever K_a and K are estimated from oral drug absorption data. Use of computer methods do not ensure against flip-flop of the two constants estimated.

In order to unambiguously demonstrate that the steeper curve represents the elimination rate for a drug given extravascularly, the drug must be given by intravenous injection into the same patient. After intravenous injection the decline in plasma drug levels with time represents the true elimination rate. The relationship between K_a and K on the shape of the plasma drug concentration time curve for a constant dose of drug given orally is shown in Figure 7-8.

The only way to be sure of the estimates is to compare the K calculated after oral administration with the K from intravenous data.

Most of the drugs observed to have flip-flop characteristics are drugs with fast elimination, (i.e., $K > K_a$). Drug absorption of most drug solutions or fast dissolving products are essentially complete or at least half completed within an hour (i.e., absorption half-life of 0.5 or 1 hr, corresponding to a K_a of 1.38 hr^{-1} or 0.69 hr^{-1}).

Since most of the drugs used orally have longer elimination half-lives, the assumption of using the smaller slope or smaller rate constant (i.e., the terminal phase of curve Figure 7-8) as elimination constant is generally correct.

For drugs that have a large elimination rate constant ($K > 0.69\ \text{hr}^{-1}$), the chance for flip-flop of K_a and K are much greater. The drug isoproterenol, for example, has an oral elimination half-life of only a few minutes, and flip-flop of K_a and K has been noted (Portmann, 1970). Similarly, salicyluric acid was flip-flop when oral data were plotted. The K for salicyluric acid was much larger than K_a.[1] Many experimental drugs show flip-flop of K and K_a, whereas few of the marketed oral drugs do. The drugs with a large K are usually considered as unsuitable for an oral drug product due to their large elimination rate constant, corresponding to a very short elimination half-life.

Determination of K_a by Plotting Percent of Drug Unabsorbed Versus Time (Wagner–Nelson Method). After a single oral dose of a drug the total drug dose should be completely accounted for in the amount present in the body, the amount in the urine, and the amount in the gut. Therefore, dose (D_0) is expressed as follows:

$$D_0 = D_{GI} + D_B + D_u \tag{7.25}$$

Let $\text{Ab} = D_B + D_u$ = amount of drug absorbed and Ab^∞ = amount of drug absorbed at $t = \infty$. At any time the fraction of drug absorbed would be $\text{Ab}/\text{Ab}^\infty$, and the fraction of drug unabsorbed would be $1 - (\text{Ab}/\text{Ab}^\infty)$. The amount of drug excreted at any time t can be calculated as follows:

$$D_u = KV_d[\text{AUC}]_0^t \tag{7.26}$$

The amount of drug in the body (D_B) at any time $= C_pV_d$. At any time t the amount of drug absorbed (Ab) is as follows:

$$\text{Ab} = C_pV_d + KV_d[\text{AUC}]_0^t \tag{7.27}$$

At $t = \infty$, $C_p^\infty = 0$ (i.e., plasma concentration is negligible), and the total amount of drug absorbed is

$$\text{Ab}^\infty = 0 + KV_d[\text{AUC}]_0^\infty \tag{7.28}$$

The fraction of drug absorbed at any time is

$$\frac{\text{Ab}}{\text{Ab}^\infty} = \frac{C_pV_d + KV_d[\text{AUC}]_0^t}{KV_d[\text{AUC}]_0^\infty} \tag{7.29}$$

$$\frac{\text{Ab}}{\text{Ab}^\infty} = \frac{C_p + K[\text{AUC}]_0^t}{K[\text{AUC}]_0^\infty} \tag{7.30}$$

The fraction unabsorbed at any time t is

$$1 - \frac{\text{Ab}}{\text{Ab}^\infty} = 1 - \frac{C_p + K[\text{AUC}]_0^t}{K[\text{AUC}]_0^\infty} \tag{7.31}$$

since the drug remaining in the gut at any time t is

$$D_{GI} = De^{-K_a t} \tag{7.32}$$

Therefore, the fraction of drug remaining is

$$\frac{D_{GI}}{D} = e^{-K_a t}$$

$$\log \frac{D_{GI}}{D} = \frac{-K_a t}{2.3} \tag{7.33}$$

Since D_{GI}/D is actually the fraction of drug unabsorbed, i.e., $1 - (\text{Ab}/\text{Ab}^{\infty})$, a plot of $1 - (\text{Ab}/\text{Ab}^{\infty})$ versus time gives $-K_a/2.3$ as the slope (Fig. 7-8).

The following steps should be useful in determination of K_a:

1. Plot log concentration of drug versus time.
2. Find K from the terminal part of slope when the slope $= -K/2.3$.
3. Find $[\text{AUC}]_0^t$ by plotting C_p versus t.
4. Find $K[\text{AUC}]_0^t$ by multiplying each $[\text{AUC}]_0^t$ by K.
5. Find $[\text{AUC}]_0^{\infty}$ by adding up all the [AUC] pieces, from $t = 0$ to $t = \infty$.
6. Determine the $1 - (\text{Ab}/\text{Ab}^{\infty})$ value corresponding to each time point t by using Equation 7.31.
7. Plot $1 - (\text{Ab}/\text{Ab}^{\infty})$ versus time on semilog paper, with $1 - (\text{Ab}/\text{Ab}^{\infty})$ on the logarithmic axis.

TABLE 7-1. BLOOD CONCENTRATIONS AND ASSOCIATED DATA FOR A HYPOTHETICAL DRUG

Time t_n (hr)	Concentration C_p (μg/ml)	$[\text{AUC}]_{t_{n-1}}^{t_n}$	$[\text{AUC}]_0^t$	$K[\text{AUC}]_0^t$	AB = $C_p + K[\text{AUC}]_0^t$	$\frac{\text{Ab}}{\text{Ab}^{\infty}}$	$\left(1 - \frac{\text{Ab}}{\text{Ab}^{\infty}}\right)$
0	0.	0.	0.				
1	3.13	1.57	1.57	0.157	3.287	0.331	0.6690
2	4.93	4.03	5.60	0.560	5.490	0.553	0.4470
3	5.86	5.40	10.99	1.099	6.959	0.701	0.2990
4	6.25	6.06	17.05	1.705	7.955	0.800	0.2000
5	6.28	6.23	23.31	2.331	8.610	0.868	0.1320
6	6.11	6.20	29.51	2.951	9.061	0.913	0.0366
7	5.81	5.96	35.47	3.547	9.357	0.943	0.0570
8	5.45	5.63	41.10	4.110	9.560	0.964	0.0360
9	5.06	5.26	46.35	4.635	9.695	0.977	0.0230
10	4.66	4.86	51.21	5.121			
12	3.90	8.56	59.77	5.977			
14	3.24	7.14	66.91	6.691			
16	2.67	5.92	72.83	7.283			
18	2.19	4.86	77.69	7.769			
24	1.20	10.20	87.89	8.789			
28	0.81	4.04	91.93	9.193			
32	0.54	2.72	94.65	9.465			
36	0.36	1.80	96.45	9.645			
48	0.10	2.76	99.21	9.921			

PRACTICE PROBLEMS

Drug concentrations in the blood at various times are listed in Table 7-1. Assuming the drug follows a one-compartment model, find the K_a and compare it with the K_a value obtained by the method of residuals.

Solution

The AUC is approximated by the *trapezoidal rule*. This method is fairly accurate when there are sufficient data points. The area between each time point is calculated as follows:

$$[\mathrm{AUC}]_{t_{m-1}}^{t_n} = \frac{C_{n-1} + C_n}{2}(t_n - t_{n-1}) \qquad (7.34)$$

where C_n and C_{n-1} are concentrations. For example, at $n = 6$, the [AUC] is

$$\frac{6.28 + 6.11}{2}(6 - 5) = 6.20$$

To obtain $[\mathrm{AUC}]_0^{\infty}$, simply add up all the area pieces under the curve from zero to infinity. In this case 48 hr is long enough to be considered infinity since the blood concentration has at that point already fallen to an insignificant concentration—i.e., 0.1 μg/ml. The rest of the needed information is columnized in Table 7-2. Notice that K is found from the plot of $\log C_p$ versus t. K was found to be 0.1 hr^{-1}. The plot of $1 - (\mathrm{Ab}/\mathrm{Ab}^{\infty})$ versus t on semilog paper is shown in Figure 7-9.

A more complete method of obtaining the $[\mathrm{AUC}]_0^{\infty}$ is to estimate the residual area from the last observed plasma concentration C_{p_N} at t_m to time

TABLE 7-2. EFFECTS OF THE ABSORPTION RATE CONSTANT AND ELIMINATION RATE*

Absorption Rate Constant K_a (hr^{-1})	Elimination Rate Constant K (hr^{-1})	T_{max} (hr)	C_{max} (μg/ml)	AUC (μg hr/ml)
0.1	0.2	6.93	2.50	50
0.2	0.1	6.93	5.00	100
0.3	0.1	5.49	5.77	100
0.4	0.1	4.62	6.29	100
0.5	0.1	4.02	6.69	100
0.6	0.1	3.58	6.99	100
0.3	0.1	5.49	5.77	100
0.3	0.2	4.05	4.44	50
0.3	0.3	3.33	3.68	33.3
0.3	0.4	2.88	3.16	25
0.3	0.5	2.55	2.79	20

* T_{max} = peak plasma drug concentration; C_{max} = peak drug concentration; AUC = area under the curve.

Values are based on a single oral dose (100 mg) which is 100% bioavailable ($F = 1$) and has an apparent V_d of 10 liters. The drug follows a one-compartment open model. T_{max} is calculated by Equation 7.12 and C_{max} is calculated by Equation 7.10. The AUC is calculated by the trapezoidal rule from 0 to 24 hours.

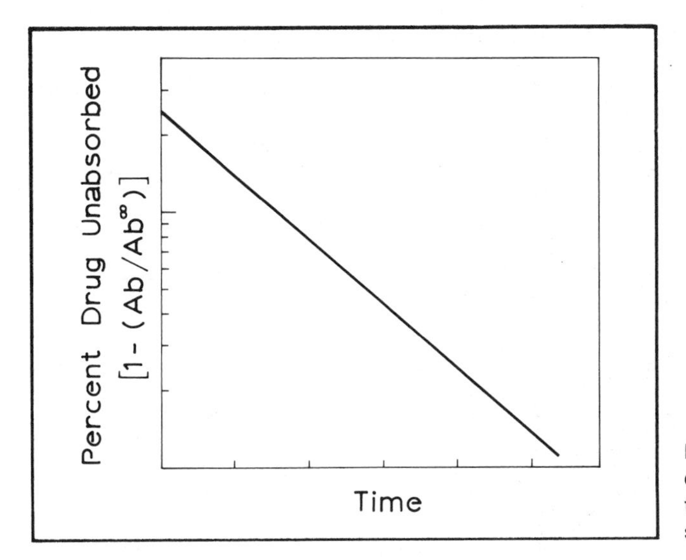

Figure 7-9. Semilog graph of data in Table 7-1 depicting the percent of drug unabsorbed versus time.

equal to infinity. This equation is

$$[\mathrm{AUC}]_t^\infty = \frac{C_{\mathrm{p}_N}}{K} \tag{7.35}$$

The total $[\mathrm{AUC}]_0^\infty$ is the sum of the areas obtained by the trapezoidal rule, i.e., $[\mathrm{AUC}]_0^t$ and the residual area $[\mathrm{AUC}]_t^\infty$ as described in the following expression:

$$[\mathrm{AUC}]_0^\infty = [\mathrm{AUC}]_0^t + [\mathrm{AUC}]_t^\infty \tag{7.36}$$

Estimation of K_a from Urinary Data. The absorption rate constant may also be estimated from urinary excretion data, using a plot of percent of drug unabsorbed versus time. For a one-compartment model

Ab = total amount of drug absorbed—i.e., the amount of drug in the body plus the amount of drug excreted

D_B = amount of drug in the body

D_u = amount of unchanged drug excreted in the urine

C_p = plasma drug concentration

C_B = body drug concentration

D_E = total amount of drug excreted (drug and metabolites)

$$\mathrm{Ab} = D_B + D_E \tag{7.37}$$

The differentiate of Equation 7.37 with respect to time gives

$$\frac{d\,\mathrm{Ab}}{dt} = \frac{dD_B}{dt} + \frac{dD_E}{dt} \tag{7.38}$$

Assuming first-order elimination kinetics with renal elimination constant, K_e,

$$\frac{dD_u}{dt} = K_e D_B = K_e V_d C_p \tag{7.39}$$

Assuming a one-compartment model,

$$V_d C_p = D_B$$

Substituting $V_d C_p$ into Equation 7.38,

$$\frac{d\,\text{Ab}}{dt} = V_d \frac{dC_p}{dt} + \frac{dD_E}{dt} \tag{7.40}$$

And rearranging Equation 7.39,

$$C_p = \frac{1}{K_e V_d}\left(\frac{dD_u}{dt}\right) \tag{7.41}$$

$$\frac{dC_p}{dt} = \frac{d/dt(dD_u/dt)}{K_e V_d} \tag{7.42}$$

Substituting for dC_p/dt into Equation 7.40 and KD_u/K_e for D_E,

$$\frac{d\,\text{Ab}}{dt} = \frac{1}{K_e}\left(\frac{dD_u}{dt}\right) + \frac{K\,dD_u}{K_e\,dt} \tag{7.43}$$

$$\frac{d\,\text{Ab}}{dt} = \frac{1}{K_e}\,\frac{(dD_u/dt)}{dt} + \frac{K}{K_e}\left(\frac{dD_u}{dt}\right) \tag{7.44}$$

When the above expression is integrated from zero to time t,

$$(\text{Ab})_t = \frac{1}{K_e}\left(\frac{dD_u}{dt}\right)_t + \frac{K}{K_e}(D_u)_t \tag{7.45}$$

At $t = \infty$ all the drug that is ultimately absorbed is expressed as Ab^∞, and $dD_u/dt = 0$. The total amount of drug absorbed is as follows:

$$\text{Ab}^\infty = \frac{K}{K_e} D_u^\infty$$

where D_u^∞ is the total amount of unchanged drug excreted in the urine.

The fraction of drug absorbed at any time t is equal to the amount of drug absorbed at this time, $(\text{Ab})_t$, divided by the total amount of drug absorbed, Ab^∞.

$$\frac{(\text{Ab})_t}{\text{Ab}^\infty} = \frac{(dD_u/dt)_t + K(D_u)_t}{KD_u^\infty} \tag{7.46}$$

A plot of the fraction of drug unabsorbed $[1 - (\text{Ab}/\text{Ab}^\infty)]$ versus time gives $-K_a/2.3$ as the slope from which the absorption rate constant is obtained.

Effect of K_a and K on C_{max}, T_{max}, and AUC. Changes in K_a and K may affect T_{max}, C_{max}, and AUC as shown in Table 7-2. If the values for K_a and K are reversed, then the same T_{max} is obtained, but the C_{max} and AUC are different. If the elimination rate constant is kept at 0.1 hr^{-1} and the K_a changes from 0.2 to 0.6 hr^{-1}

(absorption rate increases), then the T_{max} becomes shorter (from 6.93 to 3.58 hr), the C_{max} increases (from 5.00 to 6.99 μg/ml), but the AUC remains constant (100 μg hr/ml). In contrast, when the absorption rate constant is kept at 0.3 hr^{-1} and K changes from 0.1 to 0.5 hr^{-1} (elimination rate increases), then the T_{max} decreases (from 5.49 to 2.55 hr), the C_{max} decreases (from 5.77 to 2.79 μg/ml), and the AUC decreases (from 100 to 20 μg hr/ml). Graphical representations for the relationships of K_a and K on the time for peak absorption and the peak drug concentrations are shown in Figures 7-10 and 7-11.

Determination of K_a From Two-Compartment Oral Absorption Data (Loo–Riegelman Method). Plotting the percent of drug unabsorbed versus time to determine the K_a may be calculated for a drug exhibiting a two-compartment kinetic model. As in the method used previously to obtain an estimate of the K_a, no limitation is placed on the order of the absorption process. However, this method does require that the drug be given intravenously as well as orally to obtain all the necessary kinetic constants.

After oral administration of a dose of a drug that exhibits two-compartment model kinetics, the amount of drug absorbed is calculated as the sum of the amounts of drug in the central compartment (D_c) and in the tissue compartment (D_t) and the amount of drug eliminated by all routes (D_u) (Fig. 7-12):

$$\text{Ab} = D_c + D_t + D_u \tag{7.47}$$

Each of these terms may be expressed in terms of kinetics constants and plasma drug concentrations, as follows:

$$D_c = V_p C_p \tag{7.48}$$

$$D_t = V_t C_t \tag{7.49}$$

$$\frac{dD_u}{dt} = K V_p C_p$$

$$D_u = K V_p [\text{AUC}]_0^t \tag{7.50}$$

Substituting the above expressions for D_c and D_u into Equation 7.46,

$$\text{Ab} = V_p C_p + D_t + K V_p [\text{AUC}]_0^t \tag{7.51}$$

By dividing this equation by V_p to base the equation on drug concentrations, we obtain

$$\frac{\text{Ab}}{V_p} = C_p + \frac{D_t}{V_p} + K[\text{AUC}]_0^t \tag{7.52}$$

At $t = \infty$ this equation becomes

$$\frac{\text{Ab}}{V_p} + K[\text{AUC}]_0^\infty \tag{7.53}$$

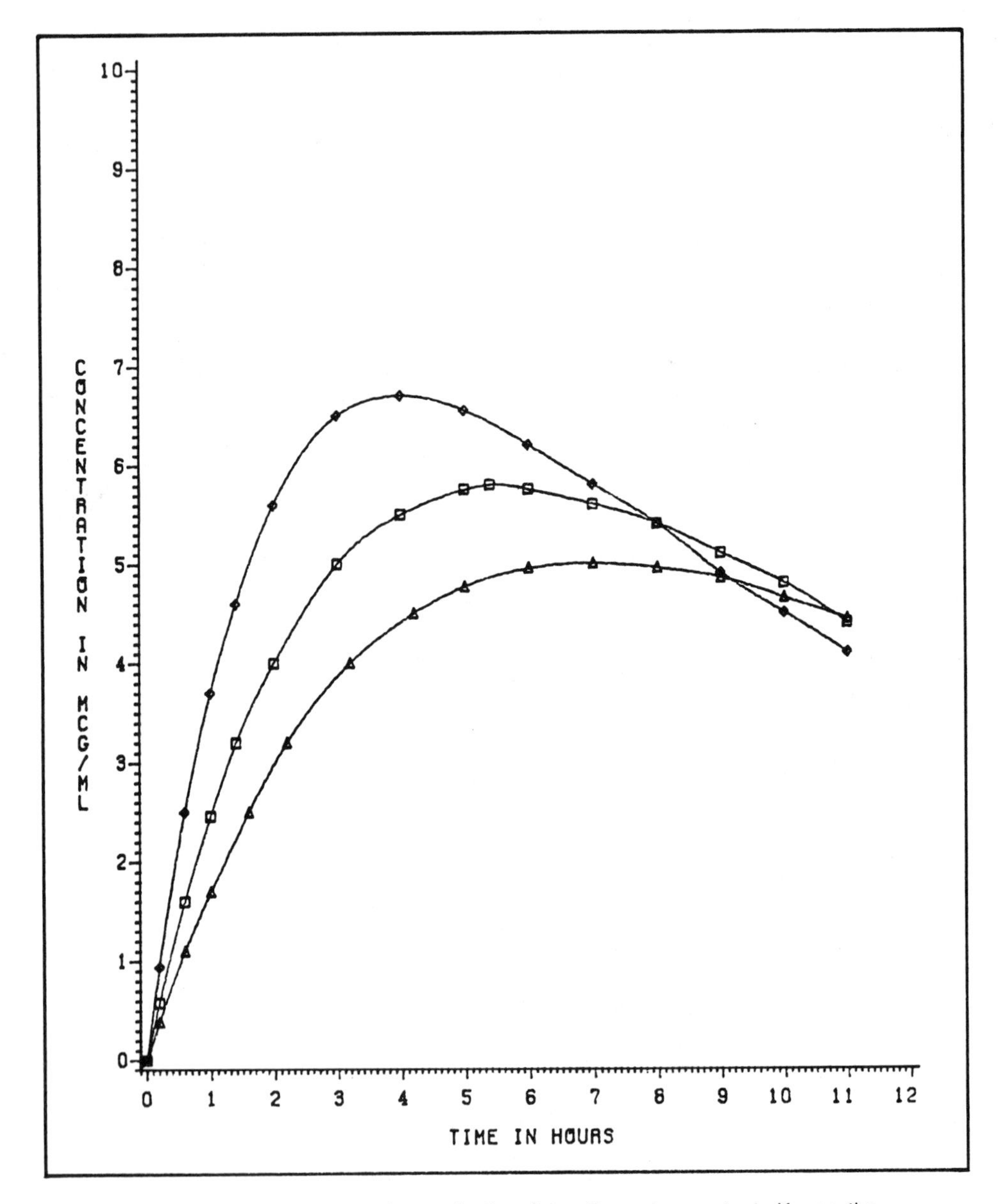

Figure 7-10. Effect of a change in the absorption rate constant, K_a, on the plasma drug concentration versus time curve. Dose of drug is 100 mg, V_d is 10 L, and K is 0.1 hr^{-1}. Δ indicates $K_a = 0.2/\text{hr}$; $\square$ indicates $K_a = 0.3/\text{hr}$; $\diamondsuit$ indicates $K_a = 0.5/\text{hr}$.

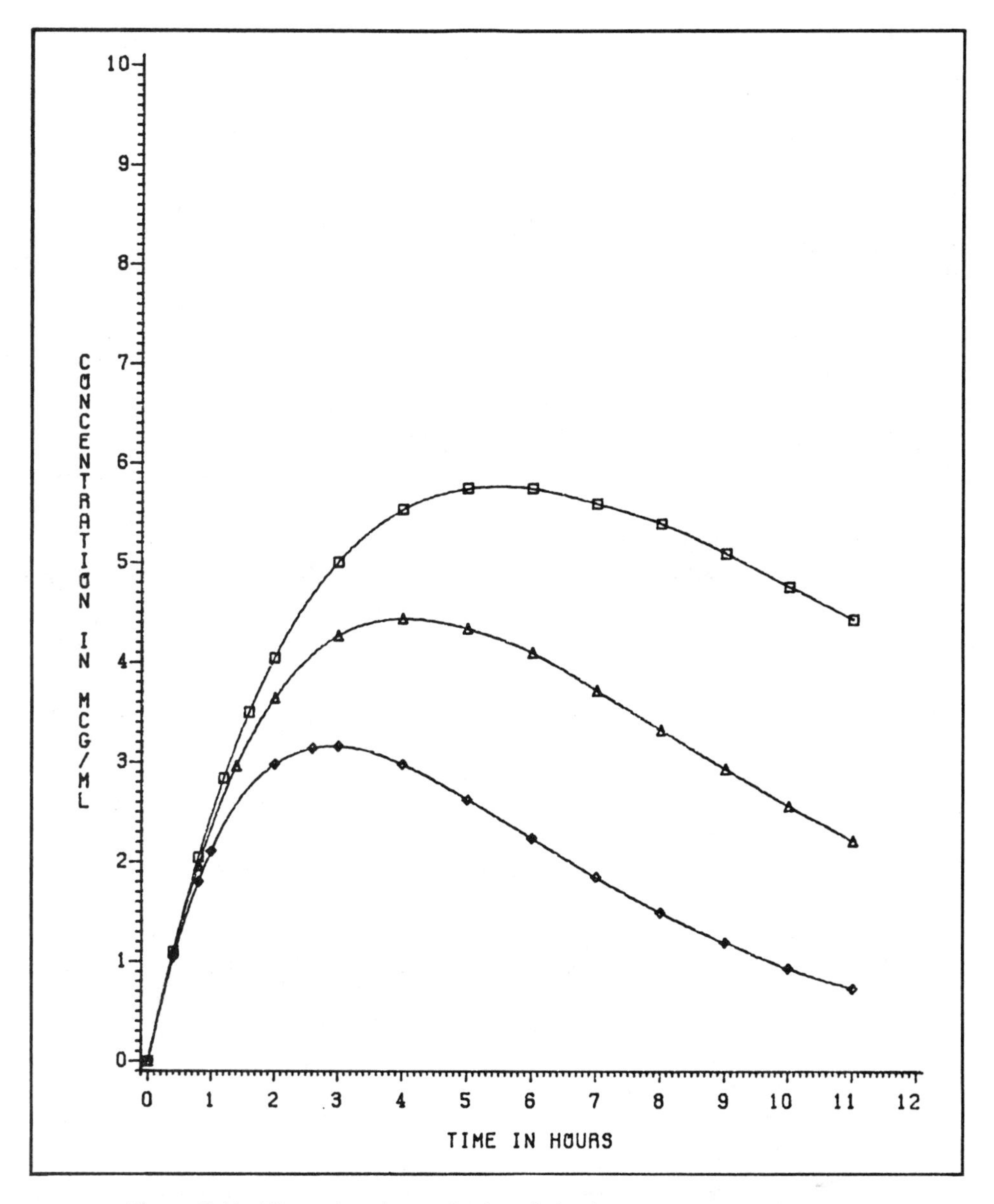

Figure 7-11. Effect of a change in the elimination rate constant, K, on the plasma drug concentration versus time curve. Dose of drug is 100 mg, V_d is 10 L, K_a is 0.1 hr^{-1}. □ indicates $K = 0.1/\text{hr}$; △ indicates $K = 0.2/\text{hr}$; ◇ indicates $K = 0.4/\text{hr}$.

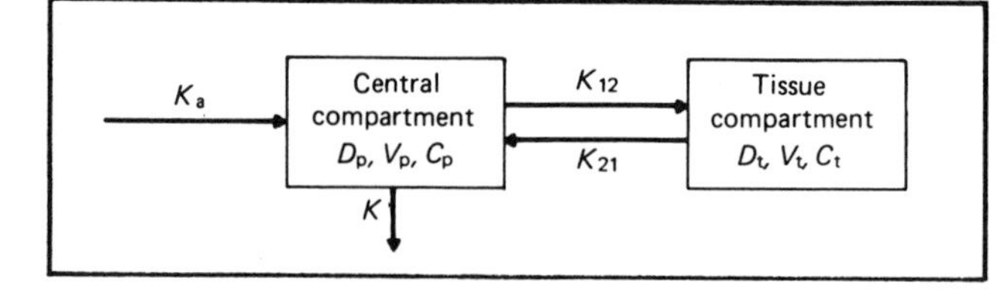

Figure 7-12. Two-compartment pharmacokinetic mode. Drug absorption and elimination occur from the central compartment.

Equation 7.52 divided by Equation 7.53 gives the fraction of drug absorbed at any time.

$$\frac{\text{Ab}}{\text{Ab}^{\infty}} = \frac{C_{\text{p}} + \dfrac{D_{\text{t}}}{V_{\text{p}}} + K[\text{AUC}]_0^t}{K[\text{AUC}]_0^{\infty}} \tag{7.54}$$

A plot of the fraction of drug unabsorbed $[1 - (\text{Ab}/\text{Ab}^{\infty})]$ versus time gives $-K_{\text{a}}/2.3$ as the slope from which the value for the absorption rate constant is obtained.

C_{p} and $K[\text{AUC}]_0^t$ are calculated from a plot of C_{p} versus time. Values for $(D_{\text{t}}/V_{\text{p}})$ can be approximated by the Loo–Riegelman method, as follows:

$$(C_{\text{t}})_{t_n} = \frac{K_{12}\Delta C_{\text{p}}\,\Delta t}{2} + \frac{K_{12}}{K_{21}}(C_{\text{p}})_{t_{n-1}}(1 - e^{-K_{21}\Delta t}) + (C_{\text{t}})_{t_{n-1}}e^{-K_{21}\Delta t} \tag{7.55}$$

where C_{t} is $D_{\text{t}}/V_{\text{p}}$, or apparent tissue concentration; t_{n} = time of sampling for sample n; t_{n-1} = time of sampling for the sampling point preceding sample n; and $(C_{\text{p}})_{t_{n-1}}$ = concentration of drug at central compartment for sample $n - 1$. Calculation of C_{t} values is shown in Table 7-3, using a typical set of oral absorption data. After calculation of C_{t} values, the percent drug unabsorbed is calculated with Equation 7.54, as shown in Table 7-4. A plot of percent drug unabsorbed versus time on a semilog graph gives a K_{a} of approximately 0.5 hr^{-1}.

For calculation of the K_{a} by this method to be possible, the drug must be given intravenously to allow evaluation of the distribution and elimination rate constants. For drugs which cannot be given by the IV route, the K_{a} cannot be calculated by the Loo–Riegelman method. For these drugs, the Wagner–Nelson method, which assumes a one-compartment model, may be used to provide an initial estimate of K_{a}. If the drug is given intravenously, there is no way of knowing whether there is any variation in the values for the elimination rate constant K and the distributive rate constants K_{12} and K_{21}. Such variations alter the rate constants. Therefore, a one-compartment model is frequently used to fit the plasma curves after an oral or intramuscular dose. The plasma level predicted from the K_{a} obtained by this method does deviate from the actual plasma level. However, in many instances this deviation is not significant.

Cumulative Relative Fraction Absorbed. The fraction of drug absorbed at any time t (Eq. 7.30) may be summed or cumulated for each time period for which a

TABLE 7-3. CALCULATION OF C_t Values*

$(C_p)_{t_n}$	$(t)_{t_n}$	ΔC_p	Δt	$\frac{(K_{12}\Delta C_p \Delta t)}{2}$	$(C_p)_{t_{n-1}}$	$(K_{12}/K_{21}) \times (1-e^{-K_{21}\Delta t})$	$(C_p)_{t_{n-1}} K_{12}/K_{21} \times (1-e^{-K_{21}\Delta t})$	$(C_t)_{t_{n-1}} e^{-K_{21}\Delta t}$	$(C_t)t_n$
3.00	0.5	3.0	0.5	0.218	0.	0.134	0.	0.	0.218
5.20	1.0	2.2	0.5	0.160	3.00	0.134	0.402	0.187	0.749
6.50	1.5	1.3	0.5	0.094	5.20	0.134	0.697	0.642	1.433
7.30	2.0	0.8	0.5	0.058	6.50	0.134	0.871	1.228	2.157
7.60	2.5	0.3	0.5	0.022	7.30	0.134	0.978	1.849	2.849
7.75	3.0	0.15	0.5	0.011	7.60	0.134	1.018	2.442	3.471
7.70	3.5	−0.05	0.5	−0.004	7.75	0.134	1.039	2.976	4.019
7.60	4.0	−0.10	0.5	−0.007	7.70	0.134	1.032	3.444	4.469
7.10	5.0	−0.50	1.0	−0.073	7.60	0.250	1.900	3.276	5.103
6.60	6.0	−0.50	1.0	−0.073	7.10	0.250	1.775	3.740	5.442
6.00	7.0	−0.60	1.0	−0.087	6.60	0.250	1.650	3.989	5.552
5.10	9.0	−0.90	2.0	−0.261	6.00	0.432	2.592	2.987	5.318
4.40	11.0	−0.70	2.0	−0.203	5.10	0.432	2.203	2.861	4.861
3.30	15.0	−1.10	4.0	−0.638	4.40	0.720	3.168	1.361	3.891

*Calculated with the following rate constants: $K_{12} = 0.29\ hr^{-1}$; $K_{21} = 0.31^{-1}$. *After Loo JCK, Riegelman S, 1968, with permission.*[2]

TABLE 7-4. CALCULATION OF PERCENTAGE UNABSORBED*

Time (hr)	$(C_p)_{t_n}$	$[AUC]_{t_{n-1}}^{t_n}$	$[AUC]_{t_0}^{t_n}$	$K[AUC]_{t_0}^{t_n}$	$(C_t)_{t_n}$	Ab/V_p	$\%Ab/V_p$	$100\%-Ab/V_p\%$
0.5	3.00	0.750	0.750	0.120	0.218	3.338	16.6	83.4
1.0	5.20	2.050	2.800	0.448	0.749	6.397	31.8	68.2
1.5	6.50	2.925	5.725	0.916	1.433	8.849	44.0	56.0
2.0	7.30	3.450	9.175	1.468	2.157	10.925	54.3	45.7
2.5	7.60	3.725	12.900	2.064	2.849	12.513	62.2	37.8
3.0	7.75	3.838	16.738	2.678	3.471	13.889	69.1	30.9
3.5	7.70	3.863	20.601	3.296	4.019	15.015	74.6	25.4
4.0	7.60	3.825	24.426	3.908	4.469	15.977	79.4	20.6
5.0	7.10	7.350	31.726	5.084	5.103	17.287	85.9	14.1
6.0	6.60	6.850	38.626	6.180	5.442	18.222	90.6	9.4
7.0	6.00	6.300	44.926	7.188	5.552	18.740	93.1	6.9
9.0	5.10	11.100	56.026	8.964	5.318	19.382	96.3	3.7
11.0	4.40	9.500	65.526	10.484	4.861	19.745	98.1	1.9
15.0	3.30	15.400	80.926	12.948	3.891	20.139	100.0	0

*$Ab/V_p = (C_p)_{t_n} + K[AUC]_{t_0}^{t_n} + (C_t)_{t_n}$

$(C_t)_{t_n} = K_{12}\Delta C_p \Delta t/2 + K_{12}/K_{21}(C_p)_{t_{n-1}}(1 - e^{-K_{21}\Delta t}) + (C_t)_{t_{n-1}} e^{-K_{21}\Delta t}$

$K = 0.16$; $K_{12} = 0.29$; $K_{21} = 0.31$

plasma drug sample was obtained. From Equation 7.30 the term Ab/Ab^{∞} becomes the cumulative relative fraction absorbed (CRFA):

$$\text{CRFA} = \frac{C_{p_t} + K[AUC]_0^t}{K[AUC]_0^{\infty}} \tag{7.56}$$

where C_{p_t} is the plasma concentration at time t.

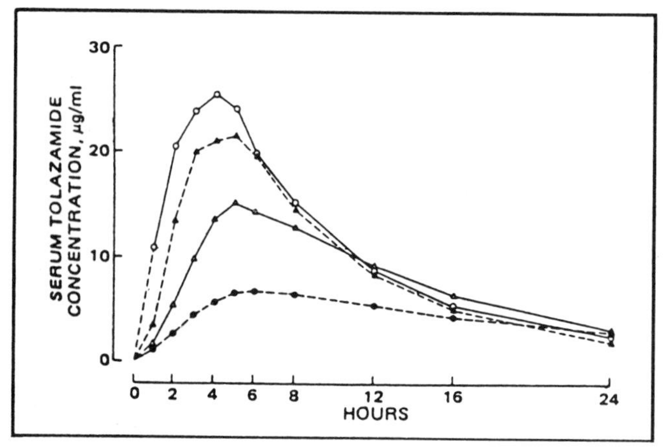

Figure 7-13. Mean serum tolazamide levels as a function of time. Key: (○) Treatment *A*; (●) Treatment *B*; (△) Treatment *C*; (▲) Treatment *D*. (*From Welling PG, et al, 1982, with permission.*[3])

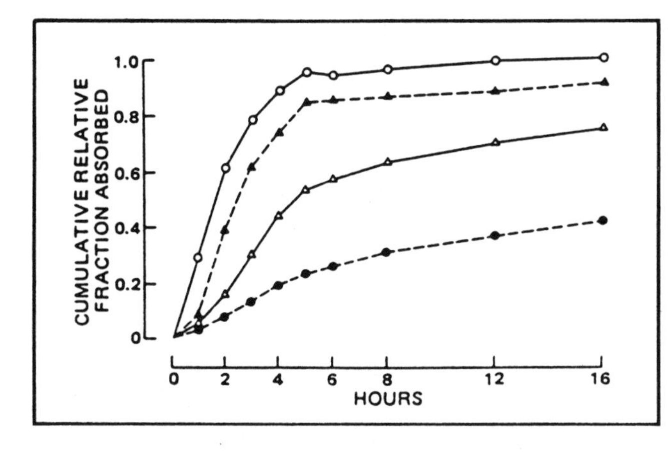

Figure 7-14. Mean cumulative relative fractions of tolazamide absorbed as a function of time. Key: (○) Treatment *A*; (●) Treatment *B*; (△) Treatment *C*; (▲) Treatment *D*. (*From Welling PG, et al, 1982, with permission.*[3])

Each fraction of drug absorbed is cumulated and plotted against the time interval in which the plasma drug sample was obtained. An example of the relationship of CRFA versus time for the absorption of tolazamide from four different drug products is shown in Figure 7-13. The data for Figure 7-14 was obtained from the serum tolazamide levels versus time curves in Figure 7-13. The CRFA versus time graph provides a visual image of the relative rates of drug absorption from various drug products. If the CRFA versus time curve is a straight line, then the drug was absorbed from the drug product at an apparent zero-order absorption rate.

Significance of Absorption Rate Constants. The systemic absorption of a drug encompasses a number of rate processes, including dissolution of the drug and transport of the drug across cellular membranes of the gut. The rate of drug absorption represents the net result of all these processes.

The calculation of K_a is useful in designing a multiple-dosage regimen. Knowledge of the K_a and K allows for the prediction of peak and trough plasma drug concentrations following multiple dosing. In bioequivalence studies drug products are frequently given in chemically equivalent doses, and the respective rates of systemic absorption may not differ markedly. Therefore, for these studies t_{max}, or time of peak drug concentration, can be very useful in comparing the respective rates of absorption of a drug from chemically equivalent drug products.

QUESTIONS

1. In a study conducted by Wagner in 1967,[4] eight human subjects were each given a single oral dose of tetracycline (250 mg). Blood samples were taken periodically and the serum fraction of each sample was analyzed for the antibiotic by microbiologic assay. The following data were obtained.

Time (hr)	*Serum Concentration (μg/ml)*
1	0.7
2	1.2
3	1.4
4	1.4
6	1.1
8	0.8
10	0.6
12	0.5
16	0.3

Assuming that this drug follows a one-compartment open model, derive the appropriate kinetic parameters and give the equation that best fits the data. Plot the calculated curve and compare the theoretical values with the experimental values. Compare these values with those obtained by Wagner.

2. Name a method of drug administration that will provide a zero-order input.
3. Contrast the percent of drug unabsorbed methods for the determination of rate constant for absorption, K_a, in terms of (a) pharmacokinetic model, (b) route of drug administration, and (c) possible sources of error.
4. What is the error inherent in the measurement of K_a for an orally administered drug which follows a two-compartment model when a one-compartment model is assumed in the calculation?
5. What are the main pharmacokinetic parameters which influence (a) time for peak drug concentration and (b) peak drug concentration?
6. The plasma drug concentrations in a patient who had received a single oral dose of a drug (10 mg/kg) were determined as follows.

Time (hr)	*Concentration (μg/ml)*
0	0
2	23.7
4	35.4
6	39.6
8	39.6
10	37.2
12	33.7
14	29.7
16	25.8
18	22.1
20	18.7
22	15.8
24	13.2
26	11.0
28	9.14

Assuming that the drug is 80% absorbed, find (a) the absorption constant, K_a; (b) the elimination half-life, $t_{1/2}$; (c) the T_{max}, or time of peak drug concentration; and (d) the volume of distribution of the patient.

7. A single oral dose (100 mg) of an antibiotic was given to an adult male

patient (43 years, 72 kg). From the literature, the pharmacokinetics of this drug fits a one-compartment open model. The equation which best fits the pharmacokinetics of the drug is

$$C_p = 45(e^{-0.17t} - e^{-1.5t})$$

From the equation above, calculate (a) T_{max}, (b) $C_{p,max}$ and (c) $T_{1/2}$ for the drug in this patient. Assume C_p is in micrograms per milliliter and the first-order rate constants are in hours $^{-1}$.

8. Two drugs A and B have the following pharmacokinetic parameters; after a single oral dose of 500 mg.

Drug	K_A *(hr^{-1})*	K *(hr^{-1})*	V_d *(ml)*
A	1.0	0.2	10,000
B	0.2	1.0	20,000

Both drugs follow a one-compartment pharmacokinetic model and are 100% bioavailable.

a. Calculate the T_{max} for each drug.
b. Calculate the $C_{p,max}$ for each drug.

REFERENCES

1. Levy, G, Amsel LP, Elliot HC: Kinetics of salicyluric acid elimination in man. J Pharm Sci 58:827–29, 1969
2. Loo JCK, Riegelman S: New method for calculating the intrinsic absorption rate of drugs. J Pharm Sci 57:918–28, 1968
3. Welling PG, Patel RB, Patel UR, et al: Bioavailability of tolazamide from tablets: Comparison of in vitro and in vivo results. J Pharm Sci 71:1259, 1982
4. Wagner JG: Use of computers in pharmacokinetics. Clin Pharmacol Ther 8:201–18, 1967

BIBLIOGRAPHY

Boxenbaum HG, Kaplan SA: Potential source of error in absorption rate calculations. J Pharmacokinet Biopharm 3:257–64, 1975

Boyes R, Adams H, Duce B: Oral absorption and disposition kinetics of lidocaine hydrochloride in dogs. J Pharmacol Exp Ther 174:1–8, 1970

Dvorchik BH, Vesell ES: Significance of error associated with use of the one-compartment formula to calculate clearance of 38 drugs. Clin Pharmacol Ther 23:617–23, 1978

Portmann G: Pharmakokinetics. In Swarbrick J (ed.), Current Concepts in the Pharmaceutical Sciences, Vol. 1. Philadelphia, Lea and Febïger, 1970, Chapter 1

Wagner JG, Nelson E: Kinetic analysis of blood levels and urinary excretion in the absorptive phase after single doses of drug. J Pharm Sci 53:1392, 1964

Wagner JG, Nelson E: Percent absorbed time plots derived from blood level and/or urinary excretion data. J Pharm Sci 52:610–11, 1963

CHAPTER EIGHT

Bioavailability and Bioequivalence

Many drugs are made and marketed by more than one pharmaceutical manufacturer. The study of biopharmaceutics gives substantial evidence that the method of manufacture and the final formulation of the drug can markedly affect the bioavailability of the drug. Because of the plethora of drug products containing the same amount of active drug, physicians, pharmacists, and others who prescribe, dispense, or purchase drugs must select products which produce equivalent therapeutic effect. To facilitate such decisions, guidelines have been developed by the U.S. Food and Drug Administration. These guidelines and methods for determining drug availability are discussed in this chapter.

DEFINITIONS

- *Bioavailability*. Indicates a measurement of the rate and extent (amount) of therapeutically active drug which reaches the general circulation.
- *Bioequivalence Requirement*. A requirement imposed by the Food and Drug Administration (FDA) for in vitro and/or in vivo testing of specified drug products, which requirement must be satisfied as a condition for marketing.
- *Bioequivalent Drug Products*. Pharmaceutic equivalents or alternatives which are *not* significantly different with respect to rate and extent of absorption when administered at the same molar dose under similar experimental conditions. Some drugs may be considered pharmaceutic equivalents that are equal in extent of absorption but not in rate of absorption; this is possible when differences in the rate of absorption are considered clinically insignificant for the particular drug products. For example, aspirin and acetaminophen are well-absorbed drugs, and small differences in the rate of absorption are of very little clinical consequence.
- *Brand Name*. Trade name of the drug. This name is privately owned by the manufacturer or distributor and is used to distinguish the specific drug

product from competitors' products—e.g., Tylenol (McNeil Laboratories).

- *Chemical Name*. Name used by the organic chemist to indicate the chemical structure of the drug—e.g., *N*-acetyl-*p*-aminophenol.
- *Drug Product*. The finished dosage form (e.g., tablet or capsule) that contains the active drug ingredient, generally but not necessarily in association with inactive ingredients.
- *Drug Product Selection*. The process of choosing or selecting the drug product in a specified dosage form.
- *Equivalence*. Relation in terms of bioavailability, therapeutic response, or a set of established standards of one drug product to another drug product.
- *Generic Name*. The established, nonproprietory or common name of the active drug in a drug product—e.g., acetaminophen.
- *Generic Substitution*. The process of dispensing a different brand or unbranded drug product in place of the prescribed drug product. The substituted drug product contains the same active ingredient or therapeutic moiety as the same salt or ester in the same dosage form but is made by a different manufacturer. For example, a prescription for Motrin brand of ibuprofen might be dispensed by the pharmacist as Rufen brand of ibuprofen if generic substitution is permitted and desired by the physician.
- *Pharmaceutic Alternatives*. Drug products that contain the same therapeutic moiety or its precursor as the same salt or ester, although not necessarily in the same amounts or dosage forms. For example, drug products containing either tetracycline phosphate or tetracycline hydrochloride equivalent to 250 mg of tetracycline base can be considered pharmaceutic alternatives. However, the drug products erythromycin estolate and erythromycin stearate are different esters of erythromycin and are not considered to be pharmaceutic alternatives.
- *Pharmaceutic Equivalents*. Drug products which contain the same amount of the same active drug ingredient (i.e., same salt or ester or chemical form), but contain different inactive ingredients. *Chemical equivalents* are the same as pharmaceutic equivalents. Pharmaceutic equivalents must be identical in strength, quality, and purity as well as content uniformity, disintegration, and dissolution rates, where applicable.
- *Pharmaceutic Substitution*. The process of dispensing a pharmaceutic alternative for the prescribed drug product. For example, ampicillin suspension is dispensed in place of ampicillin capsules or tetracycline hydrochloride is dispensed in place of tetracycline phosphate. Pharmaceutic substitution generally requires the physician's approval.
- *Therapeutic Alternatives*. Drug products containing different active ingredients which are indicated for the same therapeutic or clinical objectives. Active ingredients in therapeutic alternatives are from the same pharmacologic class and are expected to have the same therapeutic effect when administered to patients for such condition of use.
- *Therapeutic Equivalents*. Drug products that contain the same therapeutically active drug and give identical effects in vivo. Therapeutically equivalent drug

products should give the same therapeutic effect and have equal potential for adverse effects under the conditions set forth on the labels of these drug products. Drug products may be considered therapeutically equivalent if they are (1) pharmaceutic equivalents, (2) bioequivalent, (3) adequately labeled, and (4) manufactured in compliance with good manufacturing practices.

- *Therapeutic Substitution*. The process of dispensing a therapeutic alternative in place of the prescribed drug product. For example, amoxicillin is dispensed for ampicillin.

PURPOSE OF BIOAVAILABILITY STUDIES

Bioavailability studies are performed for both approved active drug ingredients or therapeutic moieties not yet approved for marketing by the FDA. New formulations of active drug ingredients or therapeutic moieties must be approved prior to marketing by the FDA. The FDA in approving a drug product for marketing must ensure that the drug product is safe and effective for its labeled indications for use. Moreover, the drug product must meet all applicable standards of identity, strength, quality, and purity. To ensure that these standards are met, the FDA requires bioavailability/pharmacokinetic studies and where necessary bioequivalency requirements for all drug products.

For unmarketed drugs which do not have full NDA (New Drug Application) approval by the FDA, in vivo bioavailability studies must be performed on the drug formulation proposed for marketing. Furthermore, the essential pharmacokinetics of the active drug ingredient or therapeutic moiety must be characterized. Essential pharmacokinetic parameters including the rate and extent of systemic absorption, elimination half-life, and rates of excretion and metabolism should be established after single- and multiple-dose administration. Data from these in vivo bioavailability studies are important to establish recommended dosage regimens and to support drug labeling.

In vivo bioavailability studies are performed also for new formulations of active drug ingredients or therapeutic moieties which have full NDA approval and are approved for marketing. The purpose of these studies is to determine the bioavailability and characterize the pharmacokinetics of the new formulation, new dosage form, or new salt or ester relative to a reference formulation.

After the bioavailability and essential pharmacokinetic parameters of the active ingredient or therapeutic moiety are established, dosage regimens may be recommended in support of drug labeling.

In summary, clinical studies are useful in determining the safety and efficacy of the drug product. Bioavailability studies are useful in defining the drug product in terms of its affect on the pharmacokinetics of the drug; whereas bioequivalency studies are useful in comparing the bioavailability of a drug from various drug products. Once the drug products are demonstrated to be bioequivalent, then the efficacy of these drug products is assumed to be similar.

RELATIVE AND ABSOLUTE AVAILABILITY

The area under the drug concentration–time curve is useful as a measure of the total amount of unaltered drug that reaches the systemic circulation. The AUC is dependent on the total quantity of available drug, FD_0, divided by the elimination rate constant, K, and the apparent volume of distribution, V_d. F is the fraction of the dose absorbed; after IV administration F is equal to unity, since the entire dose is placed into the systemic circulation instantaneously. Therefore, the drug is considered to be completely available after IV administration. After oral administration of the drug, F may vary from a value of $F=0$ (no drug absorption) to $F=1$ (complete drug absorption).

Relative Availability

Relative (apparent) availability is the availability of a drug product as compared to a recognized standard. The fraction of dose systemically available from an oral drug product is difficult to ascertain. The availability of drug in the formulation is compared to the availability of drug in a standard dosage formulation, usually a solution of the pure drug evaluated in a crossover study. The relative availability of two drug products given at the same dosage level and by the same route of administration can be obtained with the following equation.

$$\text{Relative availability} = \frac{[\text{AUC}]_A}{[\text{AUC}]_B} \tag{8.1}$$

where drug product B is the recognized reference standard. This fraction may be multiplied by 100 to give *percent* relative availability.

When different doses are administered, a correction for the size of the dose is made, as in the following equation.

$$\text{Relative availability} = \frac{[\text{AUC}]_A/\text{dose } A}{[\text{AUC}]_B/\text{dose } B}$$

Urinary drug excretion data may also be used to measure relative availability, as long as the total amount of intact drug excreted in the urine is collected. The percent relative availability using urinary excretion data can be determined as follows.

$$\text{Percent relative availability} = \frac{[D_u]_A^\infty}{[D_u]_B^\infty} \cdot 100 \tag{8.2}$$

where $[D_u]^\infty$ is the total amount of drug excreted in the urine.

Absolute Availability

The absolute availability of drug in a drug product may be measured by comparing the respective AUCs after oral and IV administration. This measurement may be performed as long as V_d and K are independent of the route of administration.

Absolute availability using plasma data can be determined as follows.

$$\text{Absolute availability} = \frac{[\text{AUC}]_{\text{PO}}/\text{dose}_{\text{PO}}}{[\text{AUC}]_{\text{IV}}/\text{dose}_{\text{IV}}} \tag{8.3}$$

Absolute availability using urinary drug excretion data can be determined by the following.

$$\text{Absolute availability} = \frac{[D_{\text{u}}]_{\text{PO}}^{\infty}/\text{dose}_{\text{PO}}}{[D_{\text{u}}]_{\text{IV}}^{\infty}/\text{dose}_{\text{IV}}} \tag{8.4}$$

The absolute bioavailability is also equal to F, the fraction of the dose which is bioavailable. For drugs given vascularly such as by IV bolus injection, $F = 1$ since all the drug is completely bioavailable. For all extravascular routes of administration, $F \leq 1$. F is usually determined by Equations 8.3 or 8.4.

PRACTICE PROBLEM

The bioavailability of a new investigational drug was studied in eight volunteers. Each volunteer received either a single oral tablet containing 200 mg of the drug, 5 ml of a pure aqueous solution containing 200 mg of the drug, or a single IV bolus injection containing 50 mg of the drug. Plasma samples were obtained periodically up to 48 hr after the dose and assayed for drug concentration. The average AUC (0–48 hr) are given in the table below. From these data calculate (1) the relative bioavailability of the drug from the tablet compared to the oral solution and (2) the absolute bioavailability of the drug from the tablet.

Drug Product	*Dose (mg)*	*AUC (μg hr / ml)*	*Standard Deviation*
Oral tablet	200	89.5	19.7
Oral solution	200	86.1	18.1
IV Bolus injection	50	37.8	5.7

Solution

The relative bioavailability of the drug from the tablet is estimated using Equation 8.1. No adjustment for dose is necessary.

$$\text{Relative bioavailability} = \frac{89.5}{86.1} = 1.04$$

The relative bioavailability of the drug from the tablet is 1.04, or 104%, compared to the solution. The difference in drug bioavailability between tablet and solution is not statistically significant.

The absolute drug bioavailability from the tablet is calculated using Equation 8.3 and adjusting for the dose.

$$F = \text{absolute bioavailability} = \frac{89.5/200}{37.8/50} = 0.59$$

Since F, the fraction of dose absorbed from the tablet, was less than 1, the drug was not completely absorbed systemically. The relative bioavailability of the drug from the tablet was approximately 100% when compared to the oral solution. Often, results from bioequivalency studies demonstrate equal drug bioavailability from various oral drug products. However, the results from these bioequivalency studies should not be misinterpreted to imply that the absolute bioavailability of the drug from the oral drug products is also 100% unless the oral formulation was compared to an intravenous injection of the drug.

METHODS OF ASSESSING BIOAVAILABILITY

There are several direct and indirect methods of assessing bioavailability in humans. The selection of a method depends on the purpose of the study, the analytic method of drug measurement, and the nature of the drug product. The parameters which are useful in determining the bioavailability of a drug from a drug product include:

1. Plasma data
   a. The time of peak plasma (blood) concentration (t_{max})
   b. The peak plasma concentration ($C_{p,max}$)
   c. The area under the plasma level–time curve (AUC)
2. Urine data
   a. The cumulative amount of drug excreted in the urine (D_u)
   b. The rate of drug excretion in the urine (dD_u/dt)
   c. The time for maximum urinary excretion (t^{∞})
3. Acute pharmacologic effect
4. Clinical observation

Since the free or therapeutically active drug can be accurately quantitated in biologic fluids, plasma and urine data give the most objective information on bioavailability.

Plasma Data

t_{max}. The time of peak plasma concentration corresponds to the time required to reach maximum drug concentration after drug administration. At t_{max} absorption is maximized, and the rate of drug absorption exactly equals the rate of drug elimination (see Fig. 7-5). Absorption still proceeds after t_{max} is reached, but at a slower rate. When comparing drug products, t_{max} can be used as an approximate indication of drug absorption rate. The value for t_{max} will become smaller (i.e., indicating less time required to reach peak plasma concentration) as the absorption rate for the drug becomes more rapid. Units for t_{max} are units of time (e.g., hours, minutes).

$C_{p,max}$. The peak plasma concentration represents the maximum plasma drug concentration obtained after oral administration of drug (see Fig. 7-5). For many drugs a relationship is found between the pharmacologic effect of a drug and the plasma drug concentration. $C_{p,max}$ provides an indication that the drug is sufficiently systematically absorbed to provide a therapeutic response. In addition, $C_{p,max}$ provides warning of possibly toxic levels of drug. The units for $C_{p,max}$ are concentration units (e.g., μg/ml, ng/ml).

AUC. The area under the plasma level–time curve is a measurement of the extent of bioavailability of a drug. The AUC reflects the total amount of active drug which reaches the systemic circulation. The AUC is the area under the drug plasma level–time curve from $t = 0$ to $t = \infty$ and is equal to the amount of unchanged drug reaching the general circulation divided by the clearance:

$$[\text{AUC}]_0^\infty = \int_0^\infty C_p \, dt \tag{8.5}$$

$$[\text{AUC}]_0^\infty = \frac{FD_0}{\text{clearance}} \equiv \frac{FD_0}{KV_d} \tag{8.6}$$

where F = fraction of dose absorbed; D_0 = dose; K = elimination rate constant; and V_d = volume of distribution. The AUC is independent of the route of administration and processes of drug elimination as long as the elimination processes do not change. The AUC can be determined by a numerical integration procedure, the trapezoidal rule method, or directly by the use of a planimeter. The units for AUC

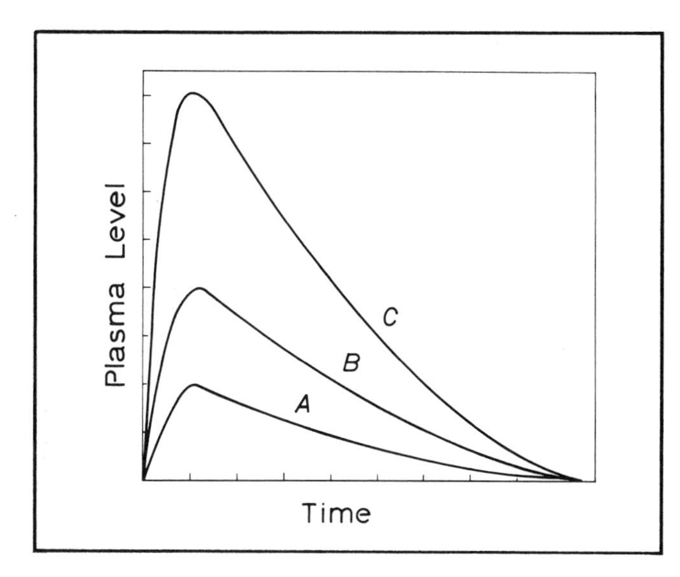

Figure 8-1. Plasma level–time curve following administration of single doses of (*A*) 250 mg; (*B*) 500 mg; and (*C*) 1000 mg of drug.

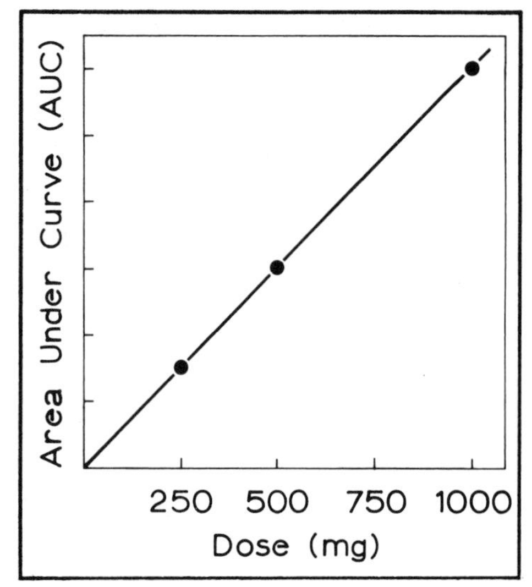

Figure 8-2. Linear relationship between AUC and dose. Data from Figure 8-1.

are concentration time (e.g., μg hr/ml).

For many drugs the AUC is directly proportional to dose. For example, if a single dose of a drug is increased from 250 to 1000 mg, the AUC will also show a fourfold increase (Figs. 8-1, 8-2).

In some cases the AUC is not directly proportional to the administered dose for all dosage levels. For example, as the dosage of drug is increased, one of the pathways for drug elimination may become saturated (Fig. 8-3). Drug elimination includes the processes of metabolism and excretion. Drug metabolism is an enzyme-dependent process. For some drugs (such as salicylate and phenytoin), continued increase of the dose causes saturation of one of the enzyme pathways for metabolism of the drug and consequent prolongation of the elimination half-life. The AUC thus increases disproportionally to the increase in dose since a smaller

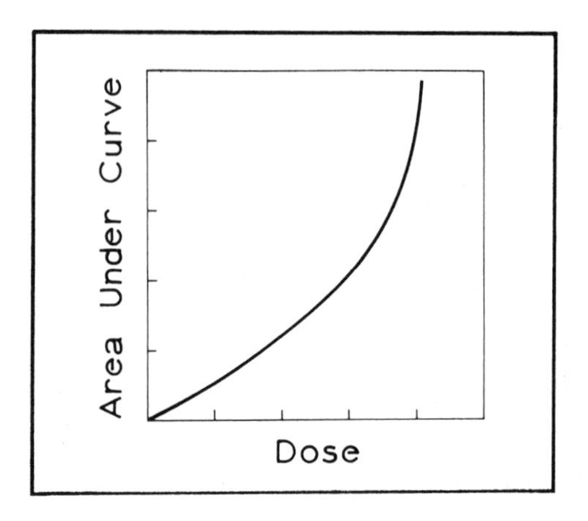

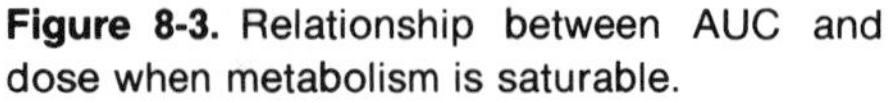

Figure 8-3. Relationship between AUC and dose when metabolism is saturable.

amount of drug is being eliminated (i.e., more drug is retained). When the AUC is not directly proportional to the dose, bioavailability of the drug is difficult to evaluate.

Urine Data

Urinary drug excretion data can be useful in estimating bioavailability. In order to obtain valid estimates, the drug must be excreted in significant quantities in the urine and complete samples of urine must be collected.

D_u^∞. The cumulative amount of drug excreted in the urine is directly related to the total amount of drug absorbed. Experimentally, urine samples are collected periodically after administration of the drug product. Each urine specimen is analyzed for free drug with a specific assay. A graph is constructed relating the cumulative drug excreted to the collection time interval (Fig. 8-4, bottom portion).

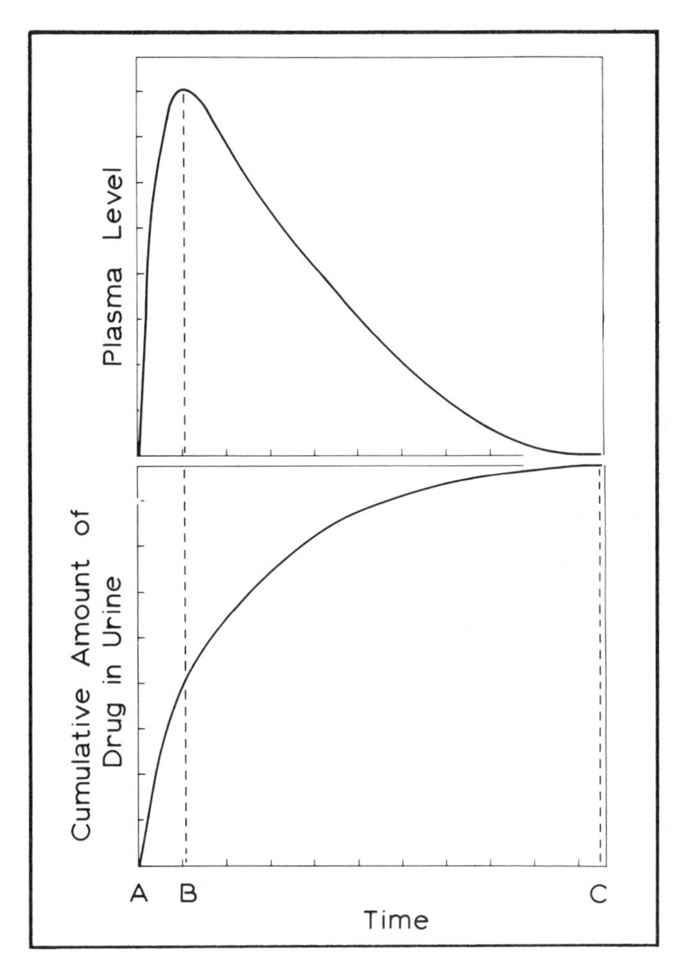

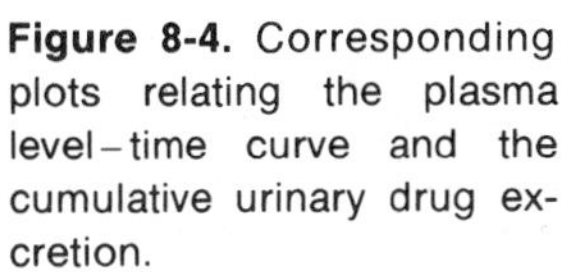
Figure 8-4. Corresponding plots relating the plasma level–time curve and the cumulative urinary drug excretion.

The relationship between the cumulative amount of drug excreted in the urine and the plasma level–time curve is shown in Figure 8-4. When the drug is essentially completely eliminated (point C), the plasma concentration approaches zero and the maximum amount of drug excreted in the urine, D_u^{∞}, is obtained.

dD_u/dt. Since most drugs are eliminated by a first-order rate process, the rate of drug excretion is dependent on the first-order elimination rate constant (K) and the concentration of drug in the plasma (C_p). In Figure 8-4 the maximum rate of drug excretion would be at point B, whereas the minimum rate of drug excretion would be at points A and C. Thus, a graph comparing the rate of drug excretion with respect to time should be identical with the plasma level–time curve for that drug (Fig. 8-5).

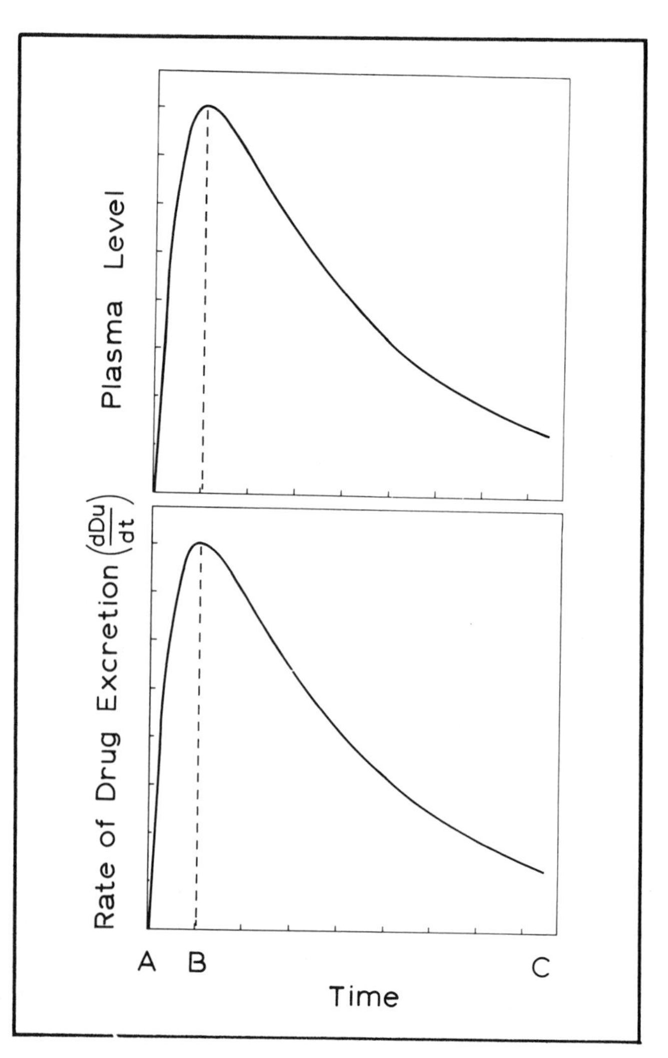

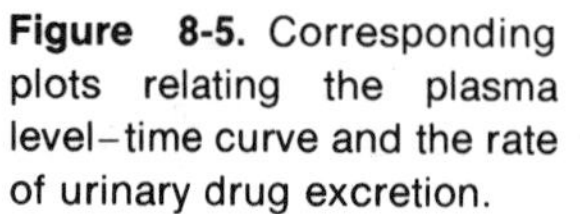
Figure 8-5. Corresponding plots relating the plasma level–time curve and the rate of urinary drug excretion.

t^{∞}. In Figures 8-4 and 8-5 the slope of the curve segment A–B is related to the rate of drug absorption, whereas point C is related to the total time required after drug administration for the drug to be absorbed and completely excreted ($t = \infty$). The t^{∞} is a useful parameter in bioequivalence studies comparing several drug products, as described later in this chapter.

Acute Pharmacologic Effect

In some cases the quantitative measurement of a drug is not available or lacks sufficient accuracy and/or reproducibility. An acute pharmacologic effect–such as effect on pupil diameter, heart rate, or blood pressure—can be useful as an index of drug bioavailability. In this case an acute pharmacologic effect–time curve is constructed. Measurements of the pharmacologic effect should be made with sufficient frequency to permit a reasonable estimate of the total area under the curve for a time period at least three times the half-life of the drug.[1]

The use of an acute pharmacologic effect to determine bioavailability may require demonstration of a dose-related response. Bioavailability may be determined by examination of the dose–response curve as well as the total area under the acute pharmacologic effect–time curve.

Clinical Response

For many years medical practitioners have observed either lack of response (therapeutic failure), good therapeutic response, or toxicity in patients receiving similar drug products.

Differences in the predicted clinical response may be due to both differences in the pharmacokinetic or pharmacodynamic behavior of the drug between individuals. Bioequivalent drug products should have the same systemic drug bioavailability and therefore the same predictable drug response. However, variable clinical responses among individuals which are unrelated to bioavailability might be due to differences in the pharmacodynamics of the drug. Differences in pharmacodynamics, which is the relationship between the drug and the receptor site, may be due to differences in receptor sensitivity to the drug. Various factors affecting pharmacodynamic drug behavior may include age, drug tolerance, drug interactions, and unknown pathophysiologic factors.

The bioavailability of a drug may be reproducible among fasted individuals on controlled studies who take the drug on an empty stomach. When the drug is used on a daily basis, however, the nature of the diet may affect the plasma drug level due to variable absorption in the presence of food or even due to a change in the metabolic clearance of the drug. Feldman et al.[2] reported that patients on a high carbohydrate diet have a much longer elimination half-life of theophylline due to the reduced metabolic clearance of the drug ($t_{1/2}$, 18.1 hr) compared to patients on normal diets ($t_{1/2}$, 6.76 hr). Previous studies demonstrated that the theophylline drug product was completely bioavailable. The higher plasma drug concentration resulting from a carbohydrate diet may subject the patient to a higher risk of drug intoxication with theophylline. The effect of food on the availability of theophylline has been reported by the FDA concerning the risk of higher theophylline plasma concentrations from a 24-hr sustained release drug product taken with food. Although most bioavailability drug studies use fasted volunteers, the diet of patients actually using the drug product may increase or decrease the bioavailability of the drug.[3]

BIOEQUIVALENCE STUDIES

The major reason for performing bioequivalence studies is that, in the past, drug products which were considered pharmaceutic equivalents did not give comparative therapeutic effects in patients. The design and evaluation of well-controlled bioequivalence studies require the cooperation of pharmacokineticists, statisticians, clinical pharmacologists, bioanalytic chemists, and others. The reader should consult the Bibliography for further information on bioavailability and bioequivalence studies. The basic guiding principle in an in vivo bioavailability study is that *no unnecessary human research be done.*

In considering a bioequivalence study, one formulation of the drug is chosen as a *reference standard* against which all other formulations of the drug are compared. The reference standard should contain the active drug of therapeutic moiety in its most bioavailable formulation (i.e., solution or suspension) and in the same quantity as in the other formulations to which it is to be compared. The reference material should be administered by the same route as the comparison formulations unless an alternative route or additional route is necessary to answer specific pharmacokinetic questions. For example, if an active drug is poorly bioavailable after oral administration, the drug may be compared after both oral and intravenous administration. When a solution or a suspension of the drug is not available, the reference standard may be a formulation currently marketed with a fully approved new drug application (NDA) for which there are valid scientific safety and efficacy data. The reference drug product should also be one that is accepted by the medical profession and that has a long history of clinical use. The reference formulation is usually the innovator's or original manufacturer's product.

For illustrative purposes, consider a drug that has been prepared at the same dosage level in three formulations, formulations A, B, and C. These formulations are given to a group of volunteers using a three-way randomized crossover design. In this experimental design all subjects receive each formulation once. From each subject plasma drug level and urinary drug excretion data are obtained. With this data we can observe the relationship between plasma and urinary excretion parameters and drug bioavailability (Fig. 8-6). First of all, the rate of drug availability from formulation A is more rapid than that from formulation B, since the t_{max} for formulation A is shorter. Since the AUC for formulation A is identical to the AUC for formulation B, the extent of bioavailability from both of these formulations is the same. Note, however, the $C_{p,max}$ is higher when the rate of drug absorption is more rapid.

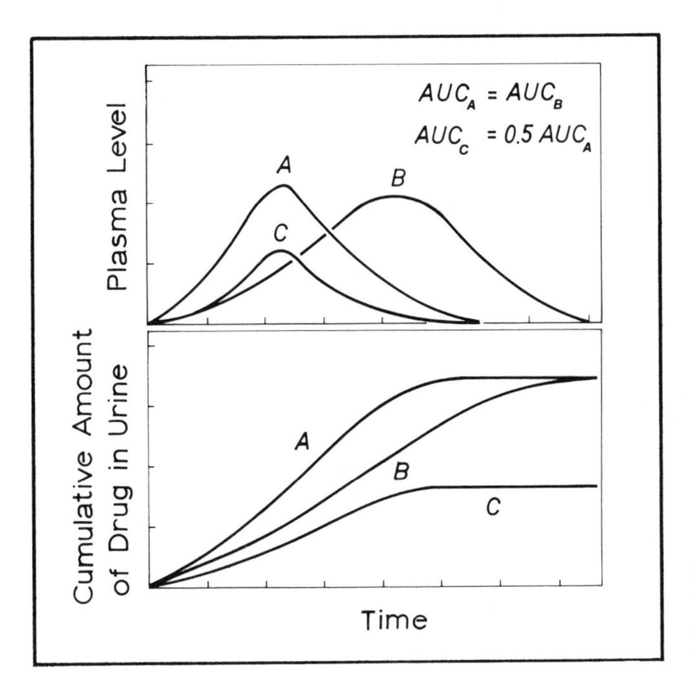

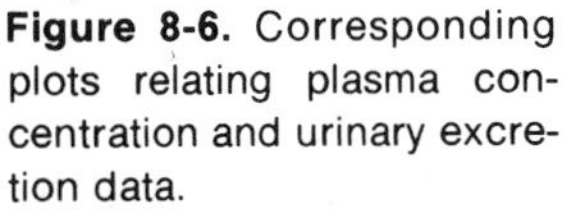
Figure 8-6. Corresponding plots relating plasma concentration and urinary excretion data.

The $C_{p,max}$ is also higher when the extent of drug bioavailability is greater as with formulation A. The rate of drug availability from formulation C is the same as that from formulation A, but the extent of drug available is less. The $C_{p,max}$ for formulation C is less than for formulation A. The decrease in $C_{p,max}$ for formulation C is proportional to the decrease in AUC in comparison to the drug plasma level data from formulation A. The corresponding urinary excretion data confirm these observations. These relationships are summarized in Table 8-1.

TABLE 8-1. RELATIONSHIP OF PLASMA LEVEL AND URINARY EXCRETION PARAMETERS TO DRUG BIOAVAILABILITY

Extent of Drug Bioavailability Decreases		Rate of Drug Bioavailability Decreases	
Parameter	***Change***	***Parameter***	***Change***
Plasma Data:			
t_{max}	Same	t_{max}	Increase
$C_{p,max}$	Decrease	$C_{p,max}$	Decrease
AUC	Decrease	AUC	Same
Urine Data:			
t^{∞}	Same	t^{∞}	Increase
$[dD_u/dt]_{max}$	Decrease	$[dD_u/dt]_{max}$	Decrease
D_u^{∞}	Decrease	D_u^{∞}	Same

Bases for Determining Bioavailability

According to the FDA, the bases for determining bioavailability include the following.

1. The in vivo bioavailability of a drug product is demonstrated if the product's rate and extent of absorption, as determined by comparison of measured parameters (e.g., concentration of the active drug ingredient in the blood, urinary excretion rates, and pharmacologic effects), are not significantly different from the reference material's.
2. Statistical techniques used should be of sufficient sensitivity to detect differences in rate and extent of absorption that are not attributable to subject variability.
3. A drug product that differs from the reference material in its rate of absorption, but not in its extent of absorption, may be considered bioavailable if the difference in the rate of absorption is intentional and appropriately reflected in the labeling and/or the rate of absorption is not detrimental to the safety and effectiveness of the drug product.

In Vitro Demonstration of Bioavailability

For certain drug products bioavailability may be demonstrated by evidence obtained in vitro in lieu of in vivo. For these drugs bioavailability is largely dependent on having the drug in the dissolved state. The rate of dissolution of the drug from the drug product is measured in vitro. Official dissolution tests are described by the United States Pharmacopeia (USP). The in vitro dissolution rate data must correlate with the in vivo bioavailability data for the drug. There are several approaches to establishing a correlation between the bioavailability of the drug in vivo and the dissolution of the drug product in vitro. An in vitro–in vivo correlation may include (1) the relationship between the percent of labeled drug content dissolved and the percent of drug systemically absorbed; (2) the relationship between the rate or amount of drug dissolved and a pharmacokinetic parameter such as T_{max}, AUC, C_{max}, K_A; (3) the relationship between the rate or amount of drug dissolved and an acute pharmacologic effect; and (4) the relationship between the mean time of in vitro dissolution and the mean residence time of the drug in vivo. There are cases in which the dissolution rate data are not adequate to ensure bioequivalence. Therefore, an in vivo bioequivalence requirement must be met.

Criteria for Establishing a Bioequivalence Requirement

Bioequivalence requirements may be imposed by the FDA on the basis of the following.

1. Evidence from well-controlled clinical trials or controlled observations in patients that various drug products do not give comparable therapeutic effects.

2. Evidence from well-controlled bioequivalence studies that such products are not bioequivalent drug products.
3. Evidence that the drug products exhibit a narrow therapeutic ratio and minimum effective concentrations in the blood, and that safe and effective use of the drug products requires careful dosage titration and patient monitoring.
4. Competent medical determination that a lack of bioequivalence would have a serious adverse effect in the treatment or prevention of a serious disease or condition.
5. Physicochemical evidence of the following:
   a. The active drug ingredient has a low solubility in water—e.g., less than 5 mg/ml.
   b. The dissolution rate of one or more such products is slow—e.g., less than 50% in 30 min when tested with a general method specified by the FDA.
   c. The particle size and/or surface area of the active drug ingredient is critical in determining its bioavailability.
   d. Certain structural forms of the active drug ingredient (e.g., polymorphic forms, conforms, solvates, complexes, and crystal modifications) dissolve poorly, thus affecting absorption.
   e. Such drug products have a high ratio of excipients to active ingredients—e.g., greater than 5 to 1.
   f. Specific inactive ingredients (e.g., hydrophilic or hydrophobic excipients and lubricants) either may be required for absorption of the active drug ingredient or therapeutic moiety or may interfere with such absorption.
6. Pharmacokinetic evidence of the following:
   a. The active drug ingredient, therapeutic moiety, or its precursor is absorbed in large part in a particular segment of the GI tract or is absorbed from a localized site.
   b. The degree of absorption of the active drug ingredient, therapeutic moiety, or its precursor is poor (e.g., less than 50%, ordinarily in comparison to an intravenous dose) even when it is administered in pure form (e.g., in solution).
   c. There is rapid metabolism of the therapeutic moiety in the intestinal wall or liver during the absorption process (first-order metabolism), so that the rate of absorption is unusually important in the therapeutic effect and/or toxicity of the drug product.
   d. The therapeutic moiety is rapidly metabolized or excreted so that rapid dissolution and absorption are required for effectiveness.
   e. The active drug ingredient or therapeutic moiety is unstable in specific portions of the GI tract and requires special coatings or formulations (e.g., buffers, enteric coatings, and film coatings) to ensure adequate absorption.
   f. The drug product is subject to dose-dependent kinetics in or near the therapeutic range, and the rate and extent of absorption are important to bioequivalence.

Criteria for Waiver of Evidence of In Vivo Bioavailability

For certain drug products the in vivo bioavailability of the drug product may be self-evident or unimportant to the achievement of the product's intended purposes. The FDA will waive the requirement for submission of in vivo evidence demonstrating the bioavailability of the drug product if the product meets one of the following criteria.

1. The drug product (a) is a solution intended solely for intravenous administration and (b) contains an active drug ingredient or therapeutic moiety combined with the same solvent and in the same concentration as in an intravenous solution that is the subject of an approved full new drug application.
2. The drug product is a topically applied preparation—e.g., a cream, ointment, or gel intended for local therapeutic effect.
3. The drug product is in an oral dosage form that is not intended to be absorbed—e.g., an antacid or a radiopaque medium.
4. The drug product meets both of the following conditions:
   a. It is administered by inhalation as a gas or vapor—e.g., a medicinal or an inhalation anesthetic.
   b. It contains an active drug ingredient or therapeutic moiety in the same dosage form as a drug product that is the subject of an approved full new drug application.
5. The drug product meets all of the following conditions:
   a. It is an oral solution, elixir, syrup, tincture, or similar other solubilized form.
   b. It contains an active drug ingredient or therapeutic moiety in the same concentration as a drug product that is the subject of an approved full new drug application.
   c. It contains no inactive ingredient that is known to significantly affect absorption of the active drug ingredient or therapeutic moiety.

Evaluation and Design of a Single-Dose Bioequivalency Study

A single-dose bioequivalency study is usually performed in normal, healthy human volunteers. The subjects should be in the fasting state (overnight fast) prior to drug administration and should fast for a 2–4-hr period after dosing. No other medication is normally given to the patient for 1 week prior to the study. Subjects are selected at random and a complete crossover design is employed in which the patient receives the drug product to be tested as well as the appropriate reference standard.

Examples of *Latin Square* crossover designs for a bioequivalency study in human volunteers [comparing three different drug formulations (A, B, C) or four different drug formulations (A, B, C, D)] are described in Tables 8-2 and 8-3.

The Latin square design plans the clinical trial so that each subject receives each drug product only once, with adequate time between medications for the elimination of the drug from the body. In this case each subject is his own control, and

TABLE 8-2. LATIN SQUARE CROSSOVER DESIGN FOR A BIOEQUIVALENCY STUDY OF THREE DRUG PRODUCTS IN SIX HUMAN VOLUNTEERS

	Drug Product		
Subject	*Study Period 1*	*Study Period 2*	*Study Period 3*
1	*A*	*B*	*C*
2	*B*	*C*	*A*
3	*C*	*A*	*B*
4	*A*	*C*	*B*
5	*C*	*B*	*A*
6	*B*	*A*	*C*

subject-to-subject variation is reduced. Moreover, variation due to time is reduced so that all patients do not receive the same drug product on the same day.

As shown in Tables 8-2 and 8-3, possible carry-over effects from any particular drug product is minimized by changing the sequence or order in which the drug products are given to the subject. Thus, drug product *B* may be followed by drug product *A*, *D*, or *C* (Table 8-3).

After each patient receives a drug product, blood samples are collected at appropriate time intervals so that a valid blood drug level–time curve may be obtained. The time intervals should be spaced so that the peak blood concentration,

TABLE 8-3. LATIN SQUARE CROSSOVER DESIGN FOR A BIOEQUIVALENCY STUDY OF FOUR DRUG PRODUCTS IN SIXTEEN HUMAN VOLUNTEERS

	Drug Product			
Subject	*Study Period 1*	*Study Period 2*	*Study Period 3*	*Study Period 4*
1	*A*	*B*	*C*	*D*
2	*B*	*C*	*D*	*A*
3	*C*	*D*	*A*	*B*
4	*D*	*A*	*B*	*C*
5	*A*	*B*	*D*	*C*
6	*B*	*D*	*C*	*A*
7	*D*	*C*	*A*	*B*
8	*C*	*A*	*B*	*D*
9	*A*	*C*	*B*	*D*
10	*C*	*B*	*D*	*A*
11	*B*	*D*	*A*	*C*
12	*D*	*A*	*C*	*B*
13	*A*	*C*	*D*	*B*
14	*C*	*D*	*B*	*A*
15	*D*	*B*	*A*	*C*
16	*B*	*A*	*C*	*D*

the total area under the curve, and the absorption and elimination phases of the curve may be described. In some cases the measurement of drug in urine samples may be necessary.

The analytical method for the measurement of the drug must be validated for accuracy, precision, and sensitivity. The use of more than one analytical method during a bioequivalency study may not be valid, since different methods may yield different values.

Data should be presented in both tabulated and graphical form for evaluation. Proper statistical evaluation should be performed on the estimated pharmacokinetic parameters. An analysis of variance (ANOVA) is needed to determine the statistical differences inherent in the pharmacokinetic parameters. A statistical difference between the pharmacokinetic parameters obtained from two or more drug products is considered significant if there is a probability of less than 1 in 20 times or 0.05 probability ($p \leq 0.05$) that these results would have happened on the basis of chance alone. The term *probability*, or p, is used to indicate the level of statistical significance. If $p > 0.05$, the differences between the two drug products are not considered significant. Several other statistical phrases such as a confidence level of

TABLE 8-4. GENERAL ELEMENTS OF A BIOAVAILABILITY STUDY SUBMISSION

A. Protocol
   1. Study objectives
   2. Study design
   3. Subject selection criteria
   4. Subject exclusion criteria
   5. Types of biological samples
      (a) Sampling times
      (b) Description of sample-handling procedures
   6. Sample inclusion and exclusion criteria
   7. Ethical consideration
      (a) Subject informed consent form
      (b) Emergency procedures

B. Data
   1. Case reports
   2. Analytical data for validation of assay method
   3. Analytical data from biological samples

C. Results
   1. Summary of individual subject data
   2. Statistical analysis along with summary statistics
      (a) For each individual's sample times
      (b) For AUC, C_{max}, absorption rate constant (K_a), and elimination rate constant (K)
      (c) For T_{max} with appropriate method
   3. Detectable differences at alpha = 0.05 and power = 0.80
   4. 95% symmetrical confidence interval
   5. Application of 75/75 rule to C_{max} and AUC

D. Summary and conclusion

From Purich E, 1980, with permission.[4]

95% or a significance level of 5% (0.05) have been used also to indicate similar statistical significance between products.

The clinical interpretation is important in evaluating the results of a bioequivalency study. A small difference between drug products, even if statistically significant, may produce very little difference in therapeutic response.

An outline for the submission of a completed bioavailability study for submission to the FDA is shown on Table 8-4. Before the study is performed, one should be sure that the study has been properly designed, the objectives are clearly defined, and the method of analysis has been validated (i.e., shown to measure precisely and accurately the plasma drug concentration). Moreover, the protocol for the study may be submitted to the FDA for discussion and approval prior to initiation of the investigation. After the study has been performed, the results are statistically and pharmacokinetically analyzed. These results along with case reports and various data supporting the validity of the analytical method are included in the submission. The Biopharmaceutics Branch of the FDA, after receiving the completed study, will review the study in detail according to the outline presented in Table 8-5. If necessary, an FDA investigator might inspect both the clinical and analytical facilities used for the study and audit the raw data which was used in support of the bioavailability study. The FDA will then make a decision to approve the bioavailability of the drug product.

QUESTIONS

1. An antibiotic was formulated into two different oral dosage forms, *A* and *B*. Biopharmaceutic studies revealed different antibiotic blood level curves for each drug product (Fig. 8-7). Each drug product was given in the same dose as the others. Explain how the various possible formulation factors could have caused the differences in blood levels. *Give examples* where possible. How would the corresponding urinary drug excretion curves relate to the plasma level–time curves?
2. You have just made a new formulation of acetaminophen. Design a protocol to compare your drug product against the acetaminophen drug products on the market. What criteria would you use for proof of bioequivalence for your new formulation? How would you determine if the

TABLE 8-5. GENERAL ELEMENTS OF A BIOPHARMACEUTICS REVIEW

Introduction	Determination of detectable differences
Study design	Determination of power to detect a 20% difference
Study objective(s)	at alpha = 0.05
Assay description and validation	Comments
Assay for individual samples checked	Deficiencies
Summary and analysis of data	Recommendation

From Purich E, 1980, with permission.[4]

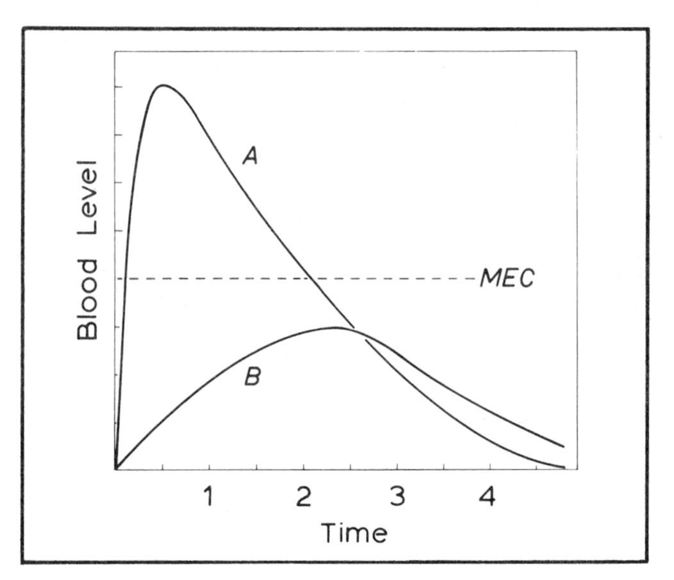

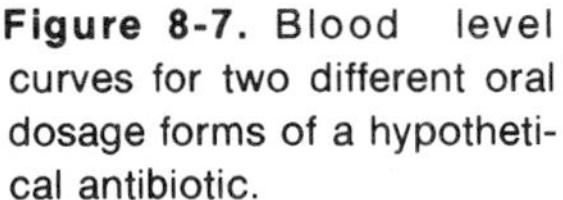
Figure 8-7. Blood level curves for two different oral dosage forms of a hypothetical antibiotic.

acetaminophen was completely (100%) systemically absorbed?

3. The data in Table 8-6 represent the average findings in antibiotic plasma samples taken from 10 humans (average weight 70 kg), tabulated in a four-way crossover design.
   a. Which of the four drug products in Table 8-6 would be preferred as a reference standard for a bioequivalency study? Why?
   b. From which oral drug product is the drug absorbed more rapidly?
   c. What is the absolute bioavailability of the drug from the oral solution?
   d. What is the relative bioavailability of the drug from the oral tablet compared to the reference standard?

TABLE 8-6. COMPARISON OF PLASMA CONCENTRATIONS OF ANTIBIOTIC, AS RELATED TO DOSAGE FORM AND TIME

		Plasma Concentration ($\mu g/ml$)		
Time After Dose (hrs)	***IV Solution* (*2 mg/kg*)**	***Oral Solution* (*10 mg/kg*)**	***Oral Tablet* (*10mg/kg*)**	***Oral Capsule* (*10mg/kg*)**
0.5	5.94	23.4	13.2	18.7
1.0	5.30	26.6	18.0	21.3
1.5	4.72	25.2	19.0	20.1
2.0	4.21	22.8	18.3	18.2
3.0	3.34	18.2	15.4	14.6
4.0	2.66	14.5	12.5	11.6
6.0	1.68	9.14	7.92	7.31
8.0	1.06	5.77	5.00	4.61
10.0	0.67	3.64	3.16	2.91
12.0	0.42	2.30	1.99	1.83
AUC$\left(\frac{\mu g}{ml} \cdot hrs\right)$	29.0	145.0	116.0	116.0

e. From the data in Table 8-6, determine:
   (1) Apparent V_d
   (2) Elimination $t_{1/2}$
   (3) First-order elimination rate constant K
   (4) Total body clearance

f. From the data above graph the cumulative urinary excretion curves which would correspond to the plasma concentration time curves.

4. Aphrodesia is a new drug manufactured by the Venus drug company. When tested in humans, the pharmacokinetics of the drug assumes a one-compartment open model with first-order absorption and first-order elimination:

$$D_{GI} \xrightarrow{K_a} D_B V_d \xrightarrow{K}$$

The drug was given in a single oral dose of 250 mg to a group of college students 21–29 years of age. Mean body weight was 60 kg. Samples of blood were obtained at various time intervals after the administration of the drug and the plasma fractions were analyzed for active drug. The following data were obtained.

Time (hr)	C_p (μg/ml)	*Time* (hr)	C_p (μg/ml)
0	0.	12	3.02
1	1.88	18	1.86
2	3.05	24	1.12
3	3.74	36	0.40
5	4.21	48	0.14
7	4.08	60	0.05
9	3.70	72	0.02

a. The minimum effective concentration of Aphrodesia in plasma is 2.3 μg/ml. What is the *onset* time of this drug?

b. The minimum effective concentration of Aphrodesia in plasma is 2.3 μg/ml. What is the *duration* of activity of this drug?

c. What is the elimination half-life of Aphrodesia in college students?

d. What is the time for peak drug concentration (t_{max}) of Aphrodesia?

e. What is the peak drug concentration ($C_{p,max}$)?

f. Assuming that the drug is 100% systemically available (i.e., fraction of drug absorbed equals unity), what is the AUC for Aphrodesia?

5. You wish to do a bioequivalency study on three different formulations of the same active drug. Lay out a "Latin square design" for the proper sequencing of these drug products in six normal healthy volunteers. What is the main reason for using a crossover design in a bioequivalency study? What is meant by a "*random*" population?

6. Four different drug products containing the same antibiotic were given to 12 volunteer adult males (age 19–28 years, average weight 73 kg) in a four-way crossover design. The volunteers were fasted 12 hr prior to taking the drug product. Urine samples were collected up to 72 hr after the administration of the drug to obtain the maximum urinary drug excretion, D_u^∞. The following data were obtained:

Drug Product	*Dose (mg/kg)*	*Cumulative Urinary Drug Excretion (D_u^∞), 0–72 hr (mg)*
IV solution	0.2	20
Oral solution	4	380
Oral tablet	4	340
Oral capsule	4	360

a. What is the *absolute* bioavailability of the drug from the *tablet*?
b. What is the *relative* bioavailability of the capsule compared to the oral solution?

7. According to the prescribing information for cimetidine (Tagamet, SKF Lab. Co.): Following IV or IM administration, 75% of the drug is recovered from the urine, after 24 hr as the parent compound. Following a single oral dose 48% of the drug is recovered from the urine after 24 hr as the parent compound. From this information what is the fraction of drug absorbed systemically from the oral dose after 24 hr?

8. Define the term *Bioequivalency Requirement*. Why does the FDA require a bioequivalency requirement for the manufacture of a generic drug product?

9. Why can we use the time for peak drug concentration (T_{max}) in a bioequivalency study for an estimate of the *rate* of drug absorption rather than calculating the K_a?

10. Ten male volunteers (18–26 years of age) weighing an average of 73 kg were given either four tablets each containing 250 mg of drug (drug product *A*) or one tablet containing 1000 mg of drug (drug product *B*). Blood levels of the drug were obtained and the data is summarized in Table 8-7.

a. State a possible reason for the difference in the time for peak drug concentration ($T_{max, A}$) after drug product *A* compared to the $T_{max, B}$ after drug product *B*. (Assume that all the tablets were made from the same formulation, i.e., the drug is in the same particle size, same salt form, same excipients, and same ratio of excipients to active drug.)
b. Draw a graph relating the cumulative amount of drug excreted in urine of patients given drug product *A* compared to the cumulative drug excreted in urine after drug product *B*. *Label axis*!
c. In a second study using the same 10 male volunteers, a 125-mg dose of the drug was given by intravenous bolus and the AUC was computed as 20 μg hr/ml. Calculate the fraction of drug systemically absorbed from drug product *B* (1×1000 mg) tablet using the data in Table 8-7.

11. After performing a bioequivalency test comparing a generic drug product to a brand name drug product, it was observed that the generic drug product had a greater bioavailability than the brand name drug product.

a. Would you approve marketing the generic drug product claiming it was superior than the brand name drug product?

TABLE 8-7. BLOOD LEVEL DATA SUMMARY FOR TWO DRUG PRODUCTS

Kinetic Variable	Unit	Drug Product A 4× 250 mg Tablet	Drug Product B 1000 mg Tablet	Statistic
Time for peak drug concentration (range)	hr	1.3 (0.7–1.5)	1.8 (1.5–2.2)	$p < 0.05$
Peak concentration (range)	μg/ml	53 (46–58)	47 (42–51)	$p < 0.05$
AUC (range)	μg hr/ml	118 (98–125)	103 (90–120)	N.S.
$t_{1/2}$	hr	3.2 (2.5–3.8)	3.8 (2.9–4.3)	N.S.

b. Would you expect *identical* pharmacologic responses to *both* drug products?

c. What therapeutic problem might arise in using the generic drug product which might not occur when using the brand name drug product?

12. The following study is from the article "Bioavailability of tolazamide from tablets: Comparison of in vitro and in vivo results" by Welling et al.[5]

Design of Study

1. *Tolazamide Formulations.* Four tolazamide tablet formulations were selected for this study. The tablet formulations were labeled *A*, *B*, *C*, and *D*. Disintegration and dissolution tests were performed by standard USP XX procedures.
2. *Subjects.* Twenty healthy adult male volunteers between the ages of 18 and 38 (mean 26 years) and weighing between 61.4 and 95.5 kg (mean 74.5 kg) were selected for the study. The subjects were randomly assigned to four groups of five each. The four treatments were administered according to a 4 × 4 Latin square design. Each treatment was separated by 1-week intervals. All subjects fasted overnight prior to

TABLE 8-8. DISINTEGRATION TIMES AND DISSOLUTION RATES OF TOLAZAMIDE TABLETS[a]

Tablet	Mean Disintegration Time[b] min (range)	Percent Dissolved in 30 min[c] (range)
A	3.8 (3.0–4.0)	103.9 (100.5–106.3)
B	2.2 (1.8–2.5)	10.9 (9.3–13.5)
C	2.3 (2.0–2.5)	31.6 (26.4–37.2)
D	26.5 (22.5–30.5)	29.7 (20.8–38.4)

[a] $n = 6$
[b] By the method of USP XX
[c] Dissolution rates in pH 7.6 buffer.
From Welling PG, et al, 1982, with permission.

TABLE 8-9. MEAN TOLAZAMIDE CONCENTRATIONS[a] IN SERUM

	Time (hr)	Treatment, μg/ml				Statistic[b]
		A	*B*	*C*	*D*	
	0	10.8 ± 7.4	1.3 ± 1.4	1.8 ± 1.9	3.5 ± 2.6	$A\overline{DCB}$
	1	20.5 ± 7.3	2.8 ± 2.8	5.4 ± 4.8	13.5 ± 6.6	$AD\overline{CB}$
	3	23.9 ± 5.3	4.4 ± 4.3	9.8 ± 5.6	20.0 ± 6.4	$\overline{AD}CB$
	4	25.4 ± 5.2	5.7 ± 4.1	13.6 ± 5.3	22.0 ± 5.4	$\overline{AD}CB$
	5	24.1 ± 6.3	6.6 ± 4.0	15.1 ± 4.7	22.6 ± 5.0	$\overline{AD}CB$
	6	19.9 ± 5.9	6.8 ± 3.4	14.3 ± 3.9	19.7 ± 4.7	$\overline{AD}CB$
	8	15.2 ± 5.5	6.6 ± 3.2	12.8 ± 4.1	14.6 ± 4.2	$\overline{ADC}B$
	12	8.8 ± 4.8	5.5 ± 3.2	9.1 ± 4.0	8.5 ± 4.1	$\overline{CAD}B$
	16	5.6 ± 3.8	4.6 ± 3.3	6.4 ± 3.9	5.4 ± 3.1	$C\overline{ADB}$
	24	2.7 ± 2.4	3.1 ± 2.6	3.1 ± 3.3	2.4 ± 1.8	$\overline{CBAD}$
C_{max}[c], μg/ml		27.8 ± 5.3	7.7 ± 4.1	16.4 ± 4.4	24.0 ± 4.5	$\overline{AD}CB$
T_{max}[d], hr		3.3 ± 0.9	7.0 ± 2.2	5.4 ± 2.0	4.0 ± 0.9	$BC\overline{DA}$
AUC_{0-24}[e], μg hr/ml		260 ± 81	112 ± 63	193 ± 70	231 ± 67	$\overline{AD}CB$

[a] Concentrations ±1 SD, $n = 20$
[b] For explanation see text
[c] Maximum concentration of tolazamide in serum
[d] Time of maximum concentration
[e] Area under the 0–24-hr serum tolazamide concentration curve calculated by trapezoidal rule
From Welling PG, et al, 1982, with permission.[5]

receiving the tolazamide tablet the following morning. The tablet was given with 180 ml of water. Food intake was allowed at 5 hr postdose. Blood samples (10 ml) were taken just prior to the dose and periodically after dosing. The serum fraction was separated from the blood and analyzed for tolazamide by high-pressure liquid chromatography.

3. *Data analysis.* Serum data was analyzed by a digital computer program using a regression analysis and by the percent of drug unabsorbed by the method of Wagner and Nelson. AUC was determined by the trapezoidal rule and an analysis of variance was determined by Tukey's method.
   a. Why was a *Latin square crossover design* used in this study?
   b. Why were the subjects *fasted* prior to taking the tolazamide tablets?
   c. Why did the authors use the Wagner–Nelson method rather than the Loo–Riegelman method for measuring the amount of drug absorbed?
   d. From the data in Table 8-8 *only*, from which tablet formulation would you expect the greatest bioavailability? *Why*?
   e. From the data in Table 8-8, did the disintegration times correlate with the dissolution times? *Why*?
   f. Does the data in Table 8-8 appear to correlate with the data in Table 8-9? *Why*?
   g. Draw the expected cumulative urinary excretion versus time curve for formulations *A* and *B*. *Label axis* and identify each curve.

h. Assuming formulation A is the *reference* formulation, what is the *relative* bioavailability of formulation D?

i. Using the data in Table 8-9 for formulation A, calculate the elimination half-life ($t_{1/2}$) for tolazamide.

REFERENCES

1. Gardner S: Bioequivalence requirements and in vivo bioavailability procedures. Fed Reg 42:1651, 1977
2. Feldman CH, Hutchinson VE, Sher TH, et al: Interaction between nutrition and theophylline metabolism in children. Ther Drug Monit 4:69–76, 1982
3. Hendles L, Iafrate RP, Weinberger M: A clinical and pharmacokinetic basis for the selection and use of slow release theophylline products. Clin Pharmacokin 9:95–135, 1984
4. Purich E: Bioavailability/bioequivalency regulations: An FDA perspective. In Albert KS (ed.), Drug Absorption and Disposition. Statistical Considerations. Washington, D.C., American Pharmaceutical Association, 1980
5. Welling PG, Patel RB, Patel UR, et al: Bioavailability of tolazamide from tablets: Comparison of in vitro and in vivo results. J Pharm Sci 71:1259–1663, 1982

BIBLIOGRAPHY

Bennett RW, Popovitch NG: Statistical inferences as applied to bioavailability data: A guide for the practicing pharmacist. Am J Hosp Pharm 34:712–23, 1977

Chodes DJ, DiSanto AR: Basics of Bioavailability. Kalamazoo, Mich., Upjohn, 1974

Dighe SV: Biopharmaceutics program. Clin Res Pract Drug Res Affairs 1:61–76, 1983

DiSanto AR, Desante KA: Bioavailability and pharmacokinetics of prednisone in humans. J Pharm Sci 64:109–12, 1975

Hendeles L, Wienberger M, Bighley L: Absolute bioavailability of oral theophylline. Am J Hosp Pharm 34:525–27, 1977

Kennedy D: Therapeutically equivalent drugs. Fed Reg 44:2932–52, 1979

Martin A, Dolusio JT (eds.): Industrial Bioavailability and Pharmacokinetics: Guidelines, Regulations and Controls. Austin, Texas, Drug Dynamics Institute, Univ. of Texas, 1977

Metzler CM: Bioavailability: A problem in equivalence. Biometrics 30:309–17, 1974

Schumacher GE: Interpretation of bioavailability data by practitioners. J Clin Pharmacol 16:554–59, 1976

Schumacher GE: Use of bioavailability data by practitioners, I: Pitfalls in interpreting the data. Am J Hosp Pharm 32:839–42, 1975

Wagner JG: An overview of the analysis and interpretation of bioavailability studies in man. Pharmacology 8:102–17, 1972

Westlake WJ: The design and analysis of comparative blood level trials. In Swarbrick J (ed.), Current Concepts in Pharmaceutical Sciences: Dosage Form Design and Bioavailability. Philadelphia, Lea and Febiger, 1973, Chap. 5

Westlake WJ: Use of statistical methods in evaluation of *in vivo* performance of dosage forms. J Pharm Sci 62:1579–89, 1973

CHAPTER NINE

Drug Clearance

Drug clearance is a measurement of drug elimination from the body without reference to the mechanism of the process. There are several definitions of clearance which are pharmacokinetically equivalent. Generally, the body or organ tissues are regarded as a compartment of fluid with a definite volume (apparent volume of distribution) in which the drug is dissolved. From this concept, clearance is defined as the volume of fluid (containing drug) which is cleared of drug per unit of time. For example, if the clearance of penicillin is 15 ml/min in a patient with an apparent volume of distribution, V_D of 12 liters, then 15 ml of the 12 liters is cleared of drug per minute.

Alternatively, clearance may be defined as the rate of drug elimination divided by the plasma drug concentration at that time point:

$$\text{Clearance} = \frac{\text{excretion rate}}{\text{plasma concentration}} = \frac{\mu\text{g/min}}{\mu\text{g/ml}} = \text{ml/min} \tag{9.1}$$

$$\text{Cl} = \frac{dD_u/dt}{C_p} \tag{9.2}$$

Multiplying both sides of the equation by C_p gives

$$\text{Cl}C_p = \frac{dD_u}{dt} \tag{9.3}$$

where dD_u/dt is the rate of drug elimination. Equation 9.3 shows that the rate of drug elimination is directly proportional to the plasma drug concentration, C_p. Clearance, however, is constant for any given plasma drug concentration. This is true as long as the rate of drug elimination is a first-order process.

Using the previous example of penicillin, assume that the plasma penicillin concentration is 10 μg/ml and 15 ml of the 12 liters (apparent volume of distribution) is cleared of drug per minute. Therefore, from Equation 9.3 the rate of drug removal is

$$\text{Rate of drug removal} = 15 \text{ ml/min} \times 10\ \mu\text{g/ml} = 150\ \mu\text{g/min}$$

Thus, 150 μg of penicillin is eliminated every minute from the body when the plasma concentration is at 10 μg/ml. Clearance, therefore, may be used to estimate the rate of drug elimination at any drug concentration.

The above example provides a means for calculating clearance. Assume that the rate of penicillin elimination is 150 μg/min, which can be measured by urinary excretion and that the plasma penicillin concentration is 10 μg/ml at this time. Using Equation 9.2, penicillin clearance may be calculated:

$$\text{Cl}_{\text{penicillin}} = 150\ \mu\text{g/min} \div 10\ \mu\text{g/ml} = 15 \text{ ml/min}$$

Clearance may also be defined as the product of the first-order elimination rate constant and the apparent volume of distribution. From Equation 9.2

$$\text{Cl} = \frac{dD_u/dt}{C_p}$$

The rate of drug elimination $(dD_u/dt) = C_p K V_d$, which may be substituted into Equation 9.2 to give Equation 9.4:

$$\text{Cl} = \frac{C_p K V_d}{C_p} \qquad \text{Cl} = KV_d \tag{9.4}$$

EXAMPLE

Determine the clearance of a drug which has an elimination half-life of 3 hr and an apparent volume of distribution of 100 ml/kg.

Solution

First determine the elimination rate constant K and then substitute properly into Equation 9.3:

$$K = \frac{0.693}{3} = 0.231 \text{ hr}^{-1}$$

$$\text{Cl} = 0.231 \text{ hr}^{-1} \times 100 \text{ ml/kg} = 23.1 \text{ ml/kg hr}$$

The clearance calculated by the equation is termed *total drug clearance* or *total body clearance*. Total body clearance is the sum total of all the clearance pathways in the body including clearance of drug through the kidney (renal clearance) and clearance of drug through the liver (hepatic clearance). Clearance may be expressed on a per kilogram body weight basis similar to the method for expressing the apparent volume of distribution on a body weight since both of these pharmacokinetic parameters are constant under normal conditions. Therefore, to obtain clearance for an individual patient, multiply the clearance per kilogram times the body weight (kg) of the patient.

MECHANISMS OF RENAL CLEARANCE

Renal excretion is a major route of elimination for many drugs. Drugs which are water soluble, have low molecular weight (≤ 300), or are slowly biotransformed by the liver will be eliminated by renal excretion. The processes by which a drug is excreted via the kidneys may include any combination of the following:

- Glomerular filtration
- Active tubular secretion
- Tubular reabsorption

Glomerular filtration is a unidirectional process which occurs for most small molecules (MW < 500), including undissociated (nonionized) and dissociated (ionized) drugs. Protein-bound drugs behave as large molecules and do not get filtered at the glomerulus. The major driving force for glomerular filtration is the hydrostatic pressure within the glomerular capillaries. The kidneys receive a large blood supply (approximately 25% of the cardiac output) via the renal artery with very little decrease in the hydrostatic pressure.

Glomerular filtration rate (GFR) is measured by using a drug that is eliminated by filtration only (i.e., it is neither reabsorbed nor secreted). Examples of such drugs are inulin and creatinine. Therefore, the clearance of inulin will be equal to the glomerular filtration rate, which is equal to 125–130 ml/min. The value for the glomerular filtration rate correlates fairly well with body surface area. Glomerular filtration of drugs is directly related to the free or non-protein-bound drug concentration in the plasma. As the free drug concentration in the plasma increases, the glomerular filtration for the drug will increase proportionately.

Active renal secretion is an active transport process. As such, active renal secretion is a carrier-mediated system which requires energy input, since the drug is transported against a concentration gradient. The carrier system is capacity limited and may be saturated. Drugs with similar structures may compete for the same carrier system. Two active renal secretion systems have been identified, systems for (1) weak acids and (2) weak bases. For example, probenecid will compete with penicillin for the same carrier system (weak acids). Active tubular secretion rate is dependent on renal plasma flow. Drugs which are commonly used to measure active tubular secretion include *p*-amino-hippuric acid (PAH) and iodopyracet (Diodrast). These substances are both filtered by the glomeruli and secreted by the tubular cells. Active secretion is extremely rapid for these drugs, and practically all the drug carried to the kidney is eliminated in a single pass. The clearance for these drugs therefore reflects the effective renal plasma flow. The effective renal plasma flow (ERPF) varies from 425 to 650 ml/min. For a drug that is excreted solely by glomerular filtration, the elimination half-life may change markedly in accordance with the binding affinity of the drug for plasma proteins. In contrast, protein binding has very little effect on the elimination half-life of a drug excreted mostly by active secretion. Since drug protein binding is reversible, the bound drug and free drug are excreted by active secretion during the first pass through the kidney. For example, some of the penicillins are extensively protein bound, but their elimination half-lives are short due to rapid elimination by active secretion.

Tubular reabsorption occurs after the drug is filtered through the glomerulus and can be active or passive. If a drug is completely reabsorbed (e.g., glucose), then the value for the clearance of the drug is approximately zero. For drugs which are partially reabsorbed, clearance values will be less than the GFR of 125–130 ml/min.

The reabsorption of drugs which are acids or weak bases is influenced by the pH of the fluid in the renal tubule (i.e., urine pH) and the pK_a of the drug. Both of these factors together determine the percentage of dissociated (ionized) and undissociated (nonionized) drug. Generally, the undissociated species is more lipid soluble (less water soluble) and has greater membrane permeability. The undissociated drug is easily reabsorbed from the renal tubule back into the body. This process of drug reabsorption can significantly reduce the amount of drug excreted, depending on the pH of the urinary fluid and the pK_a of the drug. The pK_a of the drug is a constant, but the normal urinary pH may vary from 4.5 to 8.0, depending on diet, pathophysiology, and drug intake. Vegetable diets or diets rich in carbohydrates will result in higher urinary pH, whereas diets rich in protein will result in lower urinary pH. Drugs such as ascorbic acid and antacids such as sodium carbonate may alter urinary pH when administered in large quantity. By far the most important changes in urinary pH are caused by fluids administered intravenously. Intravenous fluids such as solutions of bicarbonate or ammonium chloride are used in acid–base therapy. Excretion of these solutions may drastically change urinary pH and alter drug reabsorption.

The percentage of ionized weak acid drug corresponding to a given pH can be obtained from the Henderson–Hesselbalch equation:

$$\mathrm{pH} = \mathrm{p}K_a + \log\frac{[\text{ionized}]}{[\text{nonionized}]} \tag{9.5}$$

Rearrangement of this equation yields

$$\frac{[\text{ionized}]}{[\text{nonionized}]} = 10^{\mathrm{pH}-\mathrm{p}K_a} \tag{9.6}$$

$$\text{Percent of drug ionized} = \frac{[\text{ionized}]}{[\text{ionized}] + [\text{nonionized}]}$$

$$= \frac{10^{\mathrm{pH}-\mathrm{p}K_a}[\text{nonionized}]}{[\text{nonionized}] + 10^{\mathrm{pH}-\mathrm{p}K_a}[\text{nonionized}]}$$

$$= \frac{10^{\mathrm{pH}-\mathrm{p}K_a}}{1 + 10^{\mathrm{pH}-\mathrm{p}K_a}} \tag{9.7}$$

The percent of weak acid drug ionized in any pH environment may be calculated with Equation 9.7. For example, for acidic drugs with pK_a's of from 3 to 8, a change in urinary pH will affect the extent of dissociation (Table 9-1). The extent of dissociation is more greatly affected by changes in urinary pH with a pK_a of 5 than with a pK_a of 3. Weak acids with pK_a values of less than 2 are highly ionized at all urinary pH values and are only slightly affected by pH variations.

For a weak base drug, the Henderson–Hasselbalch equation is given as

$$\text{pH} = \text{p}K_a + \log\frac{[\text{nonionized}]}{[\text{ionized}]} \tag{9.8}$$

and

$$\text{Percent of drug ionized} = \frac{1 + 10^{\text{pH}-\text{p}K_a}}{10^{\text{pH}-\text{p}K_a}} \tag{9.9}$$

The greatest effect of urinary pH on reabsorption occurs with weak base drugs with pK_a's of 7.5–10.5.

From the Henderson–Hesselbalch relationship, a concentration ratio for the distribution of a weak acid or basic drug between urine and plasma may be derived. The urine–plasma (U: P) ratios for these drugs are as follows.

For weak acids:

$$\frac{U}{P} = \frac{1 + 10^{\text{pH urine}-\text{p}K_a}}{1 + 10^{\text{pH plasma}-\text{p}K_a}} \tag{9.10}$$

For weak bases:

$$\frac{U}{P} = \frac{1 + 10^{\text{p}K_a-\text{pH urine}}}{1 + 10^{\text{p}K_a-\text{pH plasma}}} \tag{9.11}$$

For example, amphetamine, a weak base, will be reabsorbed if the urine pH is made alkaline and more lipid-soluble nonionized species are formed. In contrast, acidification of the urine will cause the amphetamine to become more ionized (form a salt). The salt form is more water soluble and less likely to be reabsorbed and has a tendency to be excreted into the urine more quickly. In the case of weak acids (such as salicylic acid) acidification of the urine causes greater reabsorption of the drug and alkalinization of the urine causes more rapid excretion of the drug.

TABLE 9-1. EFFECT OF URINARY pH AND pK_a ON THE IONIZATION OF DRUGS

pH of Urine	Percent of Drug Ionized: pK_a 3	Percent of Drug Ionized: pK_a 5
7.4	100	99.6
5	99	50.0
4	91	9.1
3	50	0.99

PRACTICE PROBLEMS

Let $pK_a = 5$ for an acidic drug. Compare the U/P at urinary pH (a) 3; (b) 5; and (c) 7.

Solution

a. At pH = 3:

$$\frac{U}{P} = \frac{1 + 10^{3-5}}{1 + 10^{7.4-5}} = \frac{1.01}{1 + 10^{2.4}}$$

$$= \frac{1.01}{252} \approx \frac{1}{252}$$

b. At pH = 5:

$$\frac{U}{P} = \frac{1 + 10^{5-5}}{1 + 10^{7.4-5}} = \frac{2}{1 + 10^{2.4}} = \frac{2}{252}$$

c. At pH = 7:

$$\frac{U}{P} = \frac{1 + 10^{7-5}}{1 + 10^{7.4-5}} = \frac{101}{1 + 10^{2.4}} = \frac{101}{252}$$

In addition to the pH of the urine, the rate of urine flow will influence the amount of filtered drug which is reabsorbed. The normal flow of urine is approximately 1–2 ml/min. Nonpolar and nonionized drugs which are normally well reabsorbed in the renal tubules are sensitive to changes in the rate of urine flow. Drugs which increase urine flow, such as ethanol, large fluid intake, and methylxanthines (such as caffeine or theophylline) will decrease the time for drug reabsorption and promote their excretion. Thus, forced diuresis through the use of diuretics may be a useful adjunct for removing excessive drug in an intoxicated patient by increasing renal drug excretion.

Renal clearance may be measured without regard to the physiologic mechanisms involved in this process. From a physiologic viewpoint, however, renal clearance may be considered as the ratio of the sum of the glomerular filtration and active secretion rates less the reabsorption rate divided by the plasma drug concentration:

$$Cl_r = \frac{\text{filtration rate} + \text{secretion rate} - \text{reabsorption rate}}{C_p} \tag{9.12}$$

CLEARANCE RATIO

The actual physiologic process for renal clearance of a drug is not generally obtained by direct measurement. However, by comparing the clearance value for the drug to

TABLE 9-2. COMPARISON OF CLEARANCE OF A SAMPLE DRUG TO CLEARANCE OF A REFERENCE DRUG, INULIN

Clearance Ratio	Probable Mechanism of Renal Excretion
$\frac{Cl_{drug}}{Cl_{inulin}} < 1$	Drug is partially reabsorbed
$\frac{Cl_{drug}}{Cl_{inulin}} = 1$	Drug is filtered only
$\frac{Cl_{drug}}{Cl_{inulin}} > 1$	Drug is actively secreted

that of a standard reference drug (such as inulin, which is cleared through the kidney by glomerular filtration only), the physiologic clearance process for the first drug may be inferred. For example, note the clearance ratios of the renal clearance of the drug in question to the clearance of a drug such as inulin presented in Table 9-2.

DETERMINATION OF CLEARANCE

The clearance is given by the slope of the curve obtained by plotting the rate of drug excretion in urine (dD_u/dt) against C_p (see Eq. 9.3). For a drug that is excreted rapidly, dD_u/dt is large, the slope is steeper, and clearance is greater (Fig. 9-1, line A). For a drug that is excreted slowly through the kidney, the slope is smaller (Fig. 9-1, line B).

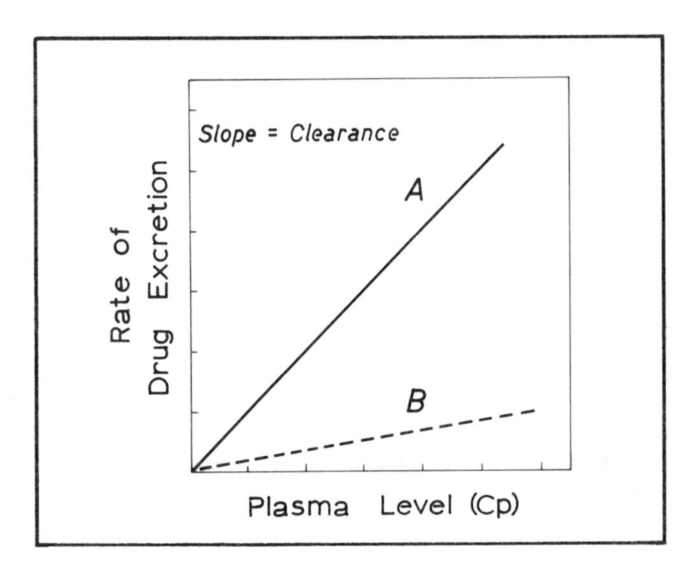

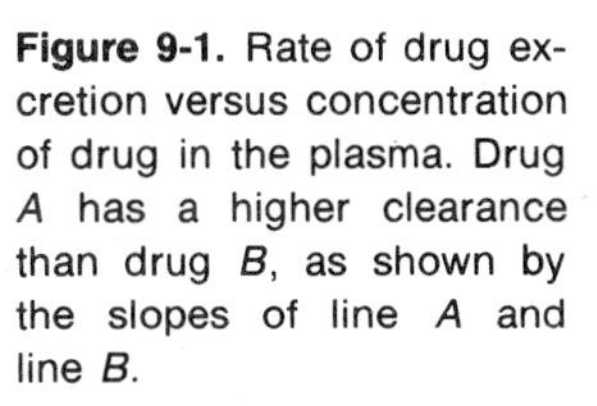
Figure 9-1. Rate of drug excretion versus concentration of drug in the plasma. Drug A has a higher clearance than drug B, as shown by the slopes of line A and line B.

By rearranging Equation 9.3 and integrating, one obtains

$$\int_0^{D_u} dD_u = \text{Cl} \int_0^t C_p \, dt \tag{9.13}$$

$$[D_u]_0^t = \text{Cl}[\text{AUC}]_0^t \tag{9.14}$$

A curve is then plotted of cumulative drug excreted in the urine versus the area under the concentration–time curve (Fig. 9-2). Clearance is obtained from the slope of the curve. The area under the curve can be estimated by the trapezoidal rule or by other measurement methods. The disadvantage of this method is that if a data point is missing, it becomes difficult to obtain the cumulative amount of drug excreted in the urine. However, if the data is complete, then the determination of clearance is more accurate by this method.

By plotting cumulative drug excreted in the urine from t_1 to t_2, $[D_u]_{t_1}^{t_2}$ versus $[\text{AUC}]_{t_1}^{t_2}$, one obtains an equation similar to that presented previously:

$$\int_{D_u^1}^{D_u^2} dD_u = \text{Cl} \int_{t_1}^{t_2} C_p \, dt \tag{9.15}$$

$$[D_u]_{t_1}^{t_2} = \text{Cl}[\text{AUC}]_{t_1}^{t_2} \tag{9.16}$$

The slope is equal to the clearance (Fig. 9-3).

Clearance rates may also be estimated by a single (nongraphical) calculation from knowledge of the $[\text{AUC}]_0^\infty$, the total amount of drug absorbed, FD_0, and the total amount of drug excreted in the urine, D_u^∞. For example, if a single IV bolus drug injection is given to a patient and the $[\text{AUC}]_0^\infty$ is obtained from the plasma

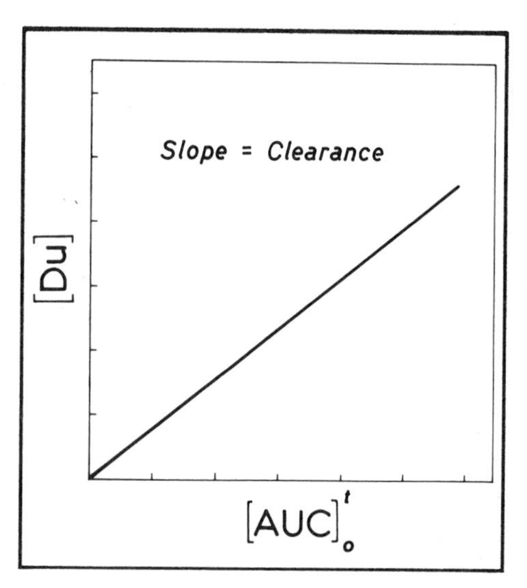

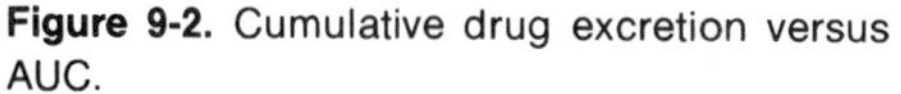
Figure 9-2. Cumulative drug excretion versus AUC.

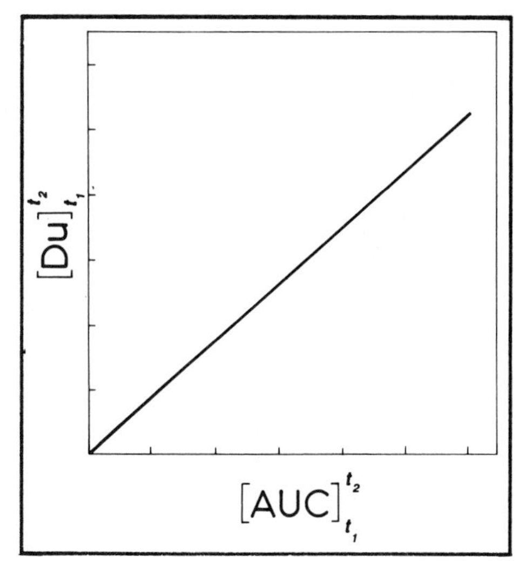

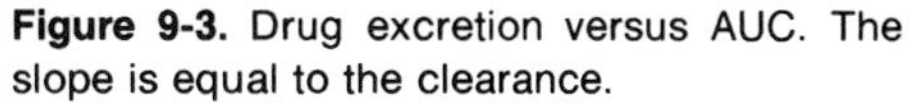
Figure 9-3. Drug excretion versus AUC. The slope is equal to the clearance.

drug level–time curve, then total body clearance is estimated by

$$\mathrm{Cl_T} = \frac{D_0}{[\mathrm{AUC}]_0^\infty} \tag{9.17}$$

If the total amount of drug excreted in the urine, D_u^∞, has been obtained, then renal clearance is calculated by

$$\mathrm{Cl_r} = \frac{D_\mathrm{u}^\infty}{[\mathrm{AUC}]_0^\infty} \tag{9.18}$$

The calculations using Equations 9.17 and 9.18 allow for rapid and easily obtainable estimates of drug clearance. However, only a single dose estimate is obtained; therefore, the calculations will not reflect nonlinear changes in the clearance rates as indicated in Figure 9-4.

Clearance can also be calculated from fitted parameters. If the volume of distribution and elimination constants are known, body clearance ($\mathrm{Cl_T}$), renal clearance ($\mathrm{Cl_r}$), and hepatic clearance ($\mathrm{Cl_h}$) can be calculated according to the following expressions.

$$\mathrm{Cl_T} = KV_\mathrm{d} \tag{9.19}$$

$$\mathrm{Cl_r} = K_\mathrm{e}V_\mathrm{d} \tag{9.20}$$

$$\mathrm{Cl_h} = K_\mathrm{m}V_\mathrm{d} \tag{9.21}$$

Total body clearance ($\mathrm{Cl_T}$) is equal to the sum of renal clearance and hepatic clearance and is based on the concept that the entire body acts as a drug-eliminating system.

$$\mathrm{Cl_T} = \mathrm{Cl_r} + \mathrm{Cl_h} \tag{9.22}$$

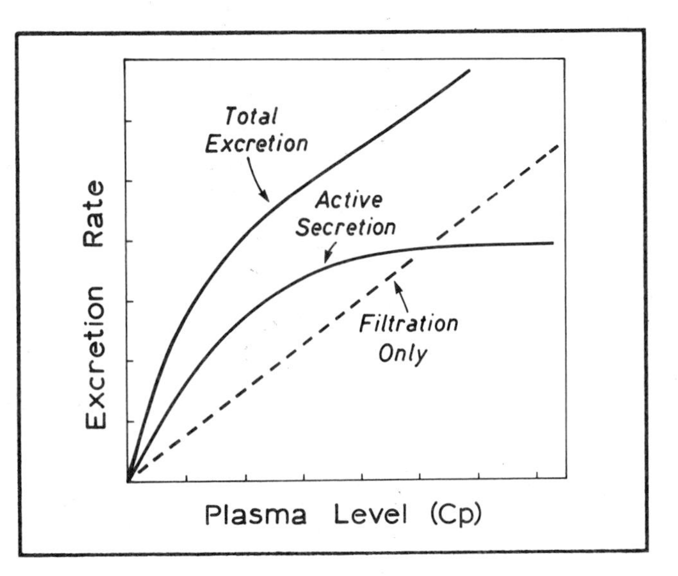

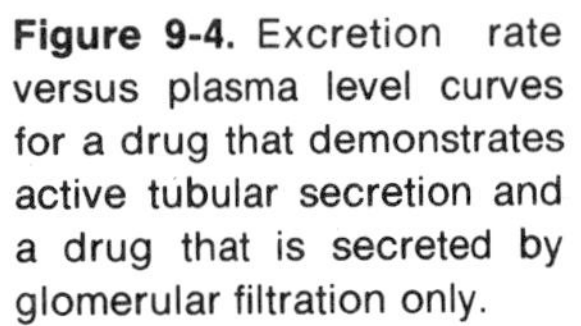
Figure 9-4. Excretion rate versus plasma level curves for a drug that demonstrates active tubular secretion and a drug that is secreted by glomerular filtration only.

PRACTICE PROBLEMS

Consider a drug which is eliminated by first-order renal excretion and hepatic metabolism. The drug follows a one-compartment model and is given in a single intravenous or oral dose (Fig. 9-5).

Working with the model presented in Figure 9-5, assume that a single dose (100 mg) of this drug is given orally. The drug is 90% systemically available. The total amount of unchanged drug recovered in the urine is 60 mg, and the total amount of metabolite recovered in the urine is 30 mg. According to the literature the elimination half-life for this drug is 3.3 hr and its apparent volume of distribution is 1000 ml. From the information given, find (a) the total body

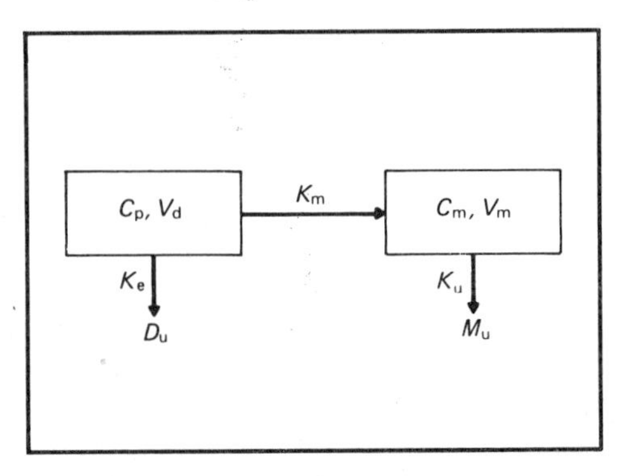

Figure 9-5. Model of a drug eliminated by first-order renal excretion and hepatic metabolism. K_e = renal excretion rate constant of parent drug; K_m = metabolism rate constant (conversion of parent drug to metabolite); K_u = renal excretion rate constant of metabolite; D_u = amount of unchanged drug in urine; M_u = amount of metabolite in urine; C_m = plasma concentration of the metabolite; C_p = plasma concentration of the parent drug; V_d = apparent volume of distribution of parent drug; and V_m = apparent volume of distribution of metabolite.

clearance; (b) the renal clearance; and (c) the nonrenal clearance of the drug.

Solution

a. Total body clearance:

$$\mathrm{Cl_T} = KV_d$$

$$\mathrm{Cl_T} = \frac{0.693}{3.3}(1000) = 210 \text{ ml/hr}$$

b. Renal clearance. First find K_e:

$$\frac{K_e}{K} = \frac{D_u^\infty}{FD_0} = \frac{D_u^\infty}{M_u^\infty + D_u^\infty} \qquad (9.23)$$

$$K_e = \left(\frac{0.693}{3.3}\right)\left(\frac{60}{30+60}\right) = 0.14 \text{ hr}^{-1}$$

Then, from Equation 9.20,

$$\mathrm{Cl_r} = K_e V_d$$

$$\mathrm{Cl_r} = (0.14)(1000) = 140 \text{ ml/hr}$$

c. Nonrenal clearance:

$$\mathrm{Cl_h} = \mathrm{Cl_T} - \mathrm{Cl_r}$$

$$\mathrm{Cl_h} = 210 - 140 = 70 \text{ ml/hr}$$

Alternatively,

$$K_m = K - K_e$$

$$= 0.21 - 0.14 = 0.07 \text{ hr}^{-1}$$

$$= K\left(\frac{M_u^\infty}{M_u^\infty + D_u^\infty}\right)$$

$$= 0.21\left(\frac{30}{30+60}\right) = 0.07 \text{ hr}^{-1}$$

Since (Eq. 9.21)

$$\mathrm{Cl_h} = K_m V_d$$

$$\mathrm{Cl_h} = (0.07)(1000) = 70 \text{ ml/hr}$$

Protein-Bound Drugs. Protein-bound drugs are not eliminated by glomerular filtration. Therefore, Equation 9.1 for the calculation of renal clearance must be modified, since only the free drug is excreted by a linear process. The bound drugs are usually excreted by active secretion, following capacity-limited kinetics. The determination of clearance which separates the two components would result in a hybrid clearance. There is no simple way to overcome this problem. Clearance values for the protein-bound drug are therefore calculated with the following equation.

$$\mathrm{Cl}_r = \frac{\text{rate of unbound drug excretion}}{\text{concentration of unbound drug in the plasma}} \tag{9.24}$$

In practice, this equation is not easily applied because the rate of drug excretion is usually determined after collecting urine samples. The drug excreted in the urine is the sum of drug excreted by active tubular secretion and by passive glomerular filtration. However, it is not possible to distinguish the amount of bound drug actively secreted from the amount of drug which is excreted by glomerular filtration. Equation 9.24 can be used for drugs that are protein bound but not actively secreted. Nonlinear drug binding would make clearance less useful due to model complication.

Equation 9.24 is also used in the calculation of free drug concentration in the plasma, where α is the percent of bound drug and $1 - \alpha$ is the fraction of free drug.

$$(1 - \alpha)C_{p,\text{total}} = C_{p,\text{free}} \tag{9.25}$$

For most drug studies the total plasma drug concentration (free plus bound drug) is used in clearance calculations. If renal clearance is corrected for the fraction of drug bound to plasma proteins using Equation 9.25, then the renal clearance for the free drug concentration will have a higher value compared to the uncorrected renal clearance using the total plasma drug concentrations.

Plasma protein binding has very little effect on the renal clearance of drugs such as penicillin which are actively secreted. For these drugs the free drug fraction is filtered at the glomerular; whereas the protein-bound drug appears to be stripped from the binding sites and actively secreted into the renal tubules.

Body Clearance for Drugs That Follow the Two-Compartment Model. Clearance is a direct measure of elimination from the central compartment regardless of the number of compartments. The central compartment consists of the plasma and highly perfused tissues in which drug equilibrates rapidly. The tissues for drug elimination, namely kidney and liver, are considered integral parts of the central compartment.

The first-order elimination rate constant K is a useful measurement for drug elimination in a one-compartment model. In multicompartment models several methods for the estimation of clearance are possible, as shown by Equations 9.26 and 9.27. The overall elimination rate constant K represents elimination from the central compartment, and total body clearance is the product of K times the volume of the central compartment, V_p. Alternatively, total body clearance may be estimated according to Equation 9.27 as the product of the elimination rate constant b times $V_{d,\beta}$. This latter method gives the same value for clearance. Other methods for calculating total body clearance considers either instantaneous clearance or steady-state clearance depending on which volume of distribution is chosen. Generally, the various calculations of total body clearance for drugs characterized by multicompartment pharmacokinetics are useful for comparison purposes. For the two-compartment model drug, body clearance can be calculated with the following equation.

$$\mathrm{Cl_T} = KV_\mathrm{p} \tag{9.26}$$

or, alternatively,

$$\mathrm{Cl_T} = bV_{\mathrm{d}_\beta} \tag{9.27}$$

To obtain renal clearance for drugs demonstrating two-compartment kinetics with metabolism and excretion, the following equation is used.

$$\mathrm{Cl_r} = K_\mathrm{e}V_\mathrm{p} \tag{9.28}$$

Fraction of Drug Excreted. For many drugs the total amount of unchanged drug, D_u^∞, excreted in the urine may be obtained by direct assay. The ratio of D_u^∞ to the fraction of the dose absorbed, FD_0, is equal to the fraction of drug excreted unchanged in the urine and is also equal to K_e/K

$$\text{Fraction of drug excreted unchanged in the urine} = f_\mathrm{u} = \frac{D_\mathrm{u}^\infty}{FD_0} = \frac{K_\mathrm{e}}{K} \tag{9.29}$$

Renal clearance may be determined from the fraction of unchanged drug excreted in the urine and the total body clearance:

$$\mathrm{Cl_r} = \frac{D_\mathrm{u}^\infty}{FD_0}\mathrm{Cl_T} \tag{9.30}$$

Equation 9.30 can also be expressed as

$$\mathrm{Cl_r} = \frac{K_\mathrm{e}}{K}\mathrm{Cl}_T \tag{9.31}$$

PRACTICE PROBLEMS

An antibiotic is given by IV bolus injection at a dose of 500 mg. The apparent volume of distribution was 21 liters and the elimination half-life was 6 hr. Urine was collected for 48 hr and 400 mg of unchanged drug was recovered. What is the fraction of the dose excreted unchanged in the urine? Calculate K, K_e, $\mathrm{Cl_T}$, $\mathrm{Cl_r}$, and $\mathrm{Cl_h}$.

Solution

Since the elimination half-life, $t_{1/2}$, for this drug is 6 hr, a urine collection for 48 hr represents $8t_{1/2}$ which allows for greater than 99% of the drug to be eliminated from the body. The fraction of drug excreted unchanged in the urine, f_u, is obtained by using Equation 9.29 and recalling that $F = 1$ for drugs given by IV bolus injections.

$$f_u = \frac{400}{500} = 0.8$$

Therefore, 80% of the absorbed dose is excreted in the urine unchanged. Calculations for K, K_e, Cl_T, Cl_r, and Cl_h are given:

$$K = \frac{0.693}{6} = 0.1155 \text{ hr}^{-1}$$

$$K_e = f_u K = (0.8)(0.1155) = 0.0924 \text{ hr}^{-1}$$

$$Cl_T = (0.1155)(21) = 2.43 \text{ liters/hr}$$

$$Cl_r = f_u\, Cl_T = (0.8)(2.43) = 1.94 \text{ liters/hr}$$

Alternatively,

$$Cl_r = K_e V_d = (0.0924)(21) = 1.94 \text{ liters/hr}$$

$$Cl_h = Cl_T - Cl_r = 2.43 - 1.94 = 0.49 \text{ liters/hr}$$

Total Body Clearance of Drugs After Intravenous Infusion. When drugs are administered by intravenous infusion, the total body clearance is obtained with the following equation.

$$Cl_T = \frac{R}{C_p^{\infty}} \qquad (9.32)$$

where C_p^{∞} is the steady-state plasma drug concentration and R is the rate of infusion. Equation 9.32 is valid for drugs that follow either the one-compartment or two-compartment open model.

Clearance for Drugs Involving Active Secretion

At low drug plasma concentrations active secretion is not saturated, and the drug is excreted by filtration and active secretion. At high concentrations the percentage of

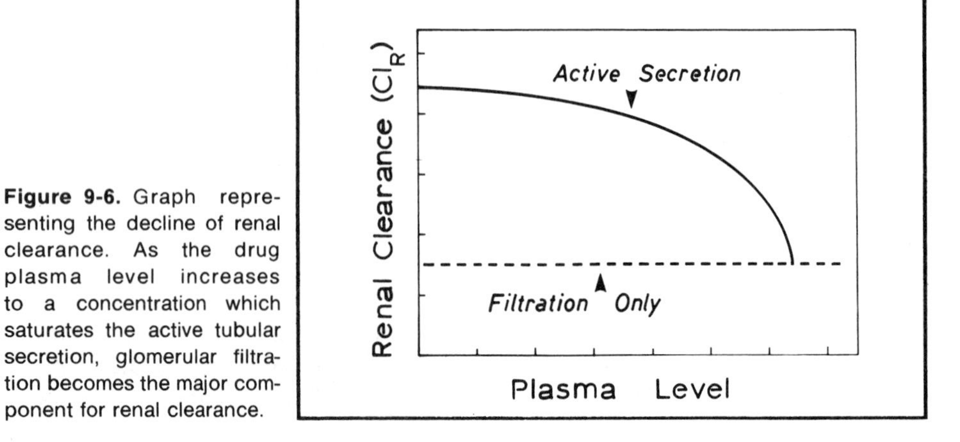

Figure 9-6. Graph representing the decline of renal clearance. As the drug plasma level increases to a concentration which saturates the active tubular secretion, glomerular filtration becomes the major component for renal clearance.

drug excreted by active secretion decreased due to saturation. Clearance decreases since excretion rate decreases (Fig. 9-4). Clearance decreases since the total excretion rate of the drug decreases to the point where it is approximately equal to the filtration rate (Fig. 9-6).

RELATIONSHIP OF CLEARANCE, $t_{1/2}$, and V_d

The half-life of a drug can be determined if the clearance and V_d are known: from Equation 9.19 we obtain

$$\mathrm{Cl}_T = KV_d$$

and

$$K = \frac{0.693}{t_{1/2}}$$

Therefore, by substitution,

$$\mathrm{Cl}_T = \frac{0.693 V_d}{t_{1/2}}$$

$$t_{1/2} = \frac{0.693 V_d}{\mathrm{Cl}_T} \quad (9.33)$$

From Equation 9.33 we see that if Cl_T decreases, which might happen in the case of renal insufficiency, the $t_{1/2}$ for the drug increases. A good relationship of V_d, K, and $t_{1/2}$ is shown in Table 9-3.

Total body clearance, Cl_T, is a useful index of measurement of drug removal and may be used preferentially to the elimination half-life, $t_{1/2}$. Total body clearance takes into account changes in both the apparent volume of distribution, V_d, and the $t_{1/2}$. In overt obesity or edematous conditions the V_d may change

TABLE 9-3. RELATIONSHIPS OF CLEARANCE, RATE CONSTANT OF ELIMINATION, AND ELIMINATION HALF-LIFE

	Medium of Distribution		
Clearance*	***Plasma Water (3000 ml)***	***Extracellular Fluid (12,000 ml)***	***Body Water (41,000 ml)***
Partial reabsorption	1.00×10^{-2}	2.50×10^{-3}	7.32×10^{-4}
(e.g., 30 ml/min)	(69 min)	(277 min)	(947 min)
Glomerular filtration	4.33×10^{-2}	1.08×10^{-2}	3.17×10^{-3}
(e.g., 130 ml/min)	(16 min)	(64 min)	(219 min)
Tubular secretion	2.17×10^{-1}	5.42×10^{-2}	1.59×10^{-2}
(e.g., 650 ml/min)	(3 min)	(13 min)	(44 min)

*Entries are values for K_e, the rate constant of elimination (in units of min^{-1}); parenthetic entries are corresponding values of the elimination half-life. The clearance given under "partial reabsorption" is arbitrary; any clearance between 0 (complete reabsorption) and 650 ml/min is possible.
From Goldstein et al., 1974, with permission.[1]

without a marked change in the $t_{1/2}$. As will be shown in Chapters 12 and 13 the V_d is important in the calculation of the loading dose; whereas, the Cl_T is important in the calculation of the maintenance dose.

Total body clearance may be calculated by the ratio $FD_0/[AUC]_0^\infty$ which is considered a model-independent method and assumes no particular pharmacokinetic model for drug elimination.

PRACTICE PROBLEMS

A new antibiotic is actively secreted by the kidney and the apparent V_d is 35 liters in the normal adult. The clearance of this drug is 650 ml/min.

1. What is the usual $t_{1/2}$ for this drug?

Solution

$$t_{1/2} = \frac{0.693(35000 \text{ ml})}{650 \text{ ml/min}}$$

$$t_{1/2} = 37.3 \text{ min}$$

2. What would be the new $t_{1/2}$ for this drug in an adult with partial renal failure whose clearance of the antibiotic was only 75 ml/min?

Solution

$$t_{1/2} = \frac{0.693(35000 \text{ ml})}{75 \text{ ml/min}}$$

$$t_{1/2} = 323 \text{ min}$$

In patients with renal impairment the $t_{1/2}$ generally changes more drastically than the V_d. The clearance given under partial reabsorption in Table 9-3 is arbitrary; any clearance between 0 (complete reabsorption) and 650 ml/min is possible.

QUESTIONS

1. Theophylline is effective in the treatment of bronchitis at a blood level of 10–20 μg/ml. At therapeutic range theophylline follows first-order kinetics. The average $t_{1/2}$ is 3.4 hr, and the range is 1.8–6.8 hr. The average volume of distribution is 30 liters.

a. What are the average, upper, and lower clearance limits for theophylline?

b. The renal clearance of theophylline is 0.36 liters/hr. What is the K_m and K_e, assuming all nonrenal clearance (Cl_{nr}) is due to metabolism?

2. A single 250-mg oral dose of an antibiotic is given to a young man (age 32 years, creatinine clearance 122 ml/min, 78 kg). From the literature, the drug is known to have an apparent V_d equal to 21% of body weight and an elimination half-life of 2 hr. The dose is normally 90% bioavailable. Urinary excretion of the unchanged drug is equal to 70% of the absorbed dose.
   a. What is the total body clearance for this drug?
   b. What is the renal clearance for this drug?
   c. What is the probable mechanism for renal clearance of this drug?
3. A drug with an elimination half-life of 1 hr was given to a male patient (80 kg) by intravenous infusion at a rate of 300 mg/hr. At 7 hr after infusion, the plasma drug concentration was 11 μg/ml.
   a. What is the total body clearance for this drug?
   b. What is the apparent V_d for this drug?
   c. If the drug is not metabolized and is eliminated only by renal excretion, what is the renal clearance of this drug?
   d. What is the probable mechanism for renal clearance of this drug?
4. In order to rapidly estimate the renal clearance of a drug in a patient, a 2-hr postdose urine sample was collected and found to contain 200 mg of drug. A midpoint plasma sample was taken (1-hr postdose) and the drug concentration in plasma was found to be 2.5 mg%. Estimate the renal clearance for this drug in the patient.
5. According to the manufacturer, the antibiotic, cephradine (Velosef, Squibb), when given by IV infusion at rate of 5.3 mg/kg hr to nine adult male volunteers (average weight 71.7 kg), a steady-state serum concentration of 17 μg/ml was measured. Calculate the average total body clearance for this drug in adults.
6. Cephradine is completely excreted unchanged in the urine, and studies have shown that probenecid given concurrently causes elevation of the serum cephradine concentration. What is the probably mechanism for the interaction of probenecid with cephradine?
7. Why is clearance used as a measurement of drug elimination rather than the excretion rate of the drug?
8. What is the advantage of using total body clearance as a measurement of drug elimination compared to using the elimination half-life of the drug?

REFERENCES

1. Goldstein A, Aronow L, Kalman SM: Principles of Drug Action. New York, Wiley, 1974

BIBLIOGRAPHY

Cafruny EJ: Renal tubular handling of drugs. Am J Med 62:490–96, 1977

Hewitt WR, Hook JB: The renal excretion of drugs. In Bridges VW, Chasseaud LF (eds.), Progress in Drug Metabolism, Vol 7, New York, Wiley, 1983, Chap. 1

Levy G: Pharmacokinetics in renal disease. Am J Med 62:461–65, 1977
Rowland M, Benet LZ, Graham GG: Clearance concepts in pharmacokinetics. J Pharm Biopharm 1:123–36, 1973
Renkin EM, Robinson RR: Glomerular filtration. N Engl J Med 290:785–92, 1974
Thomson P, Melmon K, Richardson J, et al: Lidocaine pharmacokinetics in advanced heart failure, liver disease and renal failure in humans. Ann Intern Med 78:499–508, 1973
Tucker GT: Measurement of the renal clearance of drugs. Br J Clin Pharm 12:761–70, 1981
Weiner IM, Mudge GH: Renal tubular mechanisms for excretion and organic acids and bases. Am J Med 36:743–62, 1964

CHAPTER TEN

Hepatic Elimination of Drugs

The elimination of most drugs from the body involves the processes of both metabolism (biotransformation) and excretion. The rate constant of elimination (K) is the sum of the first-order rate constant for metabolism (K_m) and the first-order rate constant for excretion (K_e).

$$K = K_e + K_m \tag{10.1}$$

Since a drug may be biotransformed to several metabolites (i.e., metabolite A, metabolite B, metabolite C, etc.), the metabolism rate constant (K_m) is the sum of the rate constants for the formation of each metabolite.

$$K_m = K_{m_A} + K_{m_B} + K_{m_C} + \cdots + K_{m_I} \tag{10.2}$$

The relationship in this equation assumes that the process of metabolism is first-order and that the substrate (i.e., drug) concentration is very low. Drug concentrations at therapeutic plasma levels for most drugs are much lower than the Michaelis–Menten constant and do not saturate the enzymes involved in metabolism.

Since these rates of elimination are considered first-order processes, the percentage of total drug metabolized may be found by the following expression.

$$\%\ \text{drug metabolized} = \frac{K_m}{K} \times 100 \tag{10.3}$$

In practice, the excretion rate constant (K_e) is easily evaluated for drugs which are primarily renal excreted. *Nonrenal drug elimination* is usually assumed to be due for the most part to hepatic metabolism. The rate constant for metabolism (K_m) is difficult to measure directly and is usually found by the difference of K and K_e.

$$K_m = K - K_e$$

PERCENT OF DRUG METABOLIZED

For most drugs the fraction of a given metabolite is constant. For example, consider a drug which has two major metabolites and is also eliminated by renal excretion (Fig. 10-1).

Assume for the drug in Figure 10-1 that 100 μM of the drug was given to a patient and the drug was completely absorbed (bioavailability factor, $F = 1$). A complete urine collection was obtained, and the quantities in parentheses indicate the amounts of each metabolite and unchanged drug which were recovered. The overall elimination half-life ($t_{1/2}$) for this drug was 2.0 hr ($K = 0.347$ hr^{-1}).

In order to determine the renal excretion rate constant, the following relationship is used.

$$\frac{K_e}{K} = \frac{D_u^\infty}{\text{total dose absorbed}} = \frac{D_u^\infty}{FD_0} \tag{10.4}$$

where D_u^∞ is the total amount of unchanged drug recovered in the urine. In this example K_e is found by proper substitution into Equation 10.4:

$$K_e = (0.347)\frac{70}{100} = 0.243 \text{ hr}^{-1}$$

To find the percent of drug eliminated by renal excretion, the following approach may be used.

$$\% \text{ drug excretion} = \frac{K_e}{K} \times 100$$

$$= \frac{0.243}{0.347} \times 100 = 70\%$$

Alternatively, since 70 μM of unchanged drug were recovered out of a total dose of 100 μM, then the percent of drug excretion may be found by the following.

$$\% \text{ drug excretion} = \frac{70}{100} \times 100 = 70\%$$

Therefore, the percent of drug metabolized is 100% minus 70%, or 30%.

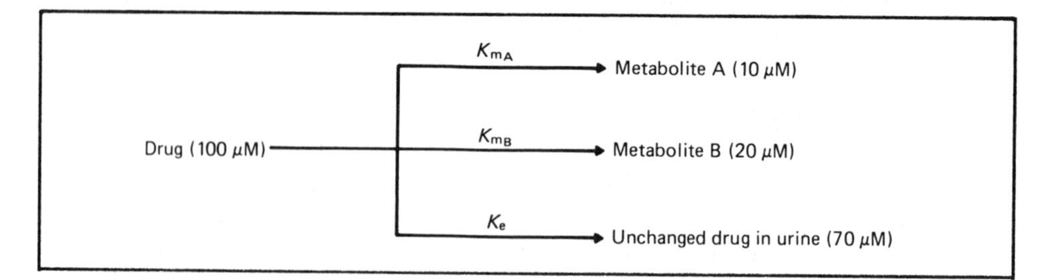

Figure 10-1. Model of a drug that has two major metabolites and is also eliminated by renal excretion.

From a clinical viewpoint, the percentages of drug excretion and metabolism constitute useful information. If the renal excretion pathway becomes impaired as in the case of certain kidney disorders, then the drug will be eliminated primarily by hepatic metabolism. The reverse is true if liver function declines. For example, if in the above situation renal excretion becomes totally impaired (i.e., $K_e \simeq 0$), the elimination $t_{1/2}$ can be determined as follows.

$$K = K_m + K_e$$

but

$$K_e \simeq 0$$

Therefore,

$$K \simeq K_m \simeq 0.104 \text{ hr}^{-1}$$

The new $t_{1/2}$ is

$$t_{1/2} = \frac{0.693}{0.104} = 6.7 \text{ hr}$$

Thus, renal impairment caused the elimination $t_{1/2}$ to be prolonged from 2 to 6.7 hr. Obviously, the dosage of this drug must be lowered to prevent the accumulation of toxic drug levels.

DRUG BIOTRANSFORMATION REACTIONS

The hepatic biotransformation enzymes play an important role for the inactivation and subsequent elimination of drugs not easily cleared through the kidney. For these drugs, such as theophylline, phenytoin, acetaminophen, and others, there is an inverse relationship between the rate of drug metabolism (biotransformation) and the elimination half-life for the drug.

For most biotransformation reactions the metabolite of the drug is more polar than the parent compound. The conversion of a drug to a more polar metabolite enables the drug to be eliminated more quickly than if the drug remained lipid soluble. A lipid-soluble drug crosses cell membranes and is easily reabsorbed by the renal tubular cells, exhibiting a consequent tendency to remain in the body. In contrast, the more polar metabolite does not cross cell membranes easily, is filtered through the glomerulus, is not readily reabsorbed, and is more rapidly excreted in the urine.

The biotransformation of drugs may be classified according to the pharmacologic activity of the metabolite or according to the biochemical mechanism for each biotransformation reaction. For most drugs biotransformation results in the formation of a more polar metabolite which is pharmacologically inactive and is eliminated more rapidly than the parent drug (Table 10-1). For some drugs the metabolite may be pharmacologically active or produce toxic effects. Prodrugs are inactive and must be biotransformed in the body to metabolites which have pharmacologic activity. Initially, prodrugs were discovered by serendipity as in the case of prontosil which is reduced to the antibacterial agent sulfanilamide. More recently prodrugs are inten-

TABLE 10-1. BIOTRANSFORMATION REACTIONS AND PHARMACOLOGIC ACTIVITY OF THE METABOLITE

Reaction		Example
Active Drug to Inactive Metabolite		
Amphetamine	deamination →	Phenylacetone
Phenobarbital	hydroxylation →	Hydroxyphenobarbital
Active Drug to Active Metabolite		
Codeine	demethylation →	Morphine
Procainamide	acetylation →	*N*-acetylprocainamide
Phenylbutazone	hydroxylation →	Oxyphenbutazone
Inactive Drug to Active Metabolite		
Hetacillin	hydrolysis →	Ampicillin
Sulfasalazine	azoreduction →	Sulfapyridine
Active Drug to Reactive Intermediate		
Acetaminophen	aromatic → hydroxylation	Reactive metabolite (hepatic necrosis)
Benzo[*a*]pyrene	aromatic → hydroxylation	Reactive metabolite (carcinogenic)

tionally designed to improve stability and absorption or to prolong the duration of activity. For example, the antiparkinsonian agent levodopa crosses the blood–brain barrier and is decarboxylated in the brain to l-dopamine, a pharmacologically active neurotransmitter. The neurotransmitter, l-dopamine, does not easily penetrate the blood–brain barrier into brain and therefore cannot be used as a therapeutic agent.

Pathways of drug biotransformation may be divided into two major groups of reactions, phase I and phase II reactions. Phase I or asynthetic reactions include oxidation, reduction, and hydrolysis, whereas phase II or synthetic reactions include conjugations. A partial list of these reactions is presented in Table 10-2. In addition, a number of drugs which resemble natural biochemical molecules are able to utilize the metabolic pathways for normal body compounds.

Usually phase I biotransformation reactions occur first and introduce or expose a functional group on the drug molecule. For example, oxygen is introduced into the phenyl group on phenylbutazone by aromatic hydroxylation to form oxyphenbutazone, a more polar metabolite. Codeine is demethylated to form morphine. In addition, the hydrolysis of esters such as aspirin or benzocaine will yield more polar products such as salicylic acid and *p*-aminobenzoic acid, respectively. For some compounds such as acetaminophen, benzo[*a*]pyrene, and other drugs containing

TABLE 10-2. SOME COMMON DRUG BIOTRANSFORMATION REACTIONS

Phase I Reactions	Phase II Reactions
Oxidation	Glucuronide conjugation
Aromatic hydroxylation	Ether glucuronide
Side chain hydroxylation	Ester glucuronide
N-, *O*-, and *S*-dealkylation	Amide glucuronide
Deamination	
Sulfoxidation, *N*-oxidation	Peptide conjugation
N-hydroxylation	Glycine conjugation (hippurate)
Reduction	
Azoreduction	Methylation
Nitroreduction	*N*-methylation
Alcohol dehydrogenase	*O*-methylation
Hydrolysis	Acetylation
Ester hydrolysis	Sulfate conjugation
Amide hydrolysis	
	Mercapturic acid synthesis

aromatic rings, reactive intermediates such as epoxides are formed during the hydroxylation reaction. These aromatic epoxides are highly reactive and will react with macromolecules possibly causing liver necrosis (acetaminophen) or cancer (benzo[*a*]pyrene). The biotransformation of salicylic acid is described in Figure 10-2 and demonstrates the variety of possible metabolites that may be formed. It should be noted that salicylic acid is also conjugated directly (phase II reaction) without a preceding phase I reaction.

Once a polar constituent is revealed or placed into the molecule, then a phase II or conjugation reaction may occur. Common examples include the conjugation of salicyclic acid with glycine to form salicyluric acid or glucuronic acid to form salicylglucuronide (Fig. 10-2).

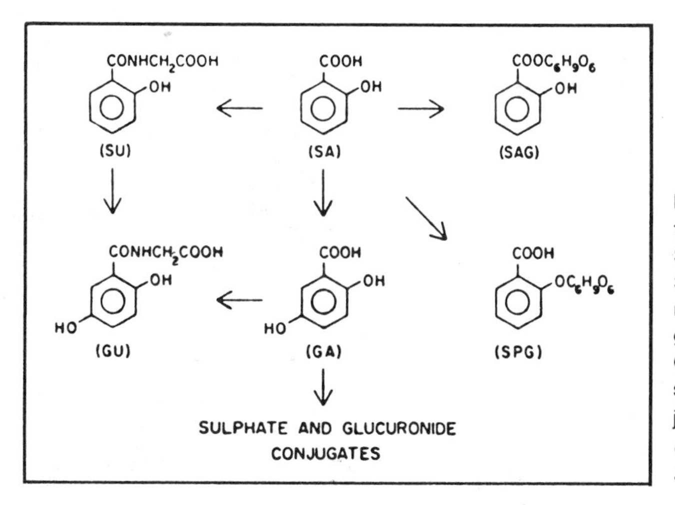

Figure 10-2. Biotransformation of salicylic acid. SA = Salicylate; SU = Salicylurate; SAG = Salicyl acyl glucuronide; SPG = Salicyl phenolic glucuronide; GA = Gentisate; GU = Gentisicyl urate; and sulfate and glucuronide conjugates. *(From Hucker HB, et al, 1980, with permission.*[1]*)*

The acetylation reaction is an important conjugation reaction for several reasons. First, the acetylated product is usually less polar than the parent drug. The acetylation of such drugs as sulfanilamide, sulfadiazine, and sulfisoxazole produces metabolites that are less water soluble and that in sufficient concentration will precipitate in the kidney tubules causing kidney damage and crystaluria. In addition, a less polar metabolite will be reabsorbed in the renal tubule and have a longer elimination half-life. For example, procainamide (elimination half-life of 3–4 hr) has an acetylated metabolite, *N*-acetylprocainamide which is biologically active and has an elimination half-life of 6–7 hr. Lastly, the *N*-acetyltransferase enzyme responsible for catalyzing the acetylation of isoniazid and other drugs demonstrates a genetic polymorphism. Two distinct subpopulations have been observed to inactivate isoniazid, including the "slow inactivators" and the "rapid inactivators."[2] Therefore, the former group may be more susceptible to adverse toxicity of isoniazide such as peripheral neuritis due to the longer elimination half-life and accumulation of the drug.

LOCATION OF DRUG BIOTRANSFORMATION ENZYMES

The major organ responsible for drug biotransformation is the liver. However, intestinal tissue, lung, and kidney also contain appreciable amounts of biotrans-

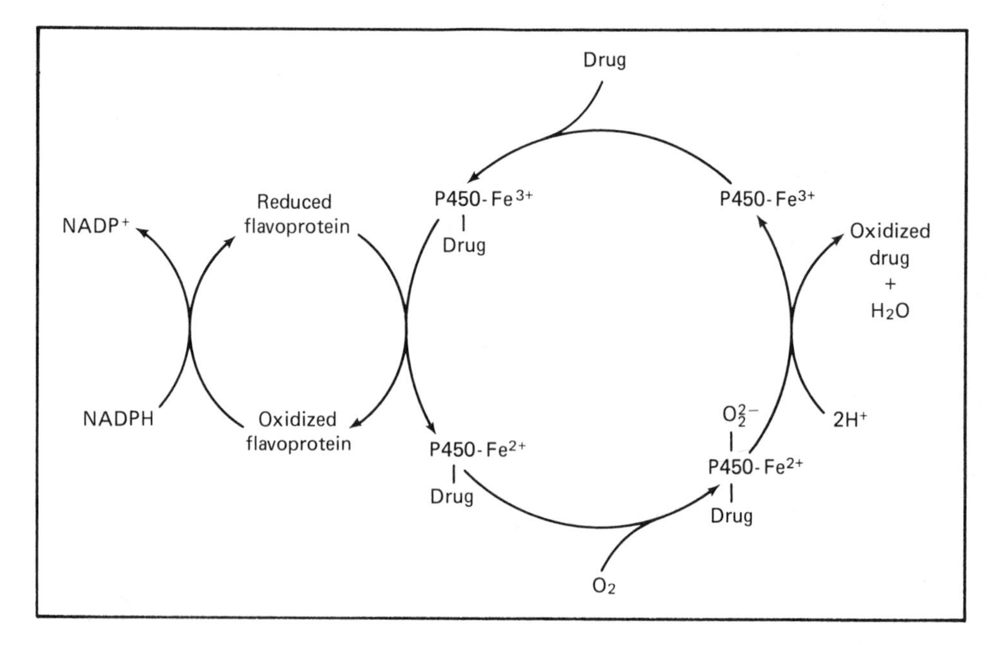

Figure 10-3. Tentative outline of the electron transport chain involving cytochrome P_{450} and the oxidation of drugs by the hepatic microsomal system. The flavoprotein appears to be NADPH–cytochrome *c* reductase, although cytochrome *c* is not involved in the reaction. (*Adapted from Hildebrandt A, Estabrook RW, 1971, with permission.*[3])

formation enzymes. Other tissues and the intestinal microflora may play a role in drug biotransformation.

On a subcellular level, the enzymes involved in drug oxidation and reduction, also known as *mixed-function oxidases*, are located on the endoplasmic reticulum. If hepatic parenchymal cells are fragmented and differentially centrifuged in an ultracentrifuge, a *microsomal fraction* or *microsome* is obtained from the post-mitochondrial supernatant. This microsomal fraction contains fragments of the endoplasmic reticulum. The mixed-function oxidase enzymes are structural enzymes which constitute an electron transport system, requiring reduced $NADPH_2$ plus molecular oxygen. Cytochrome P_{-450} is the terminal oxidase (Fig. 10-3).

The mixed-function oxidase enzymes have little specificity toward the substrate. These enzymes are largely responsible for oxidation and reduction reactions. The intrinsic enzyme activity is controlled according to genetic factors. However, mixed-function oxidase activity may become altered by various factors, including inducing agents, inhibiting agents, hepatic disease, nutritional status, and age.

FIRST-PASS EFFECTS

For some drugs the route of administration affects the metabolic rate of the compound. For example, a drug given parenterally, transdermally, or by inhalation would have a chance to distribute within the body prior to metabolism by the liver. In contrast, drugs given orally are normally absorbed in the duodenal segment of the small intestine and transported via the mesenteric vessels to the hepatic portal vein and then to the liver prior to the systemic circulation. Drugs which are highly metabolized by the liver or by the intestinal mucosal cells demonstrate poor systemic availability when given orally. This rapid metabolism of an orally administered drug prior to reaching the general circulation are termed *first-pass effects* or *presystemic elimination*.

Evidence of First-Pass Effects

First-pass effects may be suspected when there is a lack of parent or intact drug in the systemic circulation after oral administration. In such a case the AUC for a drug given orally is less than the AUC for the same dose of drug given intravenously. Due to experimental findings in animals, first-pass effects may be assumed if the intact drug appears in a cannulated hepatic portal vein but not in general circulation.

Assuming the drug is chemically stable in the gastrointestinal tract, and that drug is administered orally in solution to ensure complete absorption, the area under the plasma drug concentration curve (AUC) should be the same when the same dose is administered intravenously. Therefore, examination of the absolute bioavailability, F, may reveal evidence of drug being removed by the liver due to first-pass effects.

$$F = \frac{[\text{AUC}]_0^\infty \text{ oral}}{[\text{AUC}]_0^\infty \text{ IV}} \qquad (10.5)$$

For drugs that undergo first-pass effect, $[\mathrm{AUC}]_0^\infty$ oral is smaller than $[\mathrm{AUC}]_0^\infty$ IV and F is less than 1. A drug like isoproterenol or nitroglycerin would have an F value less than 1 since these drugs undergo significant first-pass effects.

Liver Extraction Ratio

Since there are many other reasons for a drug to have a reduced F value, the extent of first-pass effect is not very precisely measured from the F value. The liver extraction ratio (ER) provides a direct measurement of drug removal from the liver after oral administration of a drug.

$$\mathrm{ER} = \frac{C_a - C_v}{C_a} \tag{10.6}$$

where C_a is the drug concentration in the blood entering the liver and C_v is the drug concentration leaving the liver. Since C_a is usually greater than C_v, ER is usually less than 1. For example, for propanolol ER is about 0.7, i.e., about 70% of the drug is actually removed by the liver before it is available for general distribution to the body. By contrast, if the drug is injected intravenously, most of the drug would be distributed before reaching the liver and less of the drug would be metabolized.

Relationship Between Absolute Bioavailability and Liver Extraction

Liver ER provides a precise measurement of liver extraction of a drug orally administered. Unfortunately, the sampling of drug from the hepatic portal vein and artery is difficult. Therefore, most ER measurements for drugs are done in animals. These ER values may be quite different from that in humans. The following relationship between bioavailability and liver extraction enables a rough estimate of the extent of liver extraction:

$$F = 1 - \mathrm{ER} - F'' \tag{10.7}$$

where F is the fraction of bioavailable drug, ER is the drug fraction extracted by the liver, and F'' is the fraction of drug removed by nonhepatic process.

If F'' is assumed to be negligible, i.e., there is no loss of drug due to chemical degradation, gut metabolism, and incomplete absorption, ER may be estimated from

$$\mathrm{ER} = 1 - F \tag{10.8}$$

After substitution of Equation 10.5 into Equation 10.8

$$\mathrm{ER} = 1 - \frac{[\mathrm{AUC}]_0^\infty \text{ oral}}{[\mathrm{AUC}]_0^\infty \text{ IV}} \tag{10.9}$$

It should be pointed out that the ER obtained is a rough estimation of liver extraction for a drug. There are many other factors that may alter this estimation; the size of the dose, the formulation of the drug, and the physiologic condition of the patient all may effect the ER value obtained.

Liver ER provides valuable information in determining the oral dose of a drug when the intravenous dose is known. With the drug propanolol a much higher oral dose is necessary to produce sufficient therapeutic blood levels because of drug removal by the liver. Since liver extraction is affected by blood flow to the liver, dosing of drug with extensive liver metabolism may produce erratic plasma drug levels. Formulation of this drug into an oral dosage form would require extensive careful testings.

PROBLEM

A new 5-mg tablet of propanolol was developed and tested in volunteers. The bioavailability of propanolol from the tablet was 70% relative to an oral solution of propanolol and 21.6% relative to an intravenous dose of propanolol (absolute bioavailability). Comment on the feasibility of improving the absolute bioavailability of the propanolol tablet.

Solution

From the table of ER values (Table 10-3) the ER for propanolol is 0.6–0.8. If the product is perfectly formulated (i.e., the tablet dissolves completely and is

TABLE 10-3. PHARMACOKINETIC CLASSIFICATION OF DRUGS ELIMINATED PRIMARILY BY HEPATIC METABOLISM

Drug Class	Extraction Ratio (approx.)	Percent Bound
Flow-limited		
Lignocaine	0.83	45–80*
Propranolol	0.6–0.8	93
Pethidine (meperidine)	0.60–0.95	60
Pentazocine	0.8	—
Propoxyphene	0.95	—
Nortriptyline	0.5	95
Morphine	0.5–0.75	35
Capacity-limited, Binding-sensitive		
Phenytoin	0.03	90
Diazepam	0.03	98
Tolbutamide	0.02	98
Warfarin	0.003	99
Chlorpromazine	0.22	91–99
Clindamycin	0.23	94
Quinidine	0.27	82
Digitoxin	0.005	97
Capacity-limited, Binding-insensitive		
Theophylline	0.09	59
Hexobarbitone	0.16	—
Amylobarbitone	0.03	61
Antipyrine	0.07	10
Chloramphenicol	0.28	60–80
Thiopentone	0.28	72
Paracetamol	0.43	5*

*Concentration dependent.

From Blaschke TF, 1977, with permission.[4]

all absorbed), the fraction of drug absorbed after deducting for the fraction of drug extracted is calculated below:

$$
\begin{aligned}
F' &= 1 - \mathrm{ER} \\
&= 1 - 0.7 \qquad (\text{mean ER} = 0.7) \\
&= 0.3
\end{aligned}
$$

A similar calculation using ER of 0.6 and 0.8 would give F' of 0.4 and 0.2, respectively. Since the drug is 26% available relative to an intravenous dose, the oral tablet is within limits of the absolute bioavailability of this drug, i.e., the drug is only 20–40% available relative to an intravenous dose even if all the drug is absorbed.

It is important to note that the same tablet tested experimentally resulted in a bioavailability of 70% relative to an oral solution. In this case the relative bioavailability is higher because the drug extracted by the liver is not reflected in the relative bioavailability. In measuring the AUC of the oral solution, liver extraction resulted in a smaller AUC in the oral solution as well as in the tablet, therefore canceling out the effect of each other in calculating the relative availability of the tablet.

The following shows a method for calculating the absolute bioavailability from the relative bioavailability providing that the ER is accurately known. Using the above example,

Absolute availability of the solution = 1 − ER = 1 − 0.7 = 0.3 = 30%

Relative availability of the solution = 100%

Absolute availability of tablet = x percent

Relative availability of the tablet = 70%

$$x = \frac{30 \times 70}{100} = 21\%$$

Therefore, this product has an absolute bioavailability of 21%. The small percent of calculated and actual absolute bioavailability is due largely to liver extraction fluctuation. All calculations are performed with the assumption of linear pharmacokinetics which is generally a good approximation. When therapeutic drugs are administered, saturation may occur rapidly with some drugs, and ER may deviate significantly with changes in blood flow.

Estimation of Reduced Bioavailability Due to Liver Metabolism with Variable Blood Flow to the Liver

Blood flow to the liver plays an important role in the extent of drug metabolized after oral administration. Changes in blood flow to the liver may substantially alter the percent of drug metabolized and therefore alter the percent of bioavailable drug.

The relationship between blood flow, hepatic clearance, and percent of drug bioavailable is

$$F' = 1 - \frac{Cl_h}{Q} \quad (10.10)$$

Where Cl_h is the hepatic clearance of the drug and Q is the effective hepatic blood flow.

The usual effective hepatic blood flow is 1.5 L/min but may vary from 1 to 2 L/min depending on diet, food intake, physical activity, or drug intake.[5] This equation provides a reasonable approach for evaluating the reduced bioavailability due to first-pass effect. With the drug propoxyphene hydrochloride F' has been calculated from hepatic clearance and an assumed liver blood flow of 1.53 L/min.

$$F' = 1 - \frac{0.99}{1.53} = 0.35$$

The results were reasonable when compared with experimental values for the drug. While the equation seems to provide a convenient way of estimating the effect of liver blood flow on bioavailability, the problem is actually more complicated. A change in liver blood flow may alter hepatic clearance and F'. Large blood flow may deliver enough drug to the liver to alter the rate of metabolism. On the other hand, small blood flow may decrease the delivery of drug to the liver and become the rate-limiting step. Furthermore, the hepatic clearance of a drug is often calculated from plasma drug data rather than whole blood data. Significant nonlinearity may result to equilibration of drug by partitioning into the red blood cells.

Presystemic elimination or first-pass effects is a very important consideration for drugs that have a high extraction ratio (Table 10-3). Drugs with low extraction ratios, such as theophylline, have very little presystemic elimination as demonstrated by complete systemic absorption after oral administration. In contrast, drugs with high extraction ratios have poor bioavailability when given orally. Therefore, the oral dose must be higher than the intravenous dose to achieve the same therapeutic response. In some cases oral administration of a drug with high presystemic elimination, such as nitroglycerin, may be impractical due to very poor oral bioavailability, and thus the sublingual or transdermal routes of administration may be preferred. Furthermore, if an oral drug product is prepared that has slow dissolution characteristics or release rates, then more of the drug will be affected by first-pass effects compared to the doses of drug given in a more bioavailable form (such as a solution). In addition, drugs with high presystemic elimination tend to demonstrate more variability in drug bioavailability between individuals. Finally, the quantity and quality of the metabolites formed may vary according to the route of drug administration, which may be clinically important if one of the metabolites has pharmacologic or toxic activity.

To overcome first-pass effects, the route of administration of the drug may be changed. For example, nitroglycerin may be given sublingually or topically and xylocaine may be given parenterally to avoid the first-pass effects. Another way to overcome first-pass effects is to either enlarge the dose or change the drug product to a more rapidly absorbable dosage form. In either case a large amount of drug is presented rapidly to the liver and some of the drug will reach the general circulation in the intact state.

HEPATIC CLEARANCE

The clearance concept may be applied to any organ and is used as a measure of elimination of drug by the organ. *Hepatic clearance* may be defined as the volume of blood that perfuses the liver which is cleared of drug per unit of time. Hepatic clearance (Cl_h) is also equal to total body clearance (Cl_T) minus renal clearance (Cl_r), as follows.

$$Cl_h = Cl_T - Cl_r \tag{10.11}$$

EXAMPLE

The total body clearance for a drug is 15 ml/min kg. Renal clearance accounts for 10 ml/min kg. What is the hepatic clearance for the drug?

Solution

$$\text{Hepatic clearance} = 15 - 10 = 5 \text{ ml/min kg}$$

Sometimes the renal clearance is not known and hepatic clearance may be calculated from the percent of intact drug recovered in the urine.

EXAMPLE

The total body clearance of a drug is 10 ml/min kg. The renal clearance is not known. However, the drug is known from a urinary drug excretion study; 60% of the drug is recovered intact and 40% is recovered as metabolites. What is the hepatic clearance for the drug assuming metabolism occurs in the liver?

Solution

$$\begin{aligned} \text{Hepatic clearance} &= \text{body clearance} \times (1 - P) \\ &= 10 \times (100 - 60) \\ &= 4 \text{ ml/min kg} \end{aligned} \tag{10.12}$$

where P = percent of drug recovered intact in the urine. In the above example the metabolites are recovered completely and hepatic clearance may be obtained as total body clearance times the percent of dose recovered as metabolites. Often, however, the metabolites are not completely recovered and it is easier to use the above equation.

Relationship Between Blood Flow, Intrinsic Clearance, and Hepatic Clearance

Factors that affect the hepatic clearance of a drug include (1) blood flow to the liver, (2) intrinsic clearance, and (3) the fraction of drug bound to protein.

In experimental animals, it is possible to measure the blood flow (Q) to the liver as well as the concentration of drug in the artery (C_a) and the concentration of drug in the vein (C_v). As the arterial blood containing drug perfuses the liver, a certain portion of the drug is removed by metabolism and/or biliary excretion. Therefore, the concentration of drug in the vein is less than the concentration of drug in the artery. An *extraction ratio* may be expressed as 100% of the drug entering the liver less the relative concentration (C_v/C_a) of drug which is removed by the liver:

$$\mathrm{ER} = \frac{C_a - C_v}{C_a} \tag{10.13}$$

The ER may vary from 0 to 1.0. An ER of 0.25 means that 25% of the drug was removed by the liver. If both the ER for the liver and blood flow to the liver are known, then hepatic clearance may be calculated by the following expression.

$$\mathrm{Cl}_h = \frac{Q(C_a - C_v)}{C_a} \tag{10.14}$$

For some drugs (such as isoproterenol, lidocaine, and nitroglycerin), the extraction ratio is high (greater than 0.7) and the drug is removed by the liver almost as rapidly as the organ is perfused by blood in which the drug is contained. For drugs with very high extraction ratios the rate of drug metabolism is sensitive to changes in hepatic blood flow. Thus, an increase in blood flow to the liver will increase the rate of removal of the drug by the organ. Propranolol, a β-adrenergic blocking agent, decreases hepatic blood flow by decreasing cardiac output. In such a case the drug decreases its own clearance through the liver when given orally. Many drugs which demonstrate first-pass effects are drugs which have high extraction ratios with respect to the liver.

When the blood flow to the liver is constant, hepatic clearance is equal to the product of blood flow (Q) and the extraction ratio (E). However, the hepatic clearance of a drug is not constant; it changes with blood flow and the intrinsic clearance of the drug, as described in Equation 10.15. For drugs with low extraction ratios (e.g., theophylline, phenylbutazone, and procainamide), the hepatic clearance is less affected by hepatic blood flow. Instead, these drugs are more affected by the intrinsic activity of the mixed-function oxidases.

Intrinsic clearance (Cl_{int}) is used to described the ability of the liver to remove drug in the absence of flow limitations, reflecting the inherent activities of the mixed-function oxidases. Hepatic clearance is related to both liver blood flow and the intrinsic clearance of the liver.

$$\mathrm{Cl}_h = Q\left[\frac{\mathrm{Cl}_{int}}{Q + \mathrm{Cl}_{int}}\right] \tag{10.15}$$

Changes or alterations in mixed-function oxidase activity or biliary secretion affect the rate of drug removal by the liver. Drugs that show low extraction ratios and are eliminated primarily by metabolism demonstrate marked variation in overall elimination half-lives within a given population. For example, the elimination half-life of theophylline varies from 3 to 9 hr. This variation in $t_{1/2}$ is thought to be due to genetic differences in intrinsic hepatic enzyme activity. Moreover, the elimination half-lives of these same drugs are also affected by enzyme induction, enzyme inhibition, age of the individual, and nutritional and pathologic factors.

Clearance may also be expressed as the rate of drug removal divided by the plasma drug concentration:

$$\mathrm{Cl}_{\mathrm{h}} = \frac{\text{rate of drug removed by liver}}{C_{\mathrm{a}}} \tag{10.16}$$

Since the rate of drug removal by the liver is usually the rate of drug metabolism, Equation 10.16 may be expressed in terms of hepatic clearance and drug concentration entering the liver (C_{a}):

$$\text{Rate of liver drug metabolism} = \mathrm{Cl}_{\mathrm{h}} C_{\mathrm{a}} \tag{10.17}$$

The rate of liver drug metabolism is related to the free or unbound drug concentration. Drugs which are protein bound do not pass cell membranes easily. The free drug in the plasma does cross cell membranes and reaches the site of the mixed-function oxidase enzymes. It is often assumed that the concentration of drug in the liver surrounding the mixed-function oxidases is equal to the free drug concentration in the blood. Therefore, an increase in the free drug concentration in the blood will make more drug available for hepatic extraction.

Hepatic Clearance of a Protein-Bound Drug

The relationship of blood flow, intrinsic clearance, and protein binding is

$$\mathrm{Cl}_{\mathrm{h}} = Q\left[\frac{f_{\mathrm{u}}\mathrm{Cl}'_{\mathrm{int}}}{Q + f_{\mathrm{u}}\mathrm{Cl}'_{\mathrm{int}}}\right] \tag{10.18}$$

where f_{u} is the fraction of drug unbound in the blood and $\mathrm{Cl}'_{\mathrm{int}}$ is the intrinsic clearance of free drug. Equation 10.18 is derived by substituting $f_{\mathrm{u}}\mathrm{Cl}'_{\mathrm{int}}$ for $\mathrm{Cl}_{\mathrm{int}}$ in Equation 10.15.

From Equation 10.18, when $\mathrm{Cl}'_{\mathrm{int}}$ is very small in comparison to hepatic blood flow (i.e., $Q > \mathrm{Cl}'_{\mathrm{int}}$), then Equation 10.19 reduces to Equation 10.20:

$$\mathrm{Cl}_{\mathrm{h}} = Q\frac{f_{\mathrm{u}}\mathrm{Cl}'_{\mathrm{int}}}{Q} \tag{10.19}$$

$$\mathrm{Cl}_{\mathrm{h}} = f_{\mathrm{u}}\mathrm{Cl}'_{\mathrm{int}} = \mathrm{Cl}_{\mathrm{int}} \tag{10.20}$$

Assuming drug protein binding is constant within the therapeutic range, then $\mathrm{Cl}_{\mathrm{h}} = \mathrm{Cl}_{\mathrm{int}}$ for drugs with very low intrinsic clearances. Also, a change in $\mathrm{Cl}'_{\mathrm{int}}$ or f_{u} will cause a proportional change in Cl_{h}.

In the case where Cl_{int} for a drug is very large in comparison to flow (i.e., $Cl_{int} > Q$), then Equation 10.21 reduces to Equation 10.22:

$$Cl = Q\frac{Cl_{int}}{Cl_{int}} \tag{10.21}$$

$$Cl_h = Q \tag{10.22}$$

Thus, for drugs with a very high Cl_{int}, Cl_h is dependent on hepatic blood flow.

With drugs which are highly extracted to an unusual degree by the liver, the percent of drug that is plasma protein bound will not significantly affect the rate of metabolism, since the drug is removed from the plasma binding sites during

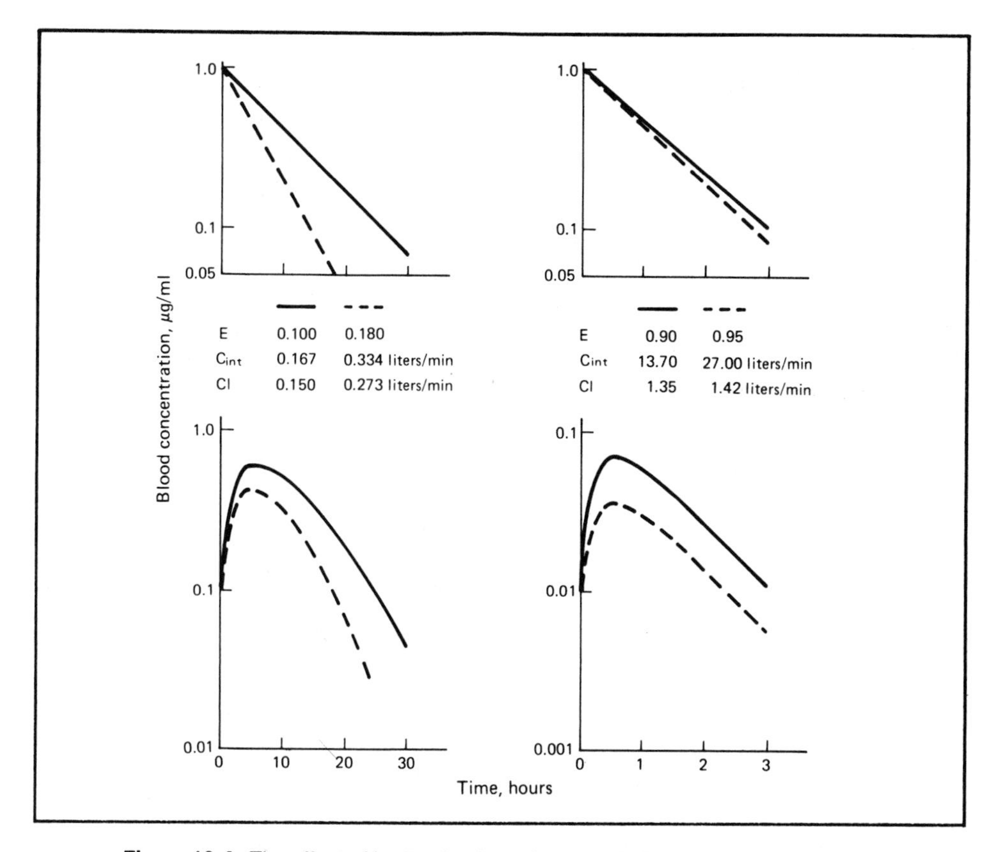

Figure 10-4. The effect of increasing hepatic total intrinsic clearance (Cl_{int}) on the total blood concentration–time curves after intravenous (upper panels) and oral (lower panels) administration of equal doses of two totally metabolized drugs. The left panels refer to a drug with an initial Cl_{int} equivalent to an extraction ratio of 0.1 at a liver blood flow of 1.5 L/min and the right panels to one with an initial extraction ratio of 0.9. The AUCs after oral administration are inversely proportional to Cl_{int}. (*From Wilkinson GR, Shand DG, 1975, with permission.*[6])

circulation through the liver. A similar situation occurs with the renal excretion of penicillin, which is actively secreted in the renal tubules. For a drug with a low hepatic extraction ratio and low plasma binding, the concentration of drug at the enzyme site will not be changed significantly when the drug is displaced from binding. For drugs highly bound to plasma proteins (more than 90%), a displacement from these binding sites will significantly increase the concentration of drug at the hepatic enzyme site and the rate of metabolism will increase.

The effects of altered hepatic intrinsic clearance and liver blood flow on the blood level–time curve have been described by Wilkinson and Shand,[6] as reproduced in Figures 10-4 and 10-5. The elimination half-life of a drug with a low

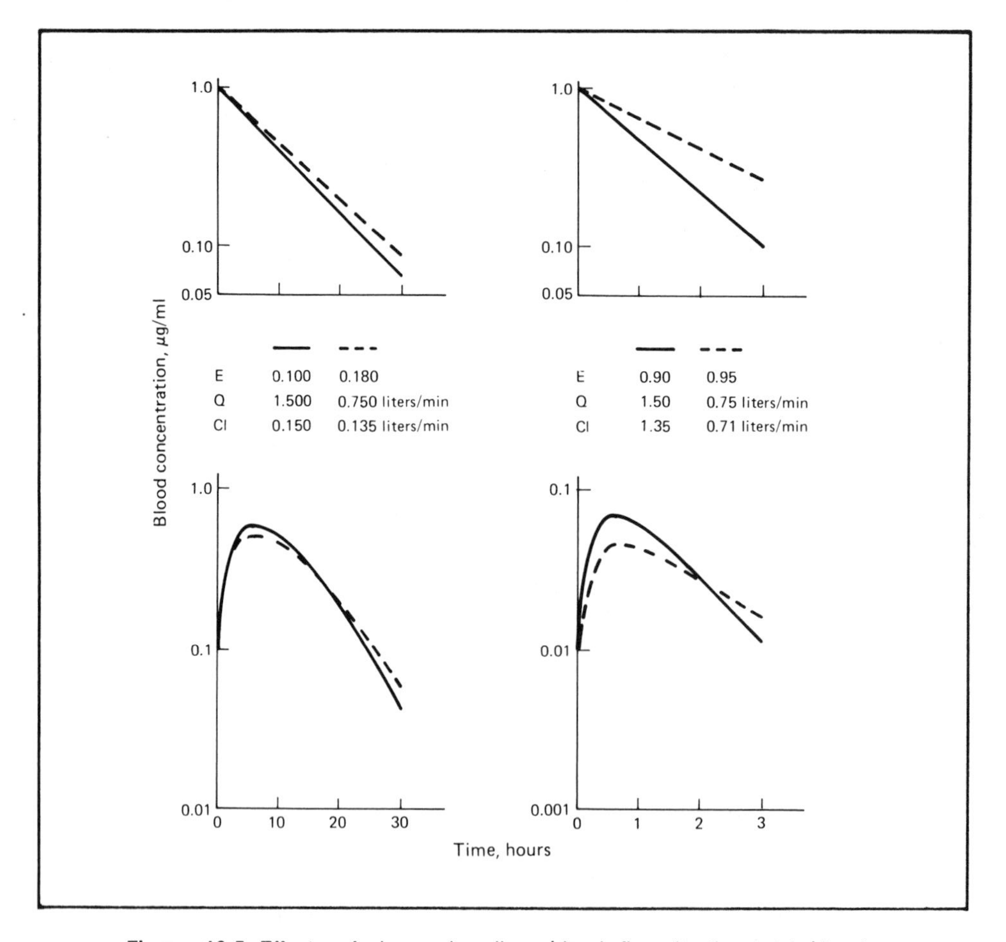

Figure 10-5. Effects of decreasing liver blood flow in the total blood concentration–time curves after intravenous (upper panels) and oral (lower panels) administration of equal doses of two totally metabolized drugs. The left panels refer to a drug with a total intrinsic clearance equivalent to an extraction ratio of 0.1 when blood flow equals 1.5 L/min, and the right panels to a drug with an intrinsic clearance equivalent to an extraction ratio of 0.9. (*From Wilkinson GR, Shand DG, 1975, with permission.*[6])

extraction ratio (0.10) and low Cl_{int} (0.167 L/min) is decreased significantly by an increase in hepatic enzyme activity—i.e., the Cl_{int} increases from 0.1 to 0.18. In contrast, when the elimination half-life of a drug already has a high extraction ratio (0.90), Cl_{int} is not markedly affected by an increase in hepatic enzyme activity (i.e., Cl_{int} increases from 13.7 to 27). However, if the drug with the high extraction ratio is given orally to patients with increased enzyme activity, a greater first-pass effect is observed, as shown by a reduction in the AUC (Fig. 10-4).

Alterations in hepatic blood flow significantly affect the elimination of drugs with high extraction ratios (e.g., propranolol) and have very little effect on the elimination of drugs with low extraction ratios (e.g., theophylline). For drugs with a lower extraction ratio any concentration of drug in the blood which perfuses the liver is more than the liver can eliminate. Consequently, small changes in hepatic blood flow do not affect the removal rate for such drugs. In contrast, drugs with high extraction ratios are removed from the blood as rapidly as they are presented to the liver. If the blood flow to the liver decreases, then the elimination of this drug is prolonged. Therefore, drugs with high extraction ratios are considered to be *flow dependent*. A number of drugs have been investigated and classified according to their extraction by the liver, as shown in Table 10-4.

TABLE 10-4. HEPATIC AND RENAL EXTRACTION RATIOS OF A NUMBER OF REPRESENTATIVE DRUGS

	Extraction Ratio		
	Low	***Intermediate***	***High***
Hepatic extraction*	Amobarbital Diazepam Digitoxin Isoniazid Phenobarbital Phenylbutazone Phenytoin Procainamide Salicylic acid Theophylline Tolbutamide Warfarin	Aspirin Quinidine Desipramine Nortriptyline	Arabinosyl-cytosine Isoproterenol Lidocaine Meperidine Morphine Nitroglycerin Pentazocine Propoxyphene Propranolol Salicylamide
Renal extraction*	Acetazolamide Chlorpropamide Diazoxide Digoxin Furosemide Gentamicin Kanamycin Phenobarbital Sulfasoxazole Tetracycline	Procainamide Quaternary ammonia compounds	(Many) Glucuronides (Many) Penicillins (Many) Sulfates (Many) Glycine conjugates

*At least 30% of the drug is eliminated by this route.
From Rowland M, 1978, p. 44, with permission.[7]

The effect of protein binding on hepatic clearance is difficult to quantitate precisely. As discussed, drug protein binding is not a factor in hepatic clearance for drugs that have high extraction ratios. These drugs are considered to be flow limited. In contrast, drugs that have low extraction ratios may be affected by plasma protein binding depending on the fraction of drug bound. For a drug that has a low extraction ratio and is less than 75–80% bound, small changes in protein binding would not produce significant changes in hepatic clearance. These drugs are considered *capacity-limited, binding-insensitive drugs*[4] and are listed on Table 10-3. Drugs highly bound to plasma protein but that have low extraction ratios are considered *capacity limited and binding sensitive* because a small displacement in the protein binding of these drugs will cause a very large increase in the free drug concentration. This large increase in free drug concentration will cause an increase in the rate of drug metabolism resulting in an overall increase in hepatic clearance. Figure 10-6 is a diagram demonstrating the relationship of protein binding, blood flow, and

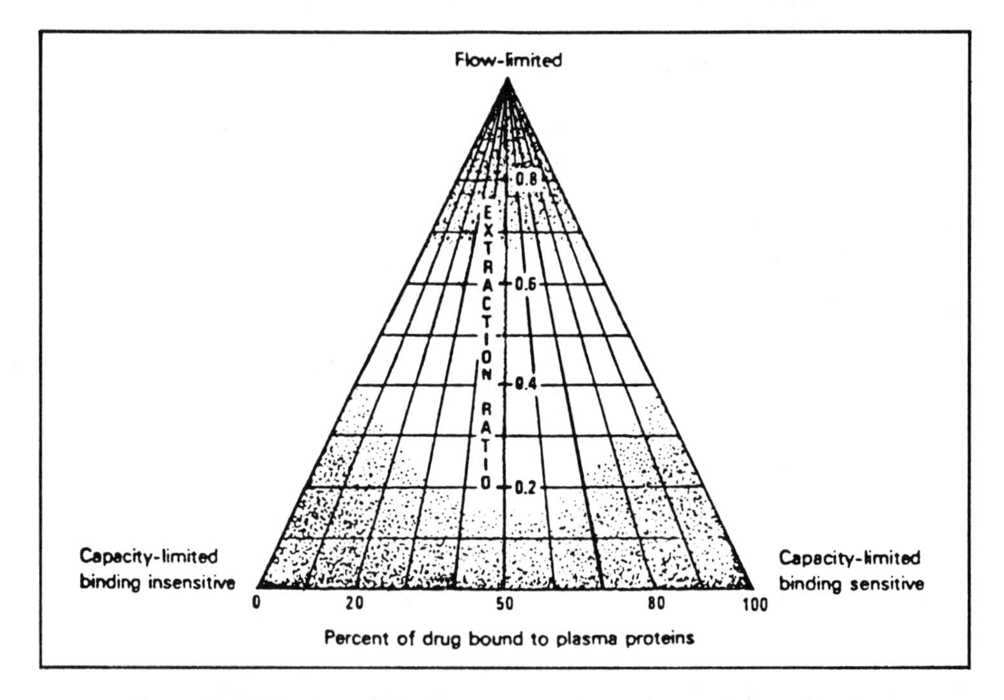

Figure 10-6. This diagram illustrates the way in which two pharmacokinetic parameters (hepatic extraction ratio and percent plasma protein binding) are used to assign a drug into one of three classes of hepatic clearance (flow-limited; capacity-limited, binding sensitive; and capacity-limited, binding insensitive). Any drug metabolized by the liver can be plotted on the triangular graph, but the classification is important only for those eliminated *primarily* by hepatic processes. The closer a drug falls to a corner of the triangle (shaded areas), the more likely it is to have the characteristic changes in disposition in liver disease as described for the three drug classes in the text. (*From Blaschke TF, 1977, with permission.*[4])

extraction. As long as the free drug concentration is greater than the intrinsic clearance, then protein binding will not affect the hepatic clearance with low intrinsic clearance.

SIGNIFICANCE OF DRUG METABOLISM

It is important to consider what fraction of the drug is eliminated by metabolism and what fraction is eliminated by excretion. Drugs which are highly metabolized (such as phenytoin, theophylline, and lidocaine) demonstrate large variations in elimination half-lives in various people. Unlike renal excretion, which is highly dependent on the glomerular filtration rate (relatively constant among different people), drug metabolism is dependent on the intrinsic activity of the biotransformation enzymes, which may be altered by genetic and environmental factors.

BILIARY EXCRETION OF DRUGS

The hepatic cells aligning the bile canaliculi are responsible for the production of bile. The production of bile appears to be an active secretion process. Separate active biliary secretion processes have been reported for organic anions, organic cations, and polar, unchanged molecules.

Physicochemical Properties

Drugs which are mainly excreted in the bile have molecular weights in excess of 500. Drugs which have molecular weights between 300 and 500 are excreted both in urine and in bile. For these drugs a decrease in one excretory route results in a compensatory increase in excretion via the other route. Compounds which have molecular weights of less than 300 are almost exclusively excreted via the kidneys into urine.

In addition to a high molecular weight, drugs excreted into bile usually require a strongly polar group. Many drugs excreted into bile are metabolites, very often glucuronide conjugates. Most metabolites are more polar than the parent drug. In addition, the formation of a glucuronide increases the molecular weight of the compound by nearly 200, as well as increasing the polarity.

Drugs excreted into the bile include the digitalis glycosides, bile salts, cholesterol, steroids, and indomethacin. Compounds which enhance bile production stimulate the biliary excretion of drugs normally eliminated by this route. Furthermore, phenobarbital, which induces many mixed-function oxidase activities, may stimulate the biliary excretion of drugs by two mechanisms, namely an increase in the formation of the glucuronide metabolite and an increase in bile flow. In contrast, compounds which decrease bile flow or pathophysiologic conditions which cause cholestasis will decrease biliary drug excretion. The route of administration may also influence the amount of the drug excreted into bile. For example, drugs given orally may be extracted by the liver into the bile to a greater extent than if the drugs were given intravenously.

Enterohepatic Circulation

A drug or its metabolite which is secreted into bile will eventually be excreted into the duodenum via the gallbladder. Subsequently, the drug or its metabolite might be excreted into the feces or be reabsorbed and become systemically available. The cycle in which the drug is absorbed, excreted into the bile, and reabsorbed is known as *enterohepatic circulation*. Some drugs excreted as a glucuronide conjugate will become hydrolized in the gut back to the parent drug by the action of a β-glucuronidase enzyme present in the intestinal bacteria. In this case the parent drug becomes available for reabsorption.

Significance of Biliary Excretion

When drug appears in the feces after oral administration, it is difficult to determine whether this presence of drug is due to biliary excretion or incomplete absorption. If the drug is given parenterally and then observed in the feces, one can assess that some of the drug was excreted in the bile. Since drug secretion into bile is an active process, it is possible to saturate this process with high drug concentrations. Moreover, other drugs may compete for the same carrier system.

Enterohepatic circulation after a single dose of drug is not as important as after multiple doses or a very high dose of drug. With a large dose or multiple doses a larger amount of drug is secreted in the bile, which drug is then reabsorbed. This reabsorption process may affect the absorption and elimination rate constants. Furthermore, the biliary secretion process may become saturated, thus altering the plasma level–time curve.

QUESTIONS

1. A drug fitting a one-compartment model was found to be eliminated from the plasma by the following pathways with the corresponding elimination rate constants.

   - Metabolism $K_m = 0.200\ \text{hr}^{-1}$
   - Kidney excretion $K_e = 0.250\ \text{hr}^{-1}$
   - Biliary excretion $K_b = 0.150\ \text{hr}^{-1}$

   a. What is the elimination half-life of this drug?
   b. What would the half-life of this drug be if biliary secretion were completely blocked?
   c. What would the half-life of this drug be if drug excretion through the kidney were completely impaired?
   d. If drug-metabolizing enzymes were induced so that the rate of metabolism of this drug *doubled*, what would the new elimination half-life be?

2. A new broad-spectrum antibiotic was administered by rapid intravenous injection to a 50-kg woman at a dose of 3 mg/kg. The apparent volume of distribution of this drug was equivalent to 5% of the body weight. The elimination half-life for this drug is 2 hr.

   a. If 90% of the unchanged drug was recovered in the urine, what is the renal excretion rate constant?
   b. Which is more important for the elimination of the drugs, renal excretion or biotransformation? Why?

3. Explain briefly:
   a. Why does a drug which has a high extraction ratio (e.g., propranolol) demonstrate greater differences between individuals after oral administration than after intravenous administration?
   b. Why does a drug with a low hepatic extraction ratio (e.g., theophylline) demonstrate greater differences between individuals after hepatic enzyme induction than a drug with a high hepatic extraction ratio?

4. A drug is being screened for antihypertensive activity. After oral administration the onset time is 0.5–1 hr. However, after intravenous administration the onset time is 6–8 hr.
   a. What reasons would you give for the differences in the onset times for oral and intravenous drug administration, respectively?
   b. Devise an experiment that would prove the validity of your reasoning.

5. Calculate the hepatic clearance for a drug with an intrinsic clearance of 40 ml/min in a normal adult patient whose hepatic blood flow is 1.5 L/min.
   a. If the patient develops congestive heart failure which reduces hepatic blood flow to 1.0 L/min but does not affect the intrinsic clearance, what is the hepatic drug clearance in this patient?
   b. If the patient was concurrently receiving medication such as phenobarbital which increased the Cl_{int} to 90 ml/min but did not alter the hepatic blood flow (1.5 L/min), what is the hepatic clearance for the drug in this patient?

6. Calculate the hepatic clearance for a drug with an intrinsic clearance of 12 L/min in a normal adult patient whose hepatic blood flow is 1.5 L/min. If this same patient develops congestive heart failure which reduces his hepatic blood flow to 1.0 L/min but does not affect intrinsic clearance, what is the hepatic drug clearance in this patient?
   a. Calculate the extraction ratio for the liver in this patient before and after congestive heart failure develops.
   b. From the above information, estimate the fraction of drug bioavailable, assuming the drug is given orally and absorption is complete.

7. Why do elimination half-lives of drugs primarily eliminated by hepatic biotransformation demonstrate greater intersubject variability than those drugs eliminated primarily by glomerular filtration?

8. A new drug demonstrates high presystemic elimination when taken orally. From which of the following drug products would the drug be most bioavailable. Why?
   a. Aqueous solution
   b. Suspension
   c. Capsule (hard gelatin)
   d. Tablet
   e. Sustained release

9. For a drug which demonstrated presystemic elimination would you expect qualitative and/or quantitative differences in the formation of metabolites from this drug given orally compared to intravenous injection? Why?

REFERENCES

1. Hucker HB, Kwan KC, Duggan DE: Pharmacokinetics and metabolism of nonsteroidal antiinflammatory agents. In Bridges JW, Chasseaud LF (eds), Progress in Drug Research, Volume 5. New York, John Wiley, 1980, Chapter 3
2. Evans DAP: Genetic variations in the acetylation of isoniazid and other drugs. Ann NY Acad Sci 151:723, 1968
3. Hildebrandt A, Estabrook RW: Evidence for the participation of cytochrome b_5 in hepatic microsomal mixed-function oxidation reactions. Arch Biochem Biophys 143:66–79, 1971
4. Blaschke TF: Protein binding and kinetics of drugs in liver diseases. Clin Pharmacokin 2:32–44, 1977
5. Rowland M: Effect of some physiologic factors on bioavailability of oral dosage forms. In Swarbrick J (ed), Current Concepts in the Pharmaceutical Sciences: Dosage Form Design and Bioavailability. Philadelphia, Lea and Febiger, 1973, Chap. 6
6. Wilkinson GR, Shand DG: A physiological approach to hepatic drug clearance. Clin Pharmacol Ther 18:377–90, 1975
7. Rowland M: Drug administration and regimens. In Melmon K, Morelli HF (eds), Clinical Pharmacology. New York, Macmillan, 1978

BIBLIOGRAPHY

Benet LZ: Effect of route of administration and distribution on drug action. J Pharm Biopharm 6:559–85, 1978

Blaschke TF: Protein binding and kinetics of drugs in liver diseases. Clin Pharmacokin 2:32–44, 1977

Geroge CF, Shand DG, Renwick (eds): Presystemic Drug Elimination. Boston, Butterworth Scientific, 1982

Gibaldi M, Perrier D: Route of administration and drug disposition. Drug Metab Rev 3:185–99, 1974

Kaplan SA, Jack ML: Physiologic and metabolic variables in bioavailability studies. In Garrett ER, Hirtz JL (eds), Drug Fate and Metabolism, Vol 3. New York, Marcel Dekker, 1979

LaDu BL, Mandel HG, Way EL: Fundamentals of Drug Metabolism and Drug Disposition. Baltimore, Williams and Wilkins, 1971

Levine WG: Biliary excretion of drugs and other xenobiotics. Prog Drug Res 25:361–420, 1980

Nies AS, Shand DG, Wilkinson GR: Altered hepatic blood flow and drug disposition. Clin Pharmacokin 1:135–56, 1976

Pang KS, Rowland M: Hepatic clearance of drugs. 1. Theoretical considerations of a "well-stirred" model and a "parallel tube" model. Influence of hepatic blood flow, plasma, and blood cell binding and the hepatocellular enzymatic activity on hepatic drug clearance. J Pharmacokin Biopharm 5:625–53, 655–80, 1977

Perrier D, Gibaldi M: Clearance and biologic half-life as indices of intrinsic hepatic metabolism. J Pharmacol Exp Ther 191:17–24, 1974

Routledge PA, Shand DG: Presystemic drug elimination. Ann Rev Pharmacol Toxicol 19:447–68, 1979

Shand DG, Kornhauser DM, Wilkinson GR: Effects of route administration and blood flow on hepatic drug elimination. J Pharmacol Exp Ther 195:425–32, 1975

Wilkinson GR: Pharmacodynamics of drug disposition: Hemodynamic considerations. Ann Rev Pharmacol 15:11–27, 1975

Wilkinson GR: Pharmacokinetics in disease states modifying body perfusion. In Benet LZ (ed), The Effect of Disease States on Drug Pharmacokinetics. Washington, D.C., American Pharmaceutical Association, 1976

Williams RT: Hepatic metabolism of drugs. Gut 13:579–85, 1972

CHAPTER ELEVEN

Protein Binding of Drugs

Many drugs interact with plasma or tissue proteins or other macromolecules such as melanin and DNA to form a drug–macromolecule complex. The formation of this complex is often named *drug protein binding*. Drug protein binding may be a reversible or an irreversible process. Irreversible drug protein binding is usually a result of chemical activation of the drug which then attaches strongly to the protein or macromolecule by covalent chemical bonding. Irreversible drug binding accounts for certain types of drug toxicity which may occur over a long time period as in the case of chemical carcinogenesis or within a relative short time period as in the case of drugs that form reactive chemical intermediates. For example, the hepatotoxicity of high doses of acetaminophen is due to the formation of reactive metabolite intermediates which interact with liver proteins.

Most drugs bind or complex with proteins by a reversible process. Reversible drug protein binding implies that the drug binds the protein with weaker chemical bonds such as hydrogen bonds or van der Waals forces. The amino acids that compose the protein chain have hydroxyl, carboxyl, or other sites available for reversible drug interactions.

The major component of plasma proteins responsible for drug binding is albumin (Table 11-1). Other proteins, such as the globulins, which may bind drugs account for only a very small proportion of the total drug plasma protein binding. Albumin is a protein with a molecular weight of 69,000 and is synthesized by the liver. In the body albumin is distributed vascularly in the plasma and extravascularly in the skin, muscle, and various other tissues. The elimination half-life for albumin is 17–18 days. Normally, the albumin concentration is maintained at a relatively constant level within the plasma compartment, approximately 3.5–4.5% (w/v). Weak acid drugs such as salicylates, phenylbutazone, and penicillins are highly bound to albumin. However, the strength of the drug binding to albumin is different for each drug. Weak base drugs such as propanolol and lidocaine also bind, particularly α_1-acid glycoprotein and lipoproteins.

Reversible drug protein binding is of major interest in pharmacokinetics. The protein-bound drug is a large complex which cannot easily cross cell membranes and

TABLE 11-1. MAJOR PROTEINS TO WHICH DRUGS BIND IN PLASMA

		Normal range of concentrations	
Protein	**Molecular weight**	***(g/L)***	***(M)***
Albumin	65,000	35–50	$5–7.5 \times 10^{-4}$
α_1-Acid glycoprotein	44,000	0.4–1.0	$0.9–2.2 \times 10^{-5}$
Lipoproteins	200,000–3,400,000	Variable	

From Tozer TN, 1984, with permission.[1]

therefore has a restricted distribution. Moreover, the protein-bound drug is pharmacologically inactive and is unavailable for therapeutic use. In contrast, the free or unbound drug crosses cell membranes and is therapeutically active. Studies which critically evaluate drug protein binding are usually performed in vitro using a purified protein such as albumin. Methods for studying protein binding, including equilibrium dialysis and ultrafiltration, make use of a semipermeable membrane which separates the protein and protein-bound drug from the free or unbound drug. By these methods the concentrations of bound drug, free drug, and total protein may be determined. Drug protein binding kinetics yield valuable information concerning proper therapeutic use of the drug and predictions of possible drug interactions.

Drug protein binding is influenced by a number of important factors, including the following:

1. The drug
   a. The physicochemical properties of the drug
   b. The total concentration of the drug in the body
2. The protein
   a. The quantity of protein available for drug protein binding
   b. The quality or physicochemical nature of the protein which is synthesized
3. The affinity between drug and protein including the magnitude of the association constant
4. Drug interactions
   a. Competition for the drug by other substances at a protein binding site
   b. Alteration of the protein by a substance which modifies the affinity of the drug for the protein; for example, aspirin acetylates lysine residues of albumin
5. The pathophysiologic condition of the patient; for example, drug protein binding may be reduced in urenic patients and in patients with hepatic disease

RELATIONSHIP OF PLASMA DRUG PROTEIN BINDING TO DISTRIBUTION AND ELIMINATION

The relationship of reversible drug protein binding in the plasma and drug distribution and elimination is shown in Figure 11-1. A decrease in protein binding that results in the increase in free drug concentration will allow more drug to cross cell

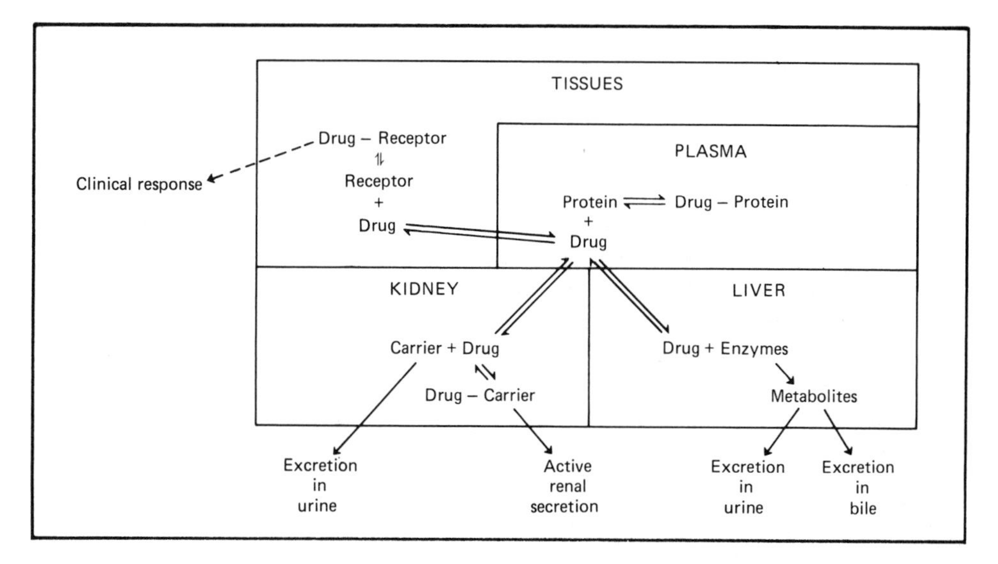

Figure 11-1. Effect of reversible drug protein binding on drug distribution and elimination. Drugs may reversibly bind with proteins. Free (nonbound) drugs penetrate cell membranes distributing into various tissues including those tissues involved in drug elimination, such as kidney and liver. Active renal secretion, which is a carrier-mediated system, may have a greater affinity for free-drug molecules compared to the plasma protein. In this case active renal drug excretion allows for rapid drug excretion despite drug protein binding. If a drug is displaced from the plasma proteins, more free drug is available for distribution into tissues and interaction with the receptors responsible for the pharmacologic response. Moreover, more free drug is available for drug elimination.

membranes and distribute into all tissues. More drug will therefore be available to interact at a receptor site to produce a more intense pharmacologic effect. Moreover, more drug will be available to those tissues involved in drug elimination including the liver and kidney.

EFFECT OF DRUG PROTEIN BINDING ON THE APPARENT VOLUME OF DISTRIBUTION

The total volume of distribution is the sum of all the volumes in the body in which the drug distributes. In terms of anatomical volumes, the drug distributes between the blood (intravascular) volume and the tissue (extravascular) volume. The apparent volume of distribution is affected by changes in the fraction of drug bound to plasma proteins. An increase in the fraction of unbound (free) drug will result in an increase in the apparent volume of distribution, as shown in the following relationship:

$$V = V_B + \frac{f_B}{f_T} V_T \qquad (11.1)$$

where V is the total volume of distribution; V_B is the volume of the blood; V_T is the volume of the tissue; f_B is the fraction of free drug in the blood; and f_T is the fraction of free drug in the tissue.

EXAMPLE

Let the apparent volume of the blood be equal to 8% of body weight, or 5.6 L in a 70-kg subject, and the apparent volume of the tissues be equal to the total body water less the blood volume, or 36.4 L. Calculate the change in the total volume of distribution for drug which is normally 97% bound to blood proteins but is suddenly displaced and is now 95% bound. Assume that the free drug concentration in the tissues is equal to the initial free drug concentration in the blood.

Initial V:

$$V = 5.6 + \frac{0.03}{0.03}(36.4) = 42 \text{ L}$$

After displacement:

$$V = 5.6 + \frac{0.05}{0.03}(36.4) = 66.3 \text{ L}$$

Thus, a small increase in the free drug concentration in the blood for a drug which is normally highly bound to plasma proteins will cause a significant increase in the total volume of distribution.

For a drug which is only 50% bound in the blood a small displacement resulting in an increase in the free drug concentration to 52% will cause only a small increase in the total volume of distribution.

Initial V:

$$V = 5.6 + \frac{0.50}{0.50}(36.4) = 42 \text{ L}$$

After displacement:

$$V = 5.6 + \frac{0.52}{0.50}(36.4) = 43.5 \text{ L}$$

Thus, the increase in the total volume of distribution due to a small increase in free drug concentration in the blood for a drug which is not highly bound to plasma proteins is probably clinically insignificant.

KINETICS OF PROTEIN BINDING

The kinetics of reversible drug–protein binding can be described by the *law of mass action*, as follows.

Protein + drug $\rightleftharpoons$ Drug–protein–complex

or

$$(P)+(D) \rightleftharpoons (PD) \tag{11.2}$$

From Equation 11.2 and the law of mass action, an association constant, K_a, can be expressed as the ratio of the molar concentration of the products and the molar concentration of the reactants.

$$K_a = \frac{(PD)}{(P)(D)} \tag{11.3}$$

The extent of the drug–protein complex formed is dependent on the association binding constant K_a. The magnitude of K_a yields information on the degree of drug protein binding. Drugs strongly bound to protein have a very large K_a and exist mostly as the drug–protein complex. With such drugs a large dose may be needed to obtain a reasonable therapeutic concentration of free drug.

Most kinetic studies in vitro use purified albumin as a standard protein source, since this protein is responsible for the major portion of plasma drug–protein binding. Experimentally, both the free drug (D) and the protein-bound drug (PD), as well as the total protein concentration $(P)+(PD)$ may be determined. To study the binding behavior of drugs, a determinable quantity r is defined, as follows.

$$r = \frac{\text{moles of drug bound}}{\text{total moles of protein}}$$

Since moles of drug bound is (PD) and the total moles of protein is $(P)+(PD)$, this equation becomes

$$r = \frac{(PD)}{(PD)+(P)} \tag{11.4}$$

According to Equation 11.3, $(PD) = K_a(P)(D)$; by substitution into Equation 11.4, the following expression is obtained:

$$r = \frac{K_a(P)(D)}{K_a(P)(D)+(P)}$$

$$r = \frac{K_a(D)}{1+K_a(D)} \tag{11.5}$$

This equation describes the simplest situation, in which 1 mol of drug binds to 1 mol of protein in a 1 : 1 complex. This case assumes only one independent binding site for each mole of drug. If there are n identical independent binding sites per protein molecule, then the following is used.

$$r = \frac{nK_a(D)}{1+K_a(D)} \tag{11.6}$$

Protein molecules are quite large compared to drug molecules and may contain more than one type of binding site for the drug. If there is more than one type of binding site and the drug binds independently on each binding site with its own association constant, then Equation 11.6 expands to the following.

$$r = \frac{n_1 K_1(D)}{1 + K_1(D)} + \frac{n_2 K_2(D)}{1 + K_2(D)} + \cdots \tag{11.7}$$

where the numerical subscripts represent different types of binding sites, the K's represent the binding constants, and the n's represent the number of binding sites per molecule of albumin.

DETERMINATION OF BINDING CONSTANTS AND BINDING SITES BY GRAPHIC METHODS

In Vitro Methods

The values for the association constants and the number of binding sites are obtained by various graphic methods. The reciprocal of Equation 11.6 gives the following equation.

$$\frac{1}{r} = \frac{1 + K_a(D)}{nK_a(D)}$$

$$\frac{1}{r} = \frac{1}{nK_a(D)} + \frac{1}{n} \tag{11.8}$$

A graph of $1/r$ versus $1/(D)$ is called a *double reciprocal plot*. The y intercept is $1/n$ and the slope is $1/nK_a$. From this graph (Fig. 11-2), the number of binding

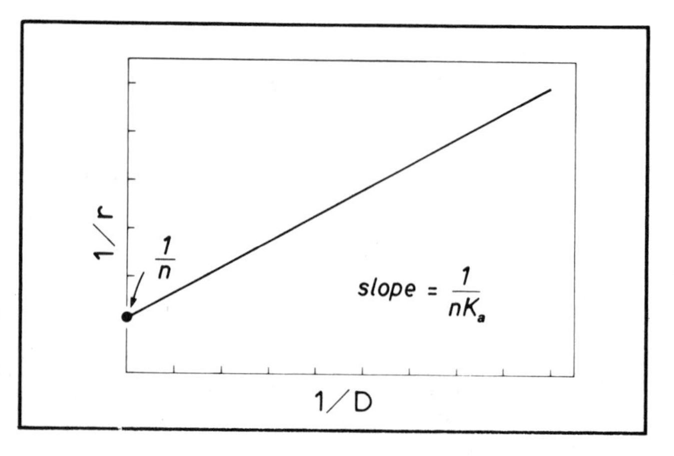

Figure 11-2. Hypothetical binding of drug to protein. The line was obtained with the double reciprocal equation.

sites may be determined from the y intercept, and the association constant may be determined from the slope if the value for n is known.

If the graph of $1/r$ versus $1/D$ does not yield a straight line, then the drug–protein binding process is probably more complex. Equation 11.6 assumes one type of binding site and no interaction among the binding sites. Frequently, Equation 11.8 is used to estimate the number of binding sites and binding constants, using computerized iteration methods.

Another graphic technique called the *Scatchard plot* is a rearrangement of Equation 11.6. The Scatchard plot spreads the data to give a better line for the estimation of the binding constants and binding sites. From Equation 11.6, we obtain

$$r = \frac{nK_a(D)}{1 + K_a(D)}$$

$$r + rK_a(D) = nK_a(D)$$

$$r = nK_a(D) - rK_a(D)$$

$$\frac{r}{(D)} = nK_a - rK_a \qquad (11.9)$$

A graph constructed by plotting $r/(D)$ versus r yields a straight line with the intercepts and slope shown in Figures 11-3 and 11-4.

Some drug–protein binding data produce Scatchard graphs of curvilinear lines (Figs. 11-5 and 11-6). The curvilinear line represents the summation of two straight lines that collectively form to the curve. The binding of salicylic acid to albumin is an example of this type of drug–protein binding in which there are at least two different, independent binding sites (n_1 and n_2), each with its own independent association constant (K_1 and K_2). Equation 11.7 best describes this type of drug protein interaction.

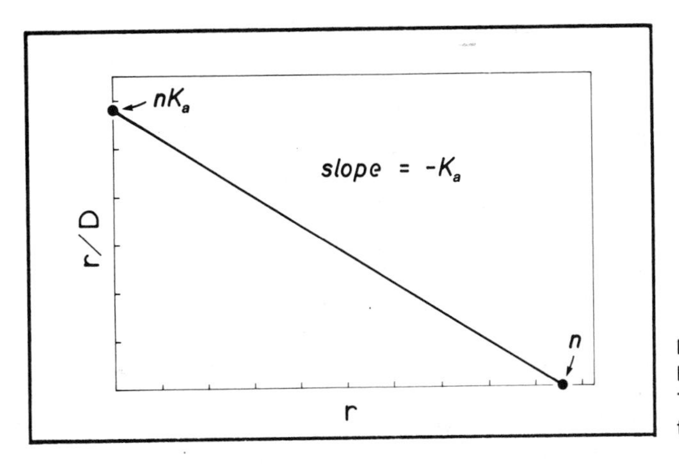

Figure 11-3. Hypothetical binding of drug to protein. The line was obtained with the Scatchard equation.

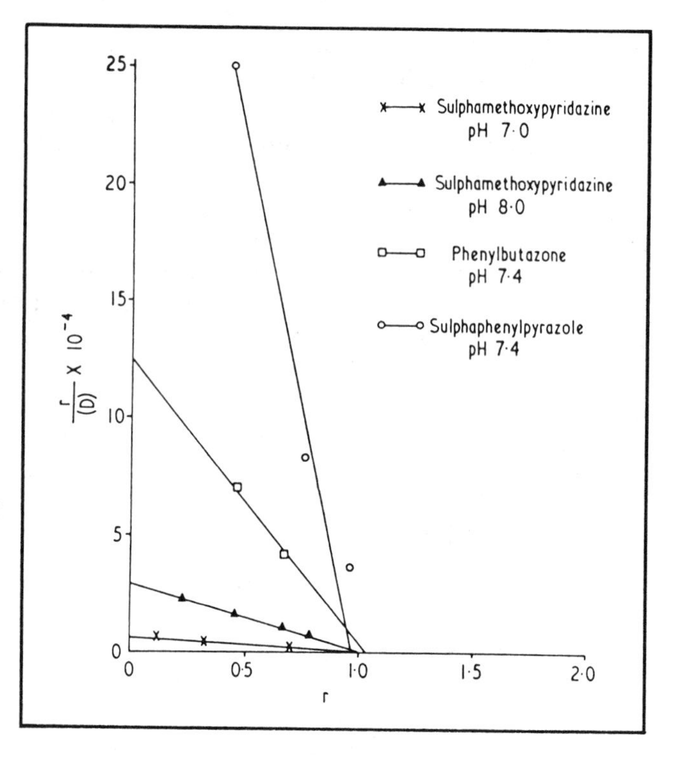

Figure 11-4. Graphic determination of number of binding sites and association constants for interaction of sulfonamides and phenylbutazone with albumin. r = Moles drug bound per mole of albumin; (D) = Concentration of unbound drug. (*From Thorp JM, 1964, with permission.*[2])

In Vivo Methods

Reciprocal and Scatchard plots cannot be used if the exact nature and amount of protein in the experimental system is unknown. The *percent of drug bound* is often used to describe the extent of drug–protein binding in the plasma. The fraction of drug bound (β) can be determined experimentally and is equal to the ratio of the concentration of bound drug $(D)_B$ and the total drug concentration of $(D)_T$ in the

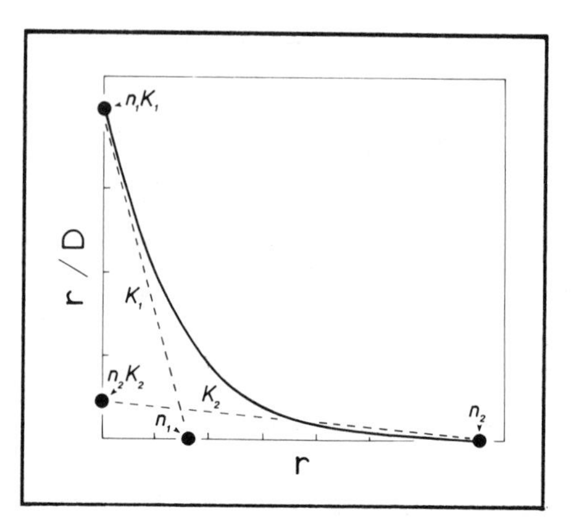

Figure 11-5. Hypothetical binding of drug to protein. The K's represent independent binding constants and the n's represent the number of binding sites per molecule of protein.

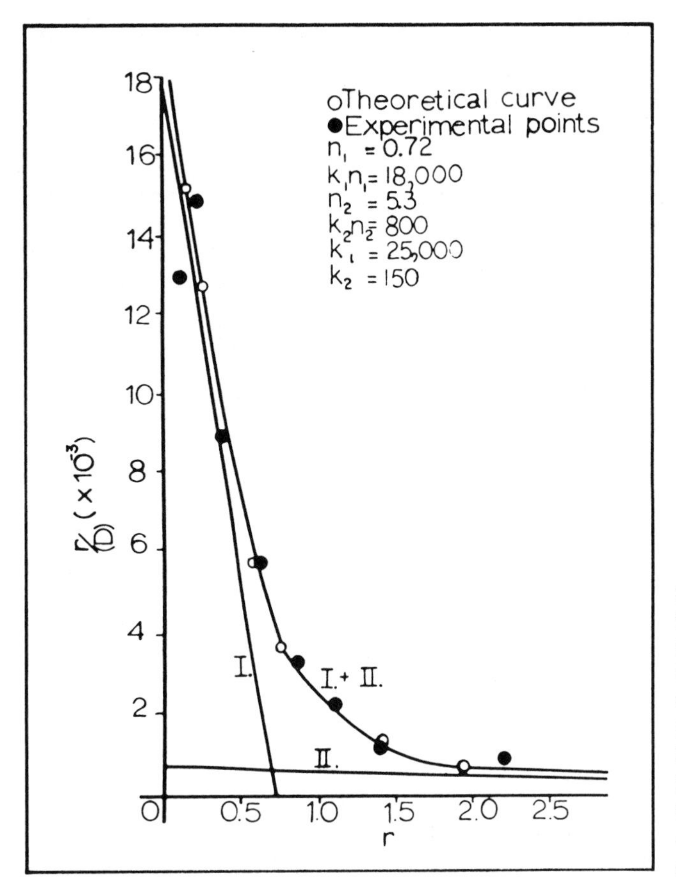

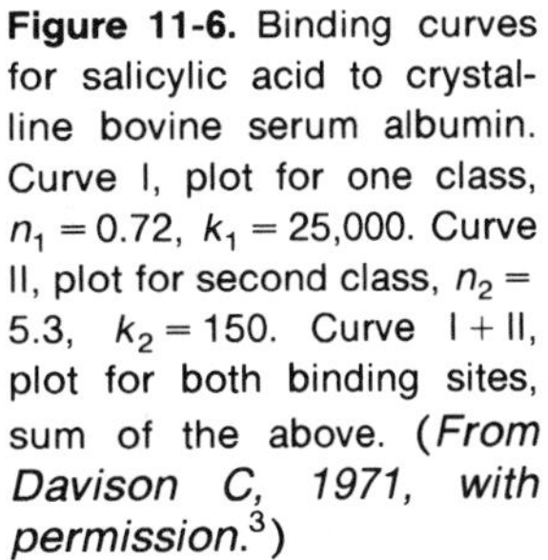
Figure 11-6. Binding curves for salicylic acid to crystalline bovine serum albumin. Curve I, plot for one class, $n_1 = 0.72$, $k_1 = 25{,}000$. Curve II, plot for second class, $n_2 = 5.3$, $k_2 = 150$. Curve I + II, plot for both binding sites, sum of the above. (*From Davison C, 1971, with permission.*[3])

plasma, as follows.

$$\beta = \frac{(D)_{\mathrm{B}}}{(D)_{\mathrm{T}}} \tag{11.10}$$

The value of the association constant can be determined even though the nature of the plasma proteins binding the drug is unknown by rearranging Equation 11.11 into Equation 11.12:

$$r = \frac{(D)_{\mathrm{B}}}{(P)_{\mathrm{T}}} = \frac{nK_{\mathrm{a}}(D)}{1 + K_{\mathrm{a}}(D)} \tag{11.11}$$

where $(D)_{\mathrm{B}}$ is the bound drug concentration; (D) is the free drug concentration; and $(P)_{\mathrm{T}}$ is the total protein concentration. Rearrangement of this equation gives the following expression, which is analogous to the Scatchard equation.

$$\frac{(D)_{\mathrm{B}}}{(D)} = nK_{\mathrm{a}}(P)_{\mathrm{T}} - K_{\mathrm{a}}(D)_{\mathrm{B}} \tag{11.12}$$

Since concentrations of both free and bound drug may be found experimentally, a graph obtained by plotting $(D)_B/(D)$ versus $(D)_B$ will yield a straight line whose slope is the association constant K_a.

Relationship Between Protein Concentration and Drug Concentration in Drug–Protein Binding

Both the concentration of drug and the concentration of protein influence the fraction of drug bound (Eq. 11.10). At a constant protein concentration (which is normally the case) the fraction of drug bound will decrease with an increase in drug concentration (Fig. 11-7).

With a constant concentration of protein, only a certain number of binding sites are available for a drug. At low drug concentrations most of the drug may be bound to the protein, whereas at high drug concentrations the protein binding sites may become saturated, with a consequent rapid increase in the free drug concentrations.

To demonstrate the relationship of the drug concentration and the protein concentration, the following expression can be derived from Equations 11.10 and 11.11.

$$\beta = \frac{1}{1 + \frac{(D)}{n(P)_T} + \frac{1}{nK_a(P)_T}} \tag{11.13}$$

From Equation 11.13, both the free drug concentration (D) and the total protein concentration (P_T) will have important effects on the fraction of drug bound. Any factors which suddenly increase the fraction of free drug concentration in the plasma will cause a change in the pharmacokinetics of the drug.

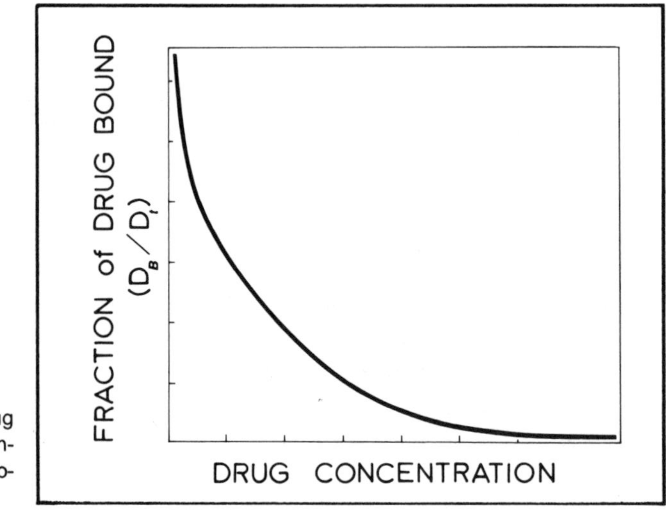

Figure 11-7. Fraction of drug bound versus drug concentration at constant protein concentration.

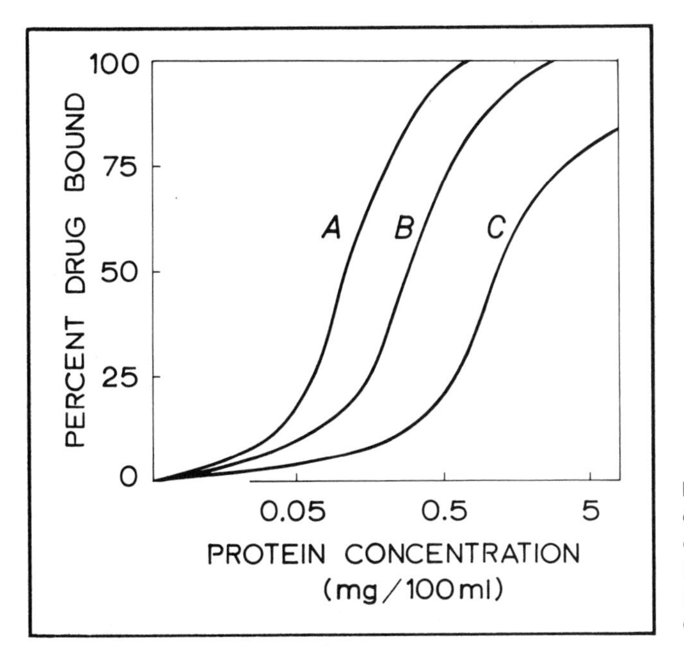

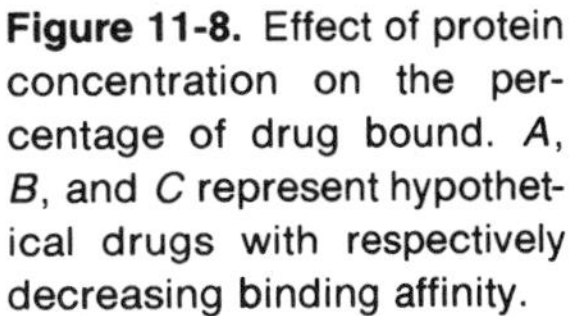
Figure 11-8. Effect of protein concentration on the percentage of drug bound. *A*, *B*, and *C* represent hypothetical drugs with respectively decreasing binding affinity.

Since protein binding is nonlinear in most cases, the percent of drug bound is dependent on the concentrations of both the drug and proteins in the plasma. In disease situations the concentration of protein may vary, thus affecting the percent of drug bound. The effect of protein concentration is demonstrated in Figure 11-8. As the protein concentration increases, the percent of drug bound increases to a maximum. The shapes of the curves are determined by the association constant of the drug–protein complex and the drug concentration.

CLINICAL SIGNIFICANCE OF DRUG–PROTEIN BINDING

Most drugs bind reversibly to plasma proteins to some extent. When the significance of the fraction of drug bound is considered, it is important to know whether the study was performed using pharmacologic or therapeutic plasma drug concentrations. As mentioned previously, the fraction of drug bound can change with plasma drug concentration and dose of drug administered. In addition, the patient's plasma protein concentration should be considered. If a patient has a low plasma protein concentration, then for any given dose of drug the concentration of free bioactive drug might be higher than anticipated. The plasma protein concentration is controlled by a number of variables, including (1) protein synthesis; (2) protein catabolism; (3) distribution of albumin between intravascular and extravascular space; and (4) excessive elimination of plasma protein, particularly albumin. A number of diseases, age, trauma, and related circumstances affect the plasma protein concentration (Table 11-2).

In some cases the *quality* of the protein may change as well as the *quantity* of protein. If qualitative protein changes occur, the affinity of the drug for the protein is

TABLE 11-2. FACTORS THAT DECREASE PLASMA PROTEIN CONCENTRATION

Mechanism	Disease State
Decreased protein synthesis	Liver disease
Increased protein catabolism	Trauma, surgery
Distribution of albumin into extravascular space	Burns
Excessive elimination of protein	Renal disease

altered. In certain liver and renal diseases there is an alteration in the quality of the plasma protein which leads to a decrease in drug-binding capacity.

The nature of drug–drug and drug–metabolite interactions is also important in drug–protein binding. In this case one drug might displace a second bound drug from the protein, causing a sudden increase in pharmacologic response due to an increase in free drug concentration.

EXAMPLE

Let us compare the percent of change in free drug concentration when two drugs, *A* (95% bound) and *B* (50% bound), are displaced by 5% from their respective binding sites by the administration of another drug (Table 11-3). For a highly bound drug *A*, an increase of 5% of free drug is actually a 100% increase in free drug level. For a weakly bound drug like drug *B*, a change of 5% in free concentration due to displacement would only cause a 10% increase in free drug level over the initially high (50%) free drug concentration. For a patient medicated with drug *B*, a 10% increase in free drug level would probably not affect the therapeutic outcome. However, a 100% increase in active drug, as occurs with drug *A*, may be toxic. Although this example is based on one drug displacing another drug, nutrients, physiologic products, and the waste products of metabolism may cause displacement from binding in a similar manner.

As illustrated by this example, displacement is most important with drugs which are more than 95% bound and have a narrow therapeutic index. Under normal circumstances only a small proportion of the total drug is active.

TABLE 11-3. COMPARISON OF EFFECTS OF 5% DISPLACEMENT ON TWO HYPOTHETICAL DRUGS

	Before Displacement	After Displacement	Percent Increase in Free Drug
Drug *A*			
Percent drug bound	95	90	
Percent drug free	5	10	+100
Drug *B*			
Percent drug bound	50	45	
Percent drug free	50	55	+10

Consequently, a small displacement of bound drug causes a disproportionate increase in the free drug concentration, which may cause drug intoxication.

With drugs that are not as highly bound to plasma proteins, a small displacement from the protein causes a transient increase in the free drug concentration, which may cause a transient increase in pharmacologic activity. However, more free drug is available for both renal excretion and hepatic biotransformation, which might be demonstrated by a decreased elimination half-life. Drug displacement from protein by a second drug can occur by competition of the second drug for similar binding sites. Moreover, any alteration of the protein structure may also change the capacity of the protein to bind drugs. For example, aspirin acetylates the lysine residue of albumin, which changes the binding capacity of this protein for certain other anti-inflammatory drugs, such as phenylbutazone.

The displacement of endogenous substances from plasma proteins by drugs is usually of little consequence. Some hormones, such as thyroid and cortisol, are normally bound to specific plasma proteins. A small displacement of these hormones rarely causes problems since physiologic feedback control mechanisms take over. However, in infants the displacement of bilirubin by drugs can cause mental retardation and even death due to the difficulty of bilirubin elimination in newborns.

Finally, the bindings of drugs to proteins can affect the duration of action of the drug. A drug which is extensively but reversibly bound to protein may have a long duration of action due to a depot effect of the drug–protein complex.

The effect of serum protein binding on the renal clearance and elimination half-life on several tetracycline analogs is shown in Table 11-4. For example, doxycycline, which is 93% bound to serum proteins, has an elimination half-life of 15.1 hours, whereas oxytetracycline, which is 35.4% bound to serum proteins, has an elimination half-life of 9.2 hours.

In contrast, a drug which is both extensively bound and actively secreted, such as penicillin, has a short elimination half-life, since active secretion takes preference in removing or stripping the drug from the proteins as the blood flows through the kidney.

TABLE 11-4. COMPARISON OF SERUM PROTEIN BINDING OF SEVERAL TETRACYCLINE ANALOGS WITH THEIR HALF-LIFE IN SERUM. RENAL CLEARANCE AND URINARY RECOVERY AFTER INTRAVENOUS INJECTION

Tetracycline Analogs	Serum Binding (%)	Half-Life (hr)	Renal Clearance (ml/min)	Urinary Recovery (%)
Oxytetracycline	35.4	9.2	98.6	70
Tetracycline	64.6	8.5	73.5	60
Demeclocycline	90.8	12.7	36.5	45
Doxycycline	93.0	15.1	16.0	45

From Kunin CM, et al, 1973, with permission.[4]

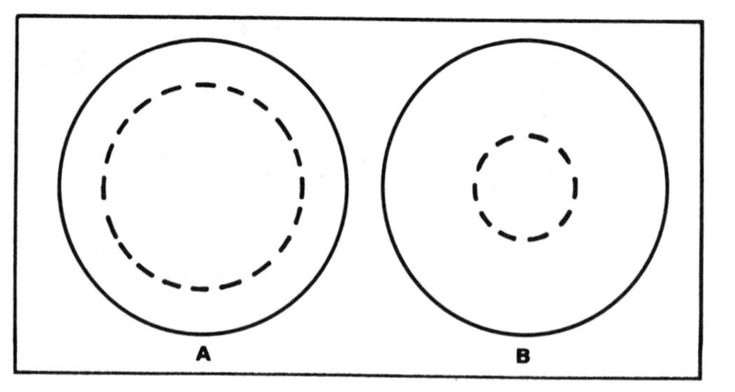

Figure 11-9. Antibiotic disc assay. (A) Antibiotic in water (10 μg/ml). (B) Antibiotic in serum (10 μg/ml).

QUESTIONS

1. Why is the zone of inhibition in an antibiotic disc assay larger for the same drug concentration (10 μg/ml) in water than in serum? See Figure 11-9.
2. Determine the number of binding sites (n) and the association constant (K) from the following data using the Scatchard equation.

r	$D(\times 10^{-4} M)$	r/D
0.40	0.33	
0.80	0.89	
1.20	2.00	
1.60	5.33	

   Can n and K have fractional values? Why?
3. Discuss the clinical significance of drug protein binding on
   a. drug elimination;
   b. drug–drug interactions;
   c. "*percent of drug bound*" data;
   d. liver disease; and
   e. kidney disease.
4. Vallner[5] (1977) reviewed the binding of drugs to albumin or plasma proteins. The following data were reported:

Drug	*Percent Drug Bound*
Tetracycline	53
Gentamycin	70
Phenytoin	93
Morphine	38

   Which drug(s) listed in the above table might be predicted to cause an adverse response due to the concurrent administration of the second drug such a sulfisoxazole (Gantrisin)? Why?

REFERENCES

1. Tozer TN: Implications of altered plasma protein binding in disease states. In Benet LZ, Massoud N, Gambertoglio JG (eds), Pharmacokinetic Basis for Drug Treatment. New

York, Raven Press, 1984
2. Thorp JM: The influence of plasma proteins on the action of drugs. In Binns TB (ed), Absorption and Distribution of Drugs. Baltimore, Williams and Wilkins, 1964
3. Davison C: Protein binding. In LaDu BN, Mandel HG, Way EL (eds), Fundamentals of Drug Metabolism and Drug Disposition. Baltimore, Williams and Wilkins, 1971
4. Kunin CM, Craig WA, Kornguth M, Monson R: Influence of binding on the pharmacologic activity of antibiotics. NY Acad Sci 226:214–24, 1973
5. Vallner JJ: Binding of drugs by albumin and plasma proteins. J Pharm Sci 66:447–65, 1977

BIBLIOGRAPHY

Anton AH, Solomon HM (eds): Drug protein binding. Ann NY Acad Sci 226:1–362, 1973

Barza M, Samuelson T, Weinstein L: Penetration of antibiotics into fibrin loci in vivo, II: Comparison of nine antibiotics—effect of dose and degree of protein binding. J Infect Dis 129:66, 1974

Birke G, Liljedahl SO, Plantin LO, Wetterfors J: Albumin catabolism in burns and following surgical procedures. Acta Chir Scand 118:353–66, 1959–1960

Coffey CJ, Bullock FJ, Schoenemann PT: Numerical solution of nonlinear pharmacokinetic equations: Effect of plasma protein binding on drug distribution and elimination. J Pharm Sci 60:1623, 1971

Gibaldi M, Levy G, McNamara PJ: Effect of plasma protein and tissue binding on the biologic half-life of drugs. Clin Pharmacol Thes 24:1–4, 1978

Greenblatt DJ, Sellers EM, Koch-Weser J: Importance of protein binding for the interpretation of serum or plasma drug concentration. J Clin Pharmacol 22:259–63, 1982

Jusko WJ: Pharmacokinetics in disease states changing protein binding. In Benet LZ (ed), The Effects of Disease States on Drug Pharmacokinetics. Washington, D.C., American Pharmaceutical Association, 1976

Jusko WJ, Gretch M: Plasma and tissue protein binding of drugs in pharmacokinetics. Drug Metab Rev 5:43–140, 1976

Koch-Wester J, Sellers EM: Binding of drugs to serum albumin. N Engl J Med 294:311–16, 526–31, 1976

Levy R, Shand D (eds): Clinical implications of drug-protein binding. Proceedings of a symposium sponsored by Syva Company. Clin Pharmacokin 9:(Suppl. 1), 1984

MacKichan JJ: Pharmacokinetic consequences of drug displacement from blood and tissue proteins. Clin Pharmacokin 9:(Suppl. 1), 32–41, 1984

Meyer MC, Gutlman DE: The bindings of drugs by plasma proteins. J Pharm Sci 57:895–918, 1968

Rothschild MA, Oratz M, Schreiber SS: Albumin metabolism. Gastroenterology 64:324–31, 1973

Rowland M: Plasma protein binding and therapeutic monitoring. Ther Drug Monitor 2:29–37, 1980

Tillemont JP, Lhoste F, Guidicelli JF: Diseases and drug protein binding. Clin Pharmacokinet 3:144–54, 1978

Tillemont JP, Zini R, d'Athier P, Vassent G: Binding of certain acidic drugs to human albumin: Theoretical and practical estimation of fundamental parameters. Eur J Clin Pharmacol 7:307–13, 1974

Wandell M, Wilcox-Thole WL: Protein binding and free drug concentrations. In Mungall DR (ed), Applied Clinical Pharmacokinetics. New York, Raven Press, 1983, pp 17–48

CHAPTER TWELVE

Intravenous Infusion

There are several advantages in giving a drug by intravenous infusion at zero order rate. First of all, in the critically ill antibiotics and drugs can often be conveniently administered by infusion in an IV bottle together with IV fluids, electrolytes, or nutrients. Second, the rate of infusion can be easily regulated to fit individual patient needs. And third, constant infusion prevents a fluctuating peak (maximum) and valley (minimum) blood level. This is desirable if the drug has a narrow therapeutic index.

The concentration of drug in the plasma by intravenous infusion at a constant rate is shown in Figure 12-1. After a while the drug accumulates to reach a plateau or steady-state level.

The plateau level is called the *steady-state concentration*, the point at which the rate of drug leaving the body and the rate of drug entering the body (infusion) are the same. The time required to reach steady-state drug concentrations in the blood is primarily dependent on the elimination half-life. The time required to reach 90%, 95%, and 99% of the steady-state concentration is shown in Table 12-1. For therapeutic purposes, more than 95% of the steady-state drug concentration in the blood is desired. This is reached in a period of time equal to six times the elimination half-life.

If the drug is given at a higher infusion rate, a higher steady-state level is obtained, but the time needed to reach steady state remains the same (Fig. 12-2).

ONE-COMPARTMENT MODEL

During infusion at a constant rate, the drug concentration at any time t can be calculated if the infusion rate (R), volume of distribution (V_d), and elimination constant (K) are known:

$$C_p = \frac{R}{V_d K}(1 - e^{-Kt}) \tag{12.1}$$

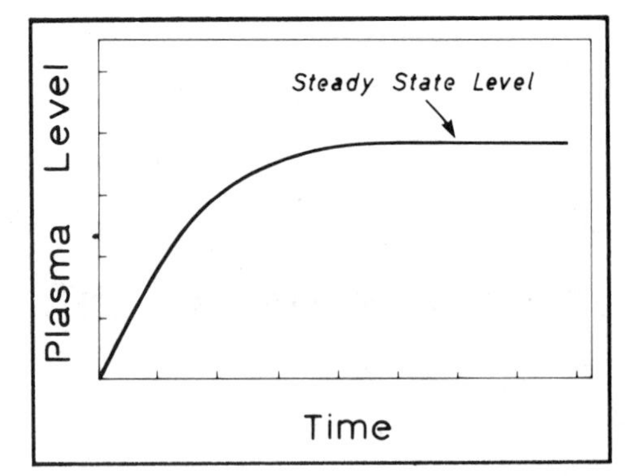

Figure 12-1. Plasma level–time curve for constant IV infusion.

If the IV infusion is stopped, then the slope of the drug elimination curve is equal to $-K/2.3$ (Fig. 12-3). Equation 12.1 shows how concentration (C_p) increases as time (t) increases. At steady state (i.e., at infinite time after infusion is started), t is very large and Equation 12.1 becomes

$$C_p = \frac{R}{V_d K}[1 - e^{-K(\infty)}]$$

Since $e^{-K(\infty)}$ approaches zero, Equation 12.1 reduces to

$$C_p^{\infty} = \frac{R}{V_d K} \qquad (12.2)$$

This equation may also be obtained with a different approach. At steady state the rate of infusion equals the rate of elimination. Therefore, the plasma drug concentration change is equal to zero:

$$\frac{dC_p}{dt} = 0$$

$$\frac{dC_p}{dt} = \frac{R}{V_d} - K(C_p) = 0$$

$$(\text{Rate in}) - (\text{rate out}) = 0$$

$$\frac{R}{V_d} = KC_p$$

$$C_p^{\infty} = \frac{R}{V_d K} \qquad (\text{Eq. 12.2})$$

TABLE 12-1. NUMBER OF $t_{1/2}$ TO REACH A FRACTION OF C_p^{∞}

Percent of C_p^{∞} Reached*	Number of Half-Lives
90	3.32
95	4.32
99	6.65

*C_p^{∞} is the steady-state drug concentration in plasma.

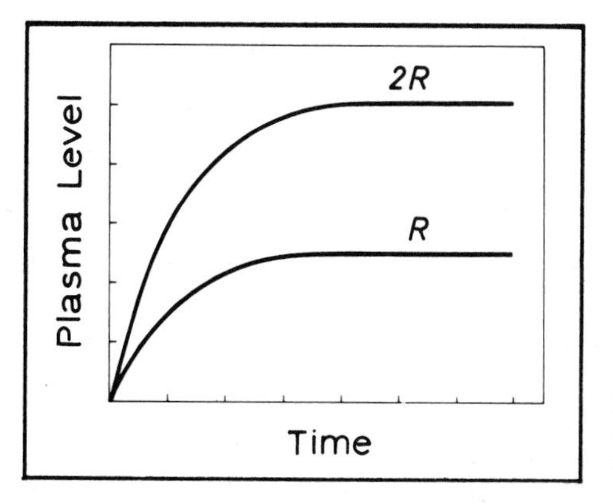

Figure 12-2. Plasma level–time curve for IV infusions given at rates of R and $2R$, respectively.

Equation 12.2 shows that the steady-state concentration (C_p^{∞}) is dependent on the volume of distribution, the elimination rate constant, and the infusion rate. Altering any one of these factors can affect steady-state concentration.

EXAMPLE 1

An antibiotic has a volume of distribution of 10 L and a K of 0.2 hr^{-1}. A steady-state plasma concentration of 10 μg/ml is desired. The infusion rate needed to maintain this concentration can be determined as follows.

Equation 12.2 can be rewritten as

$$
\begin{aligned}
R &= C_p^{\infty} V_d K \\
&= (10\ \mu\text{g/ml})(10)(1000\ \text{ml})(0.2\ \text{hr}^{-1}) \\
&= 20\ \text{mg/hr}
\end{aligned}
$$

Suppose the patient has a uremic condition and the elimination rate constant has decreased to 0.1 hr^{-1}. To maintain the steady-state concentration

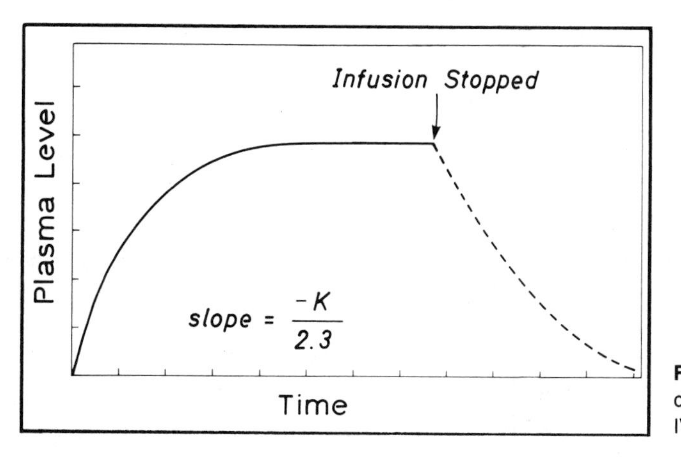

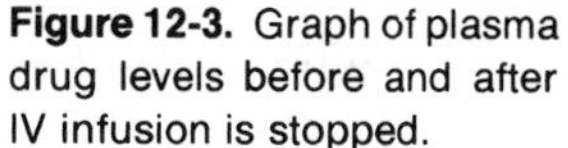
Figure 12-3. Graph of plasma drug levels before and after IV infusion is stopped.

of 10 μg/ml, we must determine a new rate of infusion as follows.

$$R = (10\ \mu\text{g/ml})(10)(1000\ \text{ml})(0.1\ \text{hr}^{-1})$$
$$= 10\ \text{mg/hr}$$

When the elimination rate decreases, then the infusion rate must decrease proportionately.

EXAMPLE 2

An infinitely long period of time is needed to reach steady-state drug levels. However, in practice it is quite acceptable to reach 99% C_p^∞ (i.e., 99% steady-state level). Using Equation 12.2, we know that steady-state level is

$$C_p^\infty = \frac{R}{V_d K}$$

and 99% steady-state level would be equal to

$$99\% \frac{R}{V_d K}$$

Substituting into Equation 12.1 for C_p, we can find out the time needed to reach steady state by solving for t:

$$99\% \frac{R}{V_d K} = \frac{R}{V_d K}(1 - e^{-Kt})$$

$$99\% = 1 - e^{-Kt}$$

$$e^{-Kt} = 1\%$$

Take the natural logarithm on both sides:

$$-Kt = \ln 0.01$$

$$t_{99\%_{ss}} = \frac{\ln 0.01}{-K} = \frac{-4.61}{-K} = \frac{4.61}{K}$$

substituting $(0.693/t_{1/2})$ for K,

$$t_{99\%_{ss}} = \frac{4.61}{(0.693/t_{1/2})} = \frac{4.61}{0.693} t_{1/2}$$

$$t_{99\%_{ss}} = 6.65 t_{1/2}$$

Notice that in the equation directly above the time needed to reach steady state is not dependent on the rate of infusion, but only on the elimination half-life. Using similar calculations, the time needed to reach any percentage of the steady-state drug concentration may be obtained (Table 12-1).

Intravenous infusion can serve as a source of data to determine total body clearance if the infusion rate and steady-state level can be determined, as with

Equation 12.2:

$$C_p^\infty = \frac{R}{V_d K}$$

$$V_d K = \frac{R}{C_p^\infty}$$

since total body clearance, Cl_T, is equal to $V_d K$,

$$Cl_T = \frac{R}{C_p^\infty} \tag{12.3}$$

EXAMPLE 3

A patient is given an antibiotic by constant infusion at the rate of 2 mg/hr for 2 weeks. Serum analysis shows a drug concentration of 10 μg/ml. The total body clearance can be determined as follows.

$$Cl_T = \frac{2000\ \mu g/hr}{10\ \mu g/ml} = 200\ ml/hr$$

TWO-COMPARTMENT MODEL DRUGS

For a drug that follows two-compartment open-model kinetics, the concentration of drug at any time t after infusion has been started depends on the rate of infusion, the volume of distribution, the elimination $t_{1/2}$, and other pharmacokinetic constants, as governed by the following equation.

$$C_p = \frac{R}{V_p K}\left(1 + \frac{b-K}{a-b}e^{-at} + \frac{K-a}{a-b}e^{-bt}\right) \tag{12.4}$$

At steady state (i.e., at $t = \infty$) the second and third terms in parentheses in Equation 12.4 drop out (i.e., are equal to zero):

$$C_p^\infty = \frac{R}{V_p K} \tag{12.5}$$

This equation shows the steady-state concentration of a drug that follows a two-compartment open model, since

$$V_p K = V_b b \tag{12.6}$$

where $V_b = \beta$ volume of distribution of the drug, and V_p = volume of the central compartment. Substituting Equation 12.6 into Equation 12.5, we obtain

$$C_p^\infty = \frac{R}{V_b b} \tag{12.7}$$

By knowing b and the steady-state level, the infusion rate, V_b, can be estimated as follows.

$$V_b = \frac{R}{C_p^{\infty} b} \tag{12.8}$$

In most cases b can be obtained easily from the terminal portion of a log concentration–time curve. The volume of distribution obtained this way can be compared with that obtained by feathering the curve. V_b is also known as $(V_D)_\beta$ (beta volume of distribution). (See Eq. 5.33, Ch. 5.)

EXAMPLE 4

The volume of the central compartment of a drug is 5 L. The overall elimination rate constant is unknown, but b is found to be 0.02 hr^{-1}. Infusing the drug at a rate of 2 mg/hr for days yields a steady serum drug concentration of 5 $\mu g/ml$. What is the V_b?

$$V_b = \frac{R}{C_p^{\infty} b}$$

$$= \frac{2000\ \mu g/hr^{-1}}{(5\ \mu g/ml)(0.02\ hr^{-1})}$$

$$= (2)(10^4\ ml) = 20\ L$$

Please note that V_b is the apparent volume of distribution of the drug and is different from V_p, volume of the central compartment.

INFUSION PLUS LOADING DOSE

The *loading dose* D_L or initial bolus dose of a drug is used to obtain steady-state concentrations as rapidly as possible. We know that the concentration of drug in the body for a one-compartment model after an IV bolus dose is described by

$$C_1 = C_0 e^{-Kt} = \frac{D_L}{V_d} e^{-Kt} \tag{12.9}$$

and concentration by infusion at the rate R is

$$C_2 = \frac{R}{V_d K}(1 - e^{-Kt}) \tag{12.10}$$

Assume an IV bolus dose D_L of the drug is given and IV infusion is started at the same time. The total concentration C_p at t hours after the start of infusion would be equal to $C_1 + C_2$ due to the sum contributions of bolus and infusion, or

$$C_p = C_1 + C_2$$

$$= \frac{D_L}{V_d}e^{-Kt} + \frac{R}{V_d K}(1 - e^{-Kt}) \qquad (12.11)$$

$$= \frac{D_L}{V_d}e^{-Kt} + \frac{R}{V_d K} - \frac{R}{V_d K}e^{-Kt}$$

$$= \frac{R}{V_d K} + \left(\frac{D_L}{V_d}e^{-Kt} - \frac{R}{V_d K}e^{-Kt}\right) \qquad (12.12)$$

Let the loading dose (D_L) equal the amount of drug in the body at steady state.

$$D_L = C_p^{\infty} V_d$$

From Equation 12.2, $C_p^{\infty} V_d = R/K$. Therefore,

$$D_L = R/K$$

Substituting $D_L = R/K$ makes the expression in parentheses in Equation 12.12 cancel out. Equation 12.12 reduces to Equation 12.2, which is the expression for C_p^{∞} on steady-state plasma concentrations:

$$C_p = \frac{R}{V_d K} + (0)$$

$$C_p^{\infty} = \frac{R}{V_d K} \qquad (C_p^{\infty} \text{ is constant at any time } t) \qquad \text{(Eq. 12.2)}$$

Therefore, if a proper IV bolus or loading dose is given, followed by an IV infusion, steady-state plasma drug concentrations are obtained immediately and maintained.

The loading dose needed to get immediate steady-state drug levels can also be found by the following approach.

Loading dose equation:

$$C_p = \frac{D_L}{V_d}e^{-Kt}$$

Infusion equation:

$$C_p = \frac{R}{KV_d}(1 - e^{-Kt})$$

Adding up the two equations yields Equation 12.13, an equation describing simultaneous infusion after a loading dose:

$$C_p = \frac{D_L}{V_d}e^{-Kt} + \frac{R}{V_d K}(1 - e^{-Kt}) \qquad (12.13)$$

By differentiating this equation at steady state, we obtain

$$\frac{dC_{\mathrm{p}}}{dt} = 0 = \frac{-D_{\mathrm{L}}K}{V_{\mathrm{d}}}e^{-Kt} + \frac{RK}{V_{\mathrm{d}}K}e^{-Kt} \tag{12.14}$$

$$0 = e^{-Kt}\left(\frac{-D_{\mathrm{L}}K}{V_{\mathrm{d}}} + \frac{R}{V_{\mathrm{d}}}\right)$$

$$\frac{D_{\mathrm{L}}K}{V_{\mathrm{d}}} = \frac{R}{V_{\mathrm{d}}}$$

$$D_{\mathrm{L}} = \frac{R}{K} = \text{loading dose} \tag{12.15}$$

In order to maintain instant steady-state level $[(dC_{\mathrm{p}}/dt) = 0]$, the loading dose should be equal to R/K (Eq. 12.15).

In Figure 12-4, curve *b* shows the blood level after a single loading dose of R/V plus infusion. Note the instant steady-state level. If the loading doses is large, the plasma drug concentration takes longer to decline to steady-state drug levels (Fig. 12-4, curve *a*). If the loading dose is low, the plasma drug concentrations will increase slowly to steady-state drug levels (Fig. 12-4, curve *c*), but more quickly than without any loading dose.

Another method for the calculation of loading dose D_{L} is based on knowledge of the desired steady-state drug concentration C_{p}^{∞} and the apparent volume of distribution V_{d} for the drug, as shown in Equation 12.16.

$$D_{\mathrm{L}} = C_{\mathrm{p}}^{\infty}V_{\mathrm{d}} \tag{12.16}$$

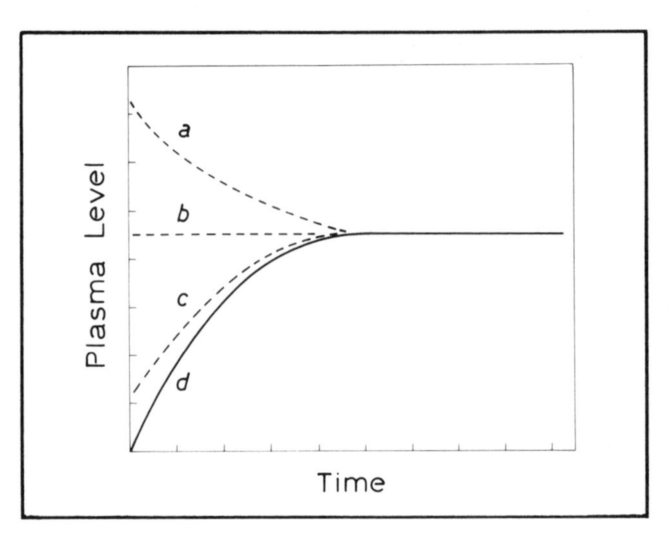

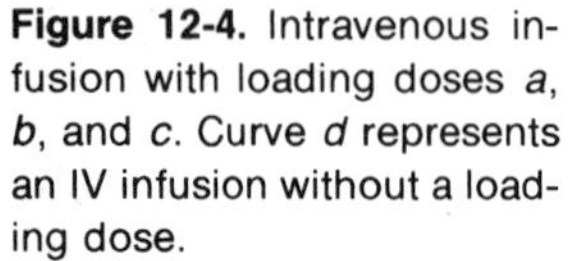

Figure 12-4. Intravenous infusion with loading doses *a*, *b*, and *c*. Curve *d* represents an IV infusion without a loading dose.

For many drugs C_p^∞ is reported in the literature as the effective therapeutic drug concentration. The V_d and the elimination half-life, $t_{1/2}$, are also available for these drugs.

PRACTICE PROBLEMS

1. A physician wants to administer an anesthetic agent at a rate of 2 mg/hr by IV infusion. The elimination rate constant is 0.1 hr^{-1} and the volume of distribution (one compartment) is 10 L. What loading dose should be recommended if the doctor wants the drug level to reach 2 $\mu g/ml$ immediately?

Solution

$$C_p^\infty = \frac{R}{V_d K} = \frac{2000}{(10 \times 10^3)(0.1)} = 2\ \mu g/ml$$

To reach C_p^∞ instantly,

$$D_L = \frac{R}{K} = \frac{2\ mg/hr}{0.1/hr} \qquad D_L = 20\ mg$$

2. What is the concentration of a drug 6 hr after administration of a loading dose of 10 mg and simultaneous infusion at 2 mg/hr (the drug has a $t_{1/2}$ of 3 hr and a volume of distribution of 10 L)?

Solution

$$K = \frac{0.693}{3} hr^{-1}$$

$$C_p = \frac{D_L}{V_d} e^{-Kt} + \frac{R}{V_d K}(1 - e^{-Kt})$$

$$C_p = \frac{10000}{10000} e^{-(0.693/3)(6)} + \frac{2000}{(10000)(0.693/3)}[1 - e^{-(0.693/3)(6)}]$$

$$C_p = 0.90\ \mu g/ml$$

3. Calculate the drug concentration in the blood after infusion has been stopped.

Solution

This concentration can be calculated in two portions (Fig. 12-3). First, one must calculate the concentration of drug during infusion, and second, one must calculate the present concentration, C_0. One then uses the IV bolus dose equation ($C = C_0 e^{-Kt}$) for calculations for any further point in time. For convenience, the two equations can be combined as follows.

$$C_p = \frac{R}{KV_d}(1 - e^{-Kb})e^{-K(t-b)} \tag{12.17}$$

where b = length of time of infusion period; t = total time (infusion and postinfusion); and $t - b$ = length of time after infusion has stopped.

4. A patient was infused for 6 hr with a drug ($K = 0.01\ \text{hr}^{-1}$; $V_d = 10$ L) at a rate of 2 mg/hr. What is the concentration of the drug in the body 2 hr after cessation of the infusion?

Solution

Using Equation 12.17,

$$C_p = \frac{2000}{(0.01)(10000)}(1 - e^{-0.01(6)})e^{-0.01(8-6)}$$

$$C_p = 1.14\ \mu\text{g/ml}$$

Alternatively,

$$C_p' = \frac{R}{KV_d}(1 - e^{-Kt})$$

$$C_p' = \frac{2000}{0.01 \times 10000}(1 - e^{-0.01(6)})$$

$$C = C_p' e^{-0.01(2)}$$

$$C = 1.14\ \mu\text{g/ml}$$

The two approaches should give the same answer.

5. An adult male asthmatic patient (78 kg, 48 years old) with a history of heavy smoking was given an IV infusion at a rate of 0.5 mg/kg hr. A loading dose of 6 mg/kg was given by IV bolus injection just prior to the start of the infusion. At 2 hr after the start of the IV infusion, the plasma theophylline concentration was measured and found to contain 5.8 μg/ml of theophylline. The apparent V_d for theophylline is 0.45 L/kg. Aminophylline is the ethylenediamine salt of theophylline and contains 80% of theophylline base.

   Since the patient was responding poorly to the aminophylline therapy, the physician wanted to increase the plasma theophylline concentration in the patient to 10 μg/ml. What dosage recommendation would you give the physician? Would you recommend another loading dose?

Solution

If no loading dose is given and the IV infusion rate is increased, the time to reach steady-state plasma drug concentrations will be about $4\text{–}5t_{1/2}$ to reach 95% of C_{ss}. Therefore, a second loading dose should be recommended to rapidly increase the plasma theophylline concentration to 10 μg/ml. The infusion rate must also be increased to maintain this desired C_p^∞.

The calculation of loading dose D_L must consider the present plasma theophylline concentration:

$$D_L = \frac{V_d(C_p \text{ desired} - C_p \text{ present})}{(S)(F)}$$

where S is the salt form of the drug and F is the fraction of drug bioavailable. For aminophylline S is equal to 0.80 and for an IV bolus injection F is equal to 1.

$$D_L = \frac{(0.45 \text{ L/kg})(78 \text{ kg})(10 - 5.8 \text{ mg/L})}{(0.80)(1)}$$

$$D_L = 184 \text{ mg aminophylline}$$

The maintenance IV infusion rate may be calculated after estimation of the patient's clearance, Cl_T. Since a loading dose and an IV infusion of 0.5 mg/hr kg was given to the patient, the plasma theophylline concentration of 5.8 mg/L is at steady-state C_p^∞. Total clearance may be estimated by

$$Cl_T = \frac{R}{C^\infty_{p,\text{present}}} = \frac{(0.6 \text{ mg/hr kg})\ (78 \text{ kg})}{5.8 \text{ mg/L}}$$

$$Cl_T = 8.07 \text{ L/hr or } 1.72 \text{ ml/min kg}$$

The usual Cl_T for adult, nonsmoking patients with uncomplicated asthma is approximately 0.65 ml/min kg. Heavy smoking is known to increase Cl_T for theophylline.

The new IV infusion rate, R', is calculated by

$$R' = C^\infty_{p,\text{desired}}\ Cl_T$$

$$R' = 10 \text{ mg/L} \times 8.07 \text{ L/hr} = 80.7 \text{ mg/hr or } 1.03 \text{ mg/hr kg}$$

INTRAVENOUS INFUSION OF TWO-COMPARTMENT MODEL DRUGS

Many drugs given by intravenous infusion follow two-compartment kinetics. For example, the respective distributions of theophylline and lidocaine in humans are described by the two-compartment open model. As with the one-compartment model drugs, intravenous infusion requires a slow build-up of drug before a stable blood level is reached. The time needed to reach a steady-state blood level depends entirely on the half-life of the drug. The equation describing plasma drug concentration as a function of time is

$$C_p = \frac{R}{V_p K}\left[1 - \left(\frac{K-b}{a-b}\right)e^{-at} - \left(\frac{a-K}{a-b}\right)e^{-bt}\right] \tag{12.18}$$

where a and b are hybrid rate constants and R is the rate of infusion. At steady state (i.e., $t = \infty$) Equation 12.18 reduces to

$$C_p^{\infty} = \frac{R}{V_p K} \tag{12.19}$$

By rearranging this equation, we get the equation needed to calculate the infusion rate for a desired steady-state plasma drug concentration.

$$R = C_p^{\infty} V_p K \tag{12.20}$$

Drugs with long half-lives require a loading dose to rapidly attain steady-state plasma drug levels. The concentration of a two-compartment drug after various loading doses is shown in Figure 12-5.

It is clinically desirable to achieve rapid therapeutic drug levels by using a loading dose. However, for drugs which follow the two-compartment pharmacokinetic model, the drug distributes slowly into extravascular tissues (compartment 2). Thus, drug equilibrium is not immediate. If a loading dose is given too rapidly, the drug may give excessively high concentrations in the plasma initially (central compartment) which decreases as equilibrium is reached (Fig. 12-5). It is not possible to maintain an instantaneous stable steady-state blood level for a two-compartment model drug with a zero-order rate of infusion. Therefore, a loading dose produces an initial blood level either slightly higher or lower than the steady-state blood level. To overcome this problem, several IV bolus injections given as short intermittent IV infusions may be used as a method for administering a loading dose to the patient.

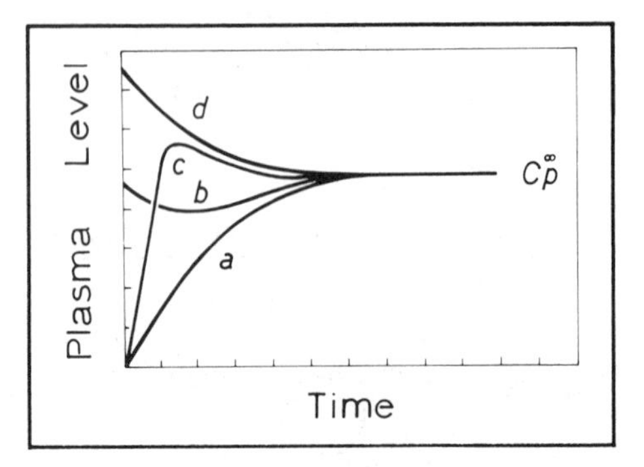

Figure 12-5. Plasma drug level after various loading doses and rates of infusion for a drug which follows a two-compartment model: (a) no loading dose; (b) loading dose = R/K (rapid infusion); (c) loading dose = R/b (slow infusion); and (d) loading dose = R/b (rapid infusion).

QUESTIONS

1. A female patient (35 years old, 65 kg) with normal renal function is to be given a drug by IV infusion. According to the literature, the elimination half-life of this drug is 7 hr and the apparent V_d is 23.1% of body weight. The pharmacokinetics of this drug assumes a first-order process. The desired steady-state plasma level for this antibiotic is 10 μg/ml.
   - **a.** Assuming no loading dose, how long after the start of the IV infusion would it take to reach 95% of the C_{ss}?
   - **b.** What is the proper loading dose for this antibiotic?
   - **c.** What is the proper infusion rate for this drug?
   - **d.** What is the total body clearance?
   - **e.** If the patient suddenly develops partial renal failure, how long would it take for a new steady-state plasma level to be established (assume that 95% of the C_p^∞ is a reasonable approximation)?
   - **f.** If the total body clearance declined 50% due to partial renal failure, what new infusion rate would you recommend to maintain the desired steady-state plasma level of 10 μg/ml?
2. An anticonvulsant drug was given as (a) a single IV dose and (b) a constant IV infusion. The serum drug concentrations are as presented in Table 12-2.
   - **a.** What is the steady-state plasma drug level?
   - **b.** What is the time for 95% steady-state plasma level?
   - **c.** What is the drug clearance?
   - **d.** What is the plasma concentration of the drug 4 hr after stopping infusion (infusion was stopped after 24 hr)?
   - **e.** What is the infusion rate for a patient weighing 75 kg to maintain a steady-state drug level of 10 μg/ml?
   - **f.** What is the plasma drug concentration 4 hr after an IV dose of 1 mg/kg followed by a constant infusion of 0.2 mg/kg hr?

TABLE 12-2. SERUM DRUG CONCENTRATIONS FOR A HYPOTHETICAL ANTICONVULSANT DRUG

	Concentration in Plasma (μg/ml)	
Time (hr)	***Single IV dose of 1 mg/kg***	***Constant IV infusion of 0.2 mg/kg hr***
0	10.0	0
2	6.7	3.3
4	4.5	5.5
6	3.0	7.0
8	2.0	8.0
10	1.35	8.6
12		9.1
18		9.7
24		9.9

3. An antibiotic is to be given by intravenous infusion. How many milliliters per minute should a sterile drug solution containing 25 mg/ml be given to a 75-kg adult male patient to achieve an infusion rate of 1 mg/kg hr?
4. An antibiotic drug is to be given to an adult male patient (75 kg, 58 years old) by intravenous infusion. The drug is supplied in sterile vials containing 30 ml of the antibiotic solution at a concentration of 125 mg/ml. What rate in milliliters per hour would you infuse this patient to obtain a steady-state concentration of 20 μg/ml? What loading dose would you suggest? Assume the drug follows the pharmacokinetics of a one-compartment open model. The apparent volume of distribution of this drug is 0.5 L/kg and the elimination half-life is 3 hr.
5. According to the manufacturer, a steady-state serum concentration of 17 μg/ml was measured when the antibiotic, cephradine (Velosef, Squibb) was given by IV infusion to nine adult male volunteers (average weight, 71.7 kg) at a rate of 5.3 mg/kg hr for 4 hr.
   a. Calculate the total body clearance for this drug.
   b. When the IV infusion was discontinued, the cephradine serum concentration decreased exponentially, declining to 1.5 μg/ml at 6.5 hr after the start of the infusion.[1] Calculate the elimination half-life.
   c. From the information above calculate the apparent volume of distribution.
   d. Cephradine is completely excreted unchanged in the urine, and studies have shown that probenecid given concurrently causes elevation of the serum cephradine concentration. What is the probable mechanism for this interaction of probenecid with cephradine?
6. Calculate the *excretion rate* at steady state for a drug given by intravenous infusion at a rate of 30 mg/hr. The C_{ss} is 20 μg/ml. If the rate of intravenous infusion were increased to 40 mg/hr, what would be the new steady-state drug concentration, C_{ss}? Would the excretion rate for the drug at the new steady state be the same? Assume first-order elimination kinetics and a one-compartment model.

REFERENCE

1. Physicians' Desk Reference. Oradell, New Jersey, Medical Economics Company, 1981, p. 1747

BIBLIOGRAPHY

Gibaldi M: Estimation of the pharmacokinetic parameters of the two-compartment open model from postinfusion plasma concentration data. J Pharm Sci 58:1133–35, 1969

Koup J, Greenblatt D, Jusko W, Smith T, Koch-Weser J: Pharmacokinetics of digoxin in normal subjects after intravenous bolus and infusion dose. J Pharmacokinet Biopharm 3:181–91, 1975

Loo J, Riegelman S: Assessment of pharmacokinetic constants from postinfusion blood curves obtained after IV infusion. J Pharm Sci 59:53–54, 1970

Loughnam PM, Sitar DS, Ogilvie RI, Neims AH: The two-compartment open system kinetic model: A review of its clinical implications and applications. J Pediatr 88:869–73, 1976

Mitenko P, Ogilvie R: Rapidly achieved plasma concentration plateaus, with observations on theophylline kinetics. Clin Pharmacol Ther 13:329–35, 1972

Riegelman JS, Loo JCK: Assessment of pharmacokinetic constants from postinfusion blood curves obtained after IV infusion. J Pharm Sci 59:53, 1970

Wagner J: A safe method for rapidly achieving plasma concentration plateaus. Clin Pharmacol Ther 16:691–700, 1974

CHAPTER THIRTEEN

Multiple-Dosage Regimens

Many drugs are given in a multiple-dosage regimen for prolonged therapeutic activity. The plasma levels of these drugs must be maintained within narrow limits to achieve maximal clinical effectiveness. Among these drugs are antibacterials, cardiotonics, anticonvulsants, and hormones. Ideally, a dosage regimen is established for each drug to provide the correct plasma level without excessive fluctuation and drug accumulation.

For certain drugs, such as antibiotics, a desirable minimum effective plasma concentration can be determined. Other drugs with narrow therapeutic indices (such as digoxin and phenytoin) require definition of the therapeutic minimum and maximum nontoxic plasma concentrations. In calculating a multiple-dosage regimen, the desired plasma concentration must be related to a therapeutic response. The two main parameters which can be adjusted in developing a dosage regimen are (a) the size of the dose of the drugs and (b) the frequency of drug administration—i.e., the time interval between doses.

DRUG ACCUMULATION

To predict the drug plasma levels during a multiple-dosage regimen, pharmacokinetic parameters are obtained from the plasma level–time curve generated by a single dose of the drug. With these parameters and knowledge of the size of the dose and dosage interval (τ) it is possible to predict the complete plasma level–time curve or the plasma level at any time after the beginning of the dosage regimen.

To calculate multiple-dosage regimens, it is necessary to decide whether successive doses of drug will have any effect on the previous dose. The principle of *superposition* assumes that early doses of drug do not affect the pharmacokinetics of subsequent doses. Therefore, the blood levels after the second, third, or nth dose will overlay or superimpose the blood level attained after the $(n-1)$th dose. In addition, the AUC ($\int_0^\infty C_p\,dt$) following the administration of a single dose equals the AUC ($\int_{t_1}^{t_2} C_p\,dt$) during a dosing interval at steady state (Fig. 13-1).

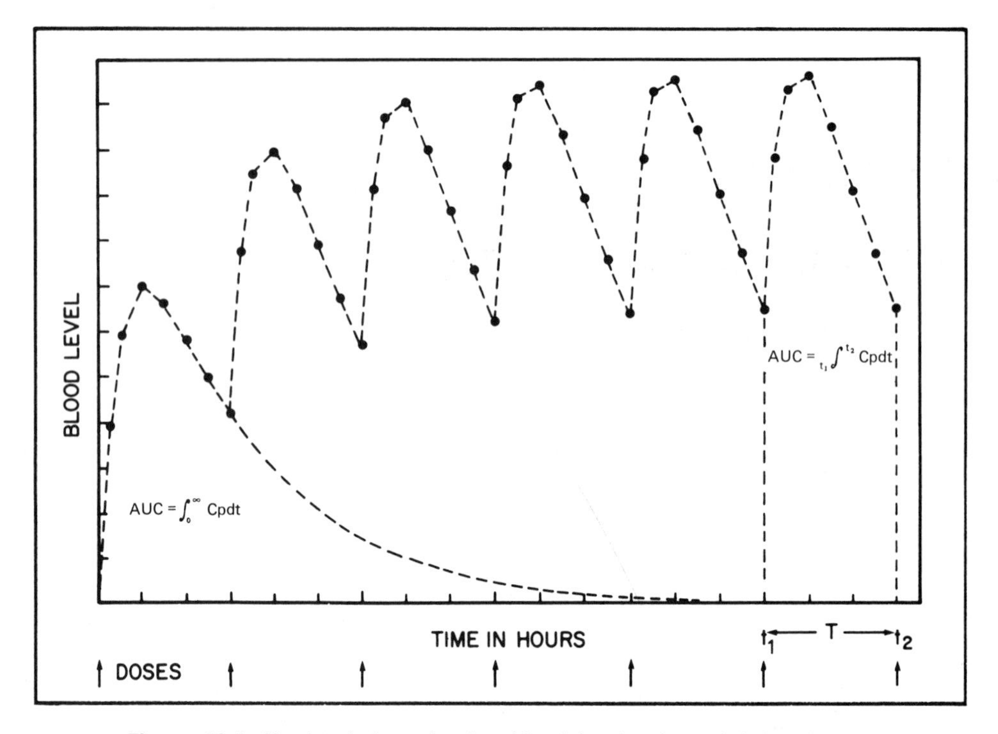

Figure 13-1. Simulated data showing blood levels after administration of multiple doses and accumulation of blood levels when equal doses are given at equal time intervals.

The principle of superposition allows one to project the plasma concentration–time curve of a drug after several consecutive doses based on the plasma drug concentration–time curve obtained after a single dose. The basic assumption is that the drug is eliminated by first-order kinetics and that the pharmacokinetics of the drug after a single dose (first dose) is not altered after taking multiple doses of the drug. From the plasma drug concentrations obtained after a single dose of drug, the plasma drug concentrations after multiple doses may be predicted as shown in Table 13-1. In Table 13-1 the plasma drug concentrations from 0 to 24 hr are measured after a single dose. A constant dose of drug is given every 4 hr and plasma drug concentrations after each dose are generated from the data after the first dose. Thus, the predicted plasma drug concentration in the patient would be the total drug concentration obtained by adding the residual drug concentration obtained after each previous dose. The superposition principle may be used to predict drug concentrations after multiple doses of many drugs. There are situations, however, for which the superposition principle does not apply. In these cases the pharmacokinetics of the drug changes after multiple dosing due to various factors, including changing pathophysiology in the patient, saturation of a drug carrier system, enzyme induction, and enzyme inhibition.

TABLE 13-1. PREDICTED PLASMA DRUG CONCENTRATIONS FOR MULTIPLE-DOSAGE REGIMEN USING THE SUPERPOSITION PRINCIPLE*

Dose Number	Time (hr)	Plasma Drug Concentration (μg/ml)						
		Dose 1	*Dose 2*	*Dose 3*	*Dose 4*	*Dose 5*	*Dose 6*	*Total*
1	0	0						0
	1	21.0						21.0
	2	22.3						22.3
	3	19.8						19.8
2	4	16.9	0					16.9
	5	14.3	21.0					35.3
	6	12.0	22.3					34.3
	7	10.1	19.8					29.9
3	8	8.50	16.9	0				25.4
	9	7.15	14.3	21.0				42.5
	10	6.01	12.0	22.3				40.3
	11	5.06	10.1	19.8				35.0
4	12	4.25	8.50	16.9	0			29.7
	13	3.58	7.15	14.3	21.0			46.0
	14	3.01	6.01	12.0	22.3			43.3
	15	2.53	5.06	10.1	19.8			37.5
5	16	2.13	4.25	8.50	16.9	0		31.8
	17	1.79	3.58	7.15	14.3	21.0		47.8
	18	1.51	3.01	6.01	12.0	22.3		44.8
	19	1.27	2.53	5.06	10.1	19.8		38.8
6	20	1.07	2.13	4.25	8.50	16.9	0	32.9
	21	0.90	1.79	3.58	7.15	14.3	21.0	48.7
	22	0.75	1.51	3.01	6.01	12.0	22.3	45.6
	23	0.63	1.27	2.53	5.06	10.1	19.8	39.4
	24	0.53	1.07	2.13	4.25	8.50	16.9	33.4

*A single oral dose of 350 mg was given and the plasma drug concentrations were measured for 0–24 hr. The same plasma drug concentrations are assumed to occur after doses 2–6. The total plasma drug concentration is the sum of the plasma drug concentrations due to each dose. For this example $V_d = 10$ L, $t_{1/2} = 4$ hr and $K_a = 1.5$ hr^{-1}. The drug is 100% bioavailable and follows the pharmacokinetics of a one-compartment open model.

If the drug is administered at a fixed dose and a fixed-dosage interval, the amount of drug in the body will increase and then plateau to a mean plasma level which is higher than the peak C_p obtained from the initial dose (Figs. 13-1 and 13-2). When the second dose is given after a time interval shorter than the time required to eliminate the previous dose, drug accumulates in the body. However, if the second dose is given after a time interval longer than the time required to eliminate the previous dose, drug will not accumulate (Table 13-1).

As repetitive equal doses are given at a constant frequency, the plasma level–time curve plateaus and a steady state is obtained. At steady state the plasma drug levels fluctuate between C_{max}^{∞} and C_{min}^{∞}. An average steady-state plasma drug concentration, C_{av}^{∞}, is obtained by dividing the AUC for a dosing period (i.e., $\int_{t_1}^{t_2} C_p\, dt$) by the dosing interval, τ, at steady state. Once steady state is obtained,

C_{max}^{∞} and C_{min}^{∞} are constant and remain unchanged from dose to dose. The C_{max}^{∞} is important in determining drug safety. The C_{max}^{∞} should always remain below the minimum toxic concentration. The C_{max}^{∞} is also a good indication of drug accumulation. If a drug produces the same C_{max}^{∞} at steady state, compared with the $(C_{n=1})_{max}$ after the first dose, then there is no drug accumulation. If C_{max}^{∞} is much larger than $(C_{n=1})_{max}$, then there is significant accumulation. Accumulation is affected by the elimination half-life of the drug and the dosing interval. The index for measuring drug accumulation R is

$$R = \frac{(C^{\infty})_{max}}{(C_{n=1})_{max}} \tag{13.1}$$

Substituting for C_{max} after the first dose and at steady state yields the following equation.

$$R = \frac{D_0/V_d[1/(1-e^{-K\tau})]}{D_0/V_d}$$

$$R = \frac{1}{1-e^{-K\tau}} \tag{13.2}$$

Equation 13.2 shows that drug accumulation measured with the R index depends on the elimination constant and the dosing interval and is independent of the dose.

For a drug given in repetitive oral doses, the time required to reach steady state is dependent on the elimination half-life of the drug and is independent of the size of the dose, the length of the dosing interval, and the number of doses. For example, if the dose or dosage interval of the drug is altered as shown in Figure 13-2, the time

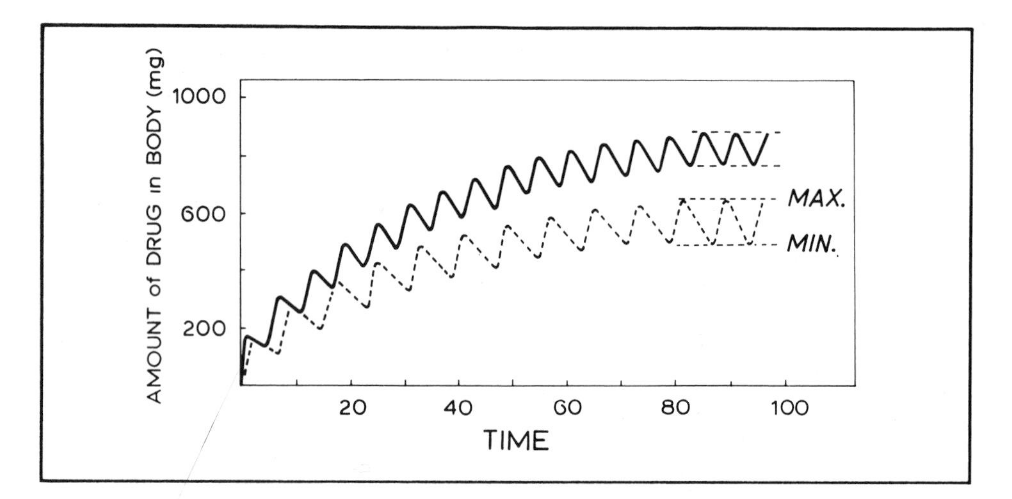

Figure 13-2. Amount of drug in the body as a function of time. Equal doses of drug were given every 6 hr (upper curve) and every 8 hr (lower curve). K_a and K remain constant.

required for the drug to reach steady state is the same, but the final steady-state plasma level changes proportionately.

An equation for the estimation of the time to reach one-half of the steady-state plasma levels or the accumulation half-life has been described by van Rossum and Tomey:[1]

$$\text{Accumulation } t_{1/2} = t_{1/2}\left(1 + 3.3 \log \frac{K_a}{K_a - K}\right) \tag{13.3}$$

For IV administration K_a is very rapid. K is very small in comparison to K_a and can be omitted in the denominator of Equation 13.3. Thus, Equation 13.3 reduces to

$$\text{Accumulation } t_{1/2} = t_{1/2}\left(1 + 3.3 \log \frac{K_a}{K_a}\right) \tag{13.4}$$

Since $K_a/K_a = 1$ and $\log 1 = 0$, the accumulation $t_{1/2}$ of a drug administered intravenously is the elimination $t_{1/2}$ of the drug. From this relationship the time to reach 50% steady-state drug concentrations is dependent on the elimination $t_{1/2}$ and not on the dose or dosage interval.

From a clinical viewpoint, the time needed to reach 90% of the steady-state plasma concentration is 3.3 times the elimination half-life, whereas the time required to reach 99% of the steady-state plasma concentration is 6.6 times the elimination half-life (Table 13-2). It should be noted from Table 13-2 that the shorter the dosage interval, the higher the steady-state drug level.

TABLE 13-2. INTERRELATION OF ELIMINATION HALF-LIFE, DOSAGE INTERVAL, MAXIMUM PLASMA CONCENTRATION, AND TIME TO REACH STEADY-STATE PLASMA CONCENTRATION*

Elimination Half-Life	Dosage Interval, τ	C_{max}^{∞} (μg/ml)	Time for C_{av}^{∞}†
0.5	0.5	200	3.3
0.5	1.0	133	3.3
1.0	0.5	341	6.6
1.0	1.0	200	6.6
1.0	2.0	133	6.6
1.0	4.0	107	6.6
1.0	10.0	100‡	6.6
2.0	1.0	341	13.2
2.0	2.0	200	13.2

*A single dose of 1000 mg of three hypothetical drugs with various elimination half-lives but equal volumes of distribution ($V_d = 10$ L) were given by multiple IV doses at various dosing intervals. All time values are in hours; (C_{max}^{∞}) = maximum steady-state concentration; C_{av}^{∞} = average steady-state plasma concentration. The maximum plasma drug concentration after the first dose of the drug is $(C_{n=1})_{max} = 100$ μg/ml.

†Time to reach 99% of steady-state plasma concentration.

‡Since the dosage interval, τ, is very large compared to the elimination half-life, no accumulation of drug occurs.

REPETITIVE INTRAVENOUS INJECTIONS

The maximum amount of drug in the body following a rapid intravenous injection is equal to the dose of the drug. For a one-compartment open model, the drug will be eliminated according to first-order kinetics:

$$D = D_0 e^{-Kt} \tag{13.5}$$

If τ is equal to the dosage interval (i.e., the time between the first dose and the next dose), then the amount of drug remaining in the body after several hours can be determined with

$$D = D_0 e^{-K\tau} \tag{13.6}$$

The fraction (f) of the dose remaining in the body is related to the elimination constant (K) and the dosage interval (τ) as follows.

$$f = \frac{D}{D_0} = e^{-K\tau} \tag{13.7}$$

With any given dose, f depends on K and τ. If τ is large, f will be smaller since D (the amount of drug remaining in the body) is smaller.

EXAMPLE

A patient receives 1000 mg every 6 hr by repetitive intravenous injection of an antibiotic with an elimination half-life of 3 hr. Assume the drug is distributed according to a one-compartment model and the volume of distribution is 20 L. Find the maximum and minimum amount of drug in the body and determine the maximum and minimum plasma concentration of the drug.

The fraction of drug remaining in the body can be found by Equation 13.7. The concentration of the drug declines to one-half after 3 hr ($t_{1/2} = 3$ hr), after which the amount of drug will again decline by one-half at the end of the next 3 hr. Therefore, at the end of 6 hr only one-quarter, or 0.25, of the original dose remains in the body. Thus f is equal to 0.25.

To use Equation 13.7, we must first find the value of K from the $t_{1/2}$:

$$K = \frac{0.693}{t_{1/2}} = \frac{0.693}{3} = 0.231 \text{ hr}^{-1}$$

The time interval, τ, is equal to 6 hr. From Equation 13.7,

$$f = e^{-(0.231)(6)}$$

$$f = 0.25$$

In this example 1000 mg of drug is given intravenously so that the amount of drug in the body is immediately increased by 1000 mg. At the end of the dosage interval (i.e., before the next dose) the amount of drug remaining in the body is 25% of the amount of drug present just after the previous dose, since $f = 0.25$. Thus, if the value of f is known, a table can be constructed relating the fraction of the dose in the body before and after rapid IV injection (Table 13-3).

TABLE 13-3. FRACTION OF THE DOSE IN THE BODY BEFORE AND AFTER INTRAVENOUS INJECTIONS OF A 1000-MG DOSE*

Number of Doses	Amount of Drug in Body	
	Before Dose	*After Dose*
1	0	1000
2	250	1250
3	312	1312
4	328	1328
5	332	1332
6	333	1333
7	333	1333
∞	333	1333

*$f = 0.25$

From Table 13-3 the maximum amount of drug in the body is 1333 mg, and the minimum amount of drug in the body is 333 mg. The difference between the maximum and minimum values, D_0, will always equal the injected dose.

$$D_{max} - D_{min} = D_0 \qquad (13.8)$$

In this example

$$1333 - 333 = 1000 \text{ mg}$$

D_{max} can also be calculated directly by the relationship

$$D_{max} = \frac{D_0}{1 - f} \qquad (13.9)$$

Substituting known data, we obtain

$$D_{max} = \frac{1000}{1 - 0.25} = 1333 \text{ mg}$$

then, from Equation 13.8,

$$D_{min} = 1333 - 1000 = 333 \text{ mg}$$

The average amount of drug in the body at steady state, D_{av}^{∞}, can be found by Equation 13.10 or 13.11. F is the fraction of dose absorbed. For IV injection F is equal to 1.0.

$$D_{av}^{\infty} = \frac{FD_0}{K\tau} \qquad (13.10)$$

$$D_{av}^{\infty} = \frac{FD_0 1.44 t_{1/2}}{\tau} \qquad (13.11)$$

Equations 13.10 and 13.11 can be used for repetitive dosing at constant time intervals and for any route of administration as long as elimination occurs from the central compartment.

Substitution of values from the example into Equation 13.11 gives

$$D_{av}^{\infty} = \frac{(1)(1000)(1.44)(3)}{6} = 720 \text{ mg}$$

The value D_{av}^{∞} is not the arithmetic mean of D_{max}^{∞} and D_{min}^{∞}. The limitation of using D_{av}^{∞} is that the fluctuations of D_{max}^{∞} and D_{min}^{∞} are not known.

In order to determine the concentration of drug in the body after multiple dosing, divide the amount of drug in the body by the volume in which it is dissolved. For a one-compartment model, the maximum, minimum, and steady-state concentrations of drug in the plasma are found by the following equations:

$$C_{max}^{\infty} = \frac{D_{max}^{\infty}}{V_d} \tag{13.12}$$

$$C_{min}^{\infty} = \frac{D_{min}^{\infty}}{V_d} \tag{13.13}$$

$$C_{av}^{\infty} = \frac{D_{av}^{\infty}}{V_d} \tag{13.14}$$

A more direct approach to finding C_{max}^{∞}, C_{min}^{∞}, and C_{av}^{∞} is as follows:

$$C_{max}^{\infty} = \frac{C_p^0}{1 - e^{-K\tau}} \tag{13.15}$$

$$C_{min}^{\infty} = \frac{C_p^0 e^{-K\tau}}{1 - e^{-K\tau}} \tag{13.16}$$

$$C_{av}^{\infty} = \frac{FD_0}{V_d K\tau} \tag{13.17}$$

For this example the values for C_{max}^{∞}, C_{min}^{∞}, and C_{av}^{∞} are 66.7, 16.7, and 36.1 μg/ml, respectively.

As mentioned, C_{av}^{∞} is not the arithmetic mean of C_{max}^{∞} and C_{min}^{∞} since plasma drug concentration decline exponentially. The C_{av}^{∞} is equal to the AUC ($\int_{t_1}^{t_2} C_p \, dt$) for a dosage interval at steady state divided by the dosage interval τ.

$$C_{av}^{\infty} = \frac{[\text{AUC}]_{t_1}^{t_2}}{\tau} \tag{13.18}$$

The AUC is related to the amount of drug absorbed divided by total body clearance, as shown in the following equation:

$$[\text{AUC}]_{t_1}^{t_2} = \frac{FD_0}{\text{Cl}_T} = \frac{FD_0}{KV_d} \tag{13.19}$$

Substitution of FD_0/KV_d for AUC in Equation 13.18 gives Equation 13.17. Equation 13.17 or 13.18 can be used to obtain the C_{av}^{∞} after a multiple-dosage regimen regardless of the route of administration.

It is sometimes desirable to know the plasma drug concentration at any time after the administration of n doses of drug. The general expression for calculating this plasma drug concentration is

$$C_p = \frac{D_0}{V_d}\left(\frac{1 - e^{-nK\tau}}{1 - e^{-K\tau}}\right)e^{-Kt} \tag{13.20}$$

where n is the number of doses given and t is the time after the nth dose.

At steady state $e^{-nK\tau}$ approaches zero and Equation 13.20 reduces to

$$C_p^{\infty} = \frac{D_0}{V_d}\left(\frac{1}{1 - e^{-K\tau}}\right)e^{-Kt} \tag{13.21}$$

where C_p^{∞} is the steady-state drug concentration at time t after the dose.

EXAMPLE

The patient in the previous example received 1000 mg of an antibiotic every 6 hr by repetitive intravenous injection. The drug has an apparent volume of distribution of 20 L and elimination half-life of 3 hr. Calculate (1) the plasma drug concentration C_p at 3 hr after the second dose and (2) the steady-state plasma drug concentration C_p^{∞} at 3 hr after the last dose.

Solution

1. The C_p at 3 hr after the second dose. Use Equation 13.20 and let $n = 2$, $t = 3$ hr, and make other appropriate substitutions:

$$C_p = \frac{1000}{20}\left(\frac{1 - e^{-(2)(0.231)(6)}}{1 - e^{-(0.231)(6)}}\right)e^{-0.231(3)}$$
$$= 31.3 \text{ mg/L}$$

2. The C_p^{∞} at 3 hr after the last dose. Since steady state is reached, use Equation 13.21 and perform the following calculation:

$$C_p^{\infty} = \frac{1000}{20}\left(\frac{1}{1 - e^{-0.231(6)}}\right)e^{-0.231(3)}$$
$$= 33.3 \text{ mg/L}$$

MULTIPLE ORAL DOSE REGIMEN

Figures 13-1 and 13-2 present typical cumulation curves for the concentration of drug in the body after multiple oral dose given at a constant dosage interval. The plasma concentration at any time during a multiple-dose regimen, assuming a one-compartment model and constant doses and dose interval, can be determined as follows.

$$C_p = \frac{FK_aD_0}{V_d(K - K_a)}\left[\left(\frac{1 - e^{-nK_a\tau}}{1 - e^{-K_a\tau}}\right)e^{-K_at} - \left(\frac{1 - e^{-nK\tau}}{1 - e^{-K\tau}}\right)e^{-Kt}\right] \tag{13.22}$$

where n = number of doses; τ = dosage interval; F = fraction of dose absorbed; and t = time after administration of n doses.

The mean plasma level at steady state, C_{av}^{∞}, is determined by a similar method employed for repeat IV injections. Equation 13.17 can be used for finding C_{av}^{∞} for any route of administration:

$$C_{av}^{\infty} = \frac{FD_0}{V_d K \tau} \qquad \text{(Eq. 13.17)}$$

Since proper evaluation of F and V_d requires IV data, the AUC of a dosing interval at steady state may be substituted in Equation 13.17 to obtain the following:

$$C_{av}^{\infty} = \frac{\int_0^{\infty} C_p \, dt}{\tau} = \frac{[\text{AUC}]_0^{\infty}}{\tau} \qquad (13.23)$$

One can see from Equation 13.17 that the magnitude of C_{av}^{∞} is directly proportional to the size of the dose and the extent of drug absorbed. Furthermore, if the dosage interval (τ) is shortened, then the value for C_{av}^{∞} will increase. The C_{av}^{∞} will be predictably higher for drugs distributed in a small V_d (e.g., plasma water) or which have long elimination half-lives than for drugs distributed in a large V_d (e.g., total body water) or have very short elimination half-lives. Since body clearance (Cl_T) is equal to KV_d, substitution into Equation 13.17 yields

$$C_{av}^{\infty} = \frac{FD_0}{Cl_T \tau} \qquad (13.24)$$

Thus, if Cl_T decreases, the C_{av}^{∞} will increase.

The C_{av}^{∞} does not give information concerning the fluctuations in plasma concentration—i.e., C_{max}^{∞} and C_{min}^{∞}. In multiple-dosage regimens C_p at any time can be obtained with Equation 13.22, where $n = n$th dose. At steady state the drug concentration can be determined by letting n equal infinity. Therefore, $e^{-nK\tau}$ becomes approximately equal to zero and Equation 13.22 becomes

$$C_p^{\infty} = \frac{K_a F D_0}{V_d (K_a - K)} \left[\left(\frac{1}{1 - e^{-K\tau}} \right) e^{-Kt} - \left(\frac{1}{1 - e^{-K_a \tau}} \right) e^{-K_a t} \right] \qquad (13.25)$$

The maximum and minimum drug concentrations (C_{max}^{∞} and C_{min}^{∞}) can be obtained with the following equations:

$$C_{max}^{\infty} = \frac{FD_0}{V_d} \left(\frac{1}{1 - e^{-K\tau}} \right) e^{-Kt_p} \qquad (13.26)$$

$$C_{min}^{\infty} = \frac{K_a F D_0}{V_d (K_a - K)} \left(\frac{1}{1 - e^{-K\tau}} \right) e^{-K\tau} \qquad (13.27)$$

The time at which maximum (peak) plasma concentration (or t_{max}) occurs following a single oral dose is

$$t_{max} = \frac{2.3}{K_a - K} \log \frac{K_a}{K} \qquad (13.28)$$

whereas the peak plasma concentration t_p following multiple doses is given by Equation 13.29.

Large fluctuations between C_{max}^{∞} and C_{min}^{∞} can be hazardous, particularly with drugs that have a narrow therapeutic index. The larger the number of divided doses, the smaller the fluctuations in plasma concentration. For example, a 500-mg dose of drug given every 6 hr will produce the same C_{av}^{∞} value as a 250-mg dose of the same drug given every 3 hr, while the C_{max}^{∞} and C_{min}^{∞} fluctuations for the latter dose will be decreased by one-half. With drugs that have a narrow therapeutic index, the dosage interval should not be longer than the elimination half-life.

EXAMPLE

An adult, male patient (46 years old, 81 kg) was given orally 250 mg of tetracycline hydrochloride every 8 hr for 2 weeks. From the literature, tetracycline hydrochloride is about 75% bioavailable and has an apparent volume of distribution of 1.5 L/kg. The elimination half-life is about 10 hr. The absorption rate constant is 0.9 hr^{-1}. From this information calculate (1) the C_{max} after the first dose; (2) the C_{min} after the first dose; (3) the plasma drug concentration C_p at 4 hr after the seventh dose; (4) the maximum plasma drug concentration at steady state, C_{max}^{∞}; (5) the minimum plasma drug concentration at steady state, C_{min}^{∞}; and (6) the average plasma drug concentration at steady state, C_{av}^{∞}.

Solution

1. The C_{max} after the first dose. The C_{max} occurs at T_{max}. Therefore, using Equation 13.28,

$$t_{max} = \frac{2.3}{0.9 - 0.07} \log 0.9/0.07$$
$$= 3.07 \text{ hr}$$

Then substitute t_{max} into the following equation for a single oral dose (one-compartment model) to obtain C_{max}:

$$C_{max} = \frac{FD_0 K_a}{V_d(K_a - K)}(e^{-Kt_{max}} - e^{-K_a t_{max}})$$
$$= \frac{(0.75)(250)(0.9)}{(121.5)(0.9 - 0.07)}(e^{-0.07(3.07)} - e^{0.9(3.07)})$$
$$= 1.28 \text{ mg/L}$$

2. The C_{min} after the first dose. The C_{min} occurs just before the administration of the next dose of drug. Therefore, set $t = 8$ hr and solve for C_{min}:

$$C_{min} = \frac{(0.75)(250)(0.9)}{(121.5)(0.9 - 0.07)}(e^{-0.07(8)} - e^{-0.9(8)})$$
$$= 0.95 \text{ mg/L}$$

3. The C_p at 4 hr after the seventh dose. The C_p may be calculated by Equation 13.22 letting $n=7$, $t=4$, $\tau=8$, and making the appropriate substitutions:

$$C_p = \frac{(0.75)(250)(0.9)}{(121.5)(0.07-0.9)}$$

$$\times\left[\left(\frac{1-e^{-(7)(0.9)(8)}}{1-e^{-0.9(8)}}\right)e^{-0.9(4)} - \left(\frac{1-e^{-(7)(0.07)(8)}}{1-e^{-(0.07)(8)}}\right)e^{-0.07(4)}\right]$$

$$= 2.86 \text{ mg/L}$$

4. The C_{max}^{∞} at steady state. The t_p at steady state is obtained from the equation

$$t_p = \frac{1}{K_a - K}\ln\left[\frac{K_a(1-e^{-K\tau})}{K(1-e^{-K_a\tau})}\right] \quad (13.29)$$

$$= \frac{1}{0.9-0.07}\ln\left[\frac{0.9(1-e^{-(0.07)(8)})}{0.07(1-e^{-(0.9)(8)})}\right]$$

$$= 2.05 \text{ hr}$$

Then C_{max}^{∞} is obtained using Equation 13.26

$$C_{max}^{\infty} = \frac{0.75(250)}{121.5}\left(\frac{1}{1-e^{-0.07(8)}}\right)e^{-0.07(2.05)}$$

$$= 3.12 \text{ mg/L}$$

5. The C_{min}^{∞} at steady state. The C_{min}^{∞} is calculated from Equation 13.27

$$C_{min}^{\infty} = \frac{(0.9)(0.75)(250)}{(121.5)(0.9-0.07)}\left(\frac{1}{1-e^{-0.07(8)}}\right)e^{-(0.07)(8)}$$

$$= 2.23 \text{ mg/L}$$

6. The C_{av}^{∞} at steady state. The C_{av}^{∞} is calculated from Equation 13.17

$$C_{av}^{\infty} = \frac{(0.75)(250)}{(121.5)(0.07)(8)}$$

$$= 2.76 \text{ mg/L}$$

LOADING DOSE

As discussed earlier, the time required for the drug to accumulate to a steady-state plasma level is dependent mainly on its elimination half-life. The time needed to reach 90% of the C_{av}^{∞} is approximately 3.3 half-lives, and the time required to reach 99% of the C_{av}^{∞} is equal to approximately 6.6 half-lives. For a drug with a half-life of

4 hr, it would take approximately 13 and 26 hr to reach 90% and 99% of the C_{av}^{∞}, respectively.

To reduce the onset time of the drug—i.e., the time it takes to achieve the minimum effective dose (assumed to be equivalent to the C_{av}^{∞})—a loading (priming) or initial dose of drug is given. The main objective of the loading dose is to achieve the C_{av}^{∞} as quickly as possible. Thereafter, a maintenance dose is given to maintain the C_{av}^{∞} so that the therapeutic effect is also maintained.

For drugs absorbed rapidly in relation to elimination ($K_a \gg K$) and which are distributed rapidly, the loading dose, D_L, can be calculated as follows:

$$\frac{D_L}{D_0} = \frac{1}{(1 - e^{-K_a\tau})(1 - e^{-K\tau})} \tag{13.30}$$

For extremely rapid absorption, as when the product of $K_a\tau$ is large or in the case of IV infusion, $e^{-K_a\tau}$ becomes approximately zero and Equation 13.30 reduces to

$$\frac{D_L}{D_0} = \frac{1}{1 - e^{-K\tau}} \tag{13.31}$$

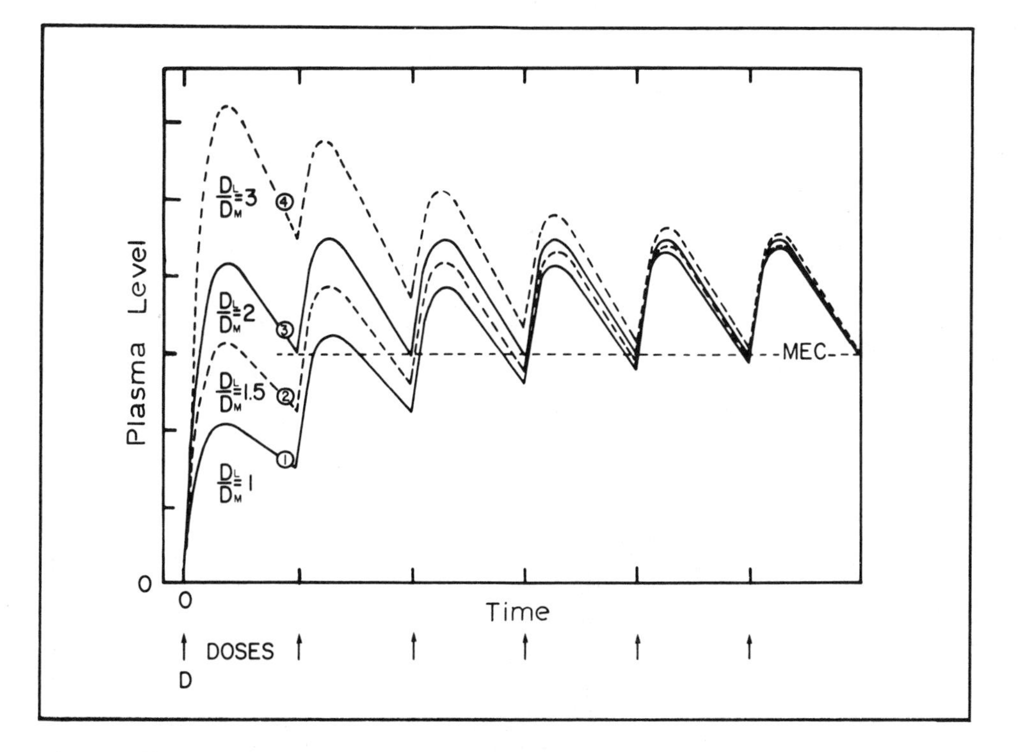

Figure 13-3. Concentration curves for dosage regimens with equal maintenance doses (D) and dosage intervals (τ) and different dose ratios. (*From Kruger-Thiemer E, 1968, with permission.*[2])

Thus the loading dose should approximate the amount of drug contained in the body during steady state. The dose ratio is equal to the loading dose divided by the maintenance dose.

$$\text{Dose ratio} = \frac{D_L}{D_0} \tag{13.32}$$

As a general rule, the dose ratio should be equal to 2.0 if the selected dosage interval is equal to the elimination half-life. Figure 13-3 shows the plasma level–time curve for dosage regimens with equal maintenance doses but different loading doses. A rapid approximation of loading dose D_L may be estimated from the following equation:

$$D_L = \frac{V_d C_{av}^{\infty}}{(S)(F)} \tag{13.33}$$

where C_{av}^{∞} is the desired plasma drug concentration; S is the salt form of the drug, and F is the fraction of drug bioavailable.

Equation 13.33 assumes very rapid drug absorption from an immediate release dosage form. The D_L calculated by this method has been used in clinical situations for which only an approximation of the D_L is needed.

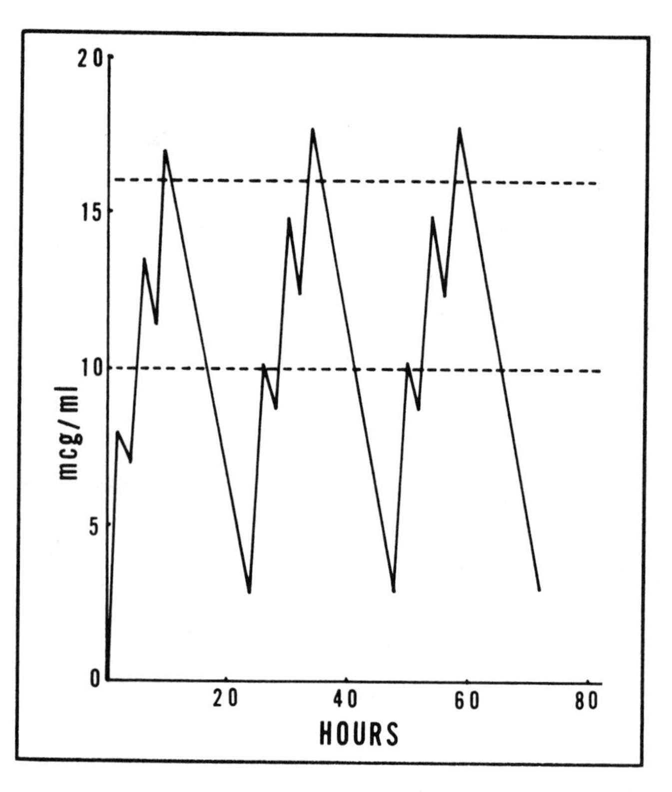

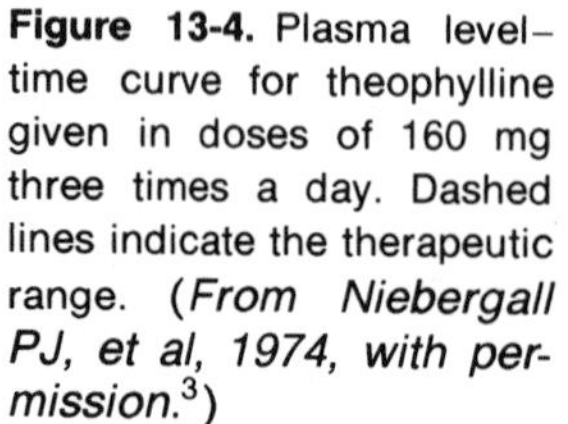

Figure 13-4. Plasma level–time curve for theophylline given in doses of 160 mg three times a day. Dashed lines indicate the therapeutic range. (*From Niebergall PJ, et al, 1974, with permission.*[3])

These calculations for loading doses are not applicable to drugs which demonstrate multicompartment kinetics. Such drugs distribute slowly into extravascular tissues, and drug equilibration may not take place until after the apparent plateau is reached in the vascular (central) compartment.

SCHEDULING OF DOSAGE REGIMEN

Predictions of steady-state plasma concentrations usually assume the drug is given at a constant dosage interval throughout a 24-hr day. Very often, however, the drug is only given during the waking hours. Niebergall et al[3] have discussed the problem of scheduling dosage regimens and have particularly warned against improper timing of the drug dosage. For example, Figure 13-4 shows the plasma levels of theophylline given three times a day. Notice that there is quite a large fluctuation between the maximum and minimum plasma levels. In comparison, procainamide was given on a 0.5-g, four-times-a-day maintenance dosage with a 1.0-g loading dose on the first day (Fig. 13-5); on the second and third days plasma levels did not reach the therapeutic range until after the second dose of drug.

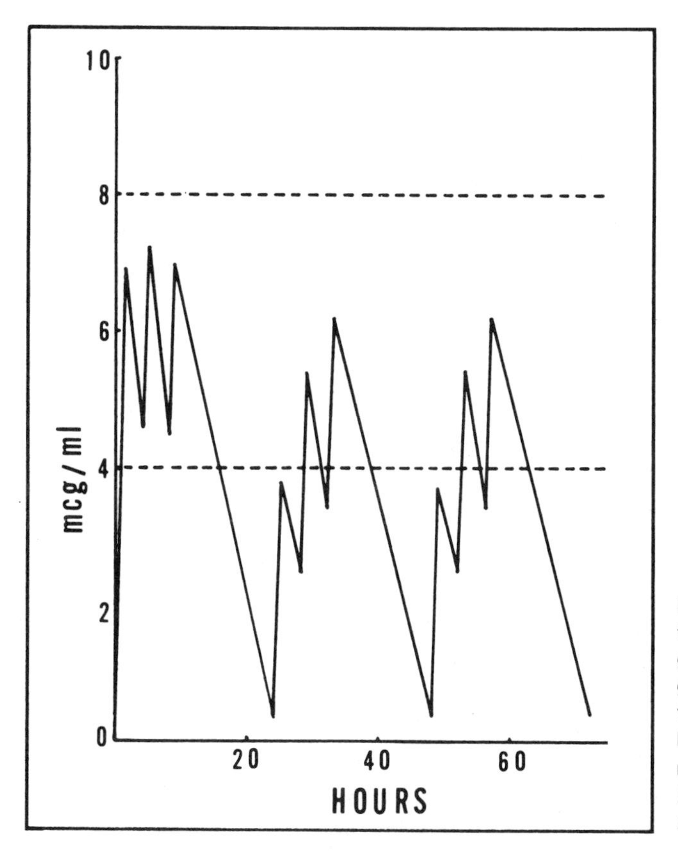

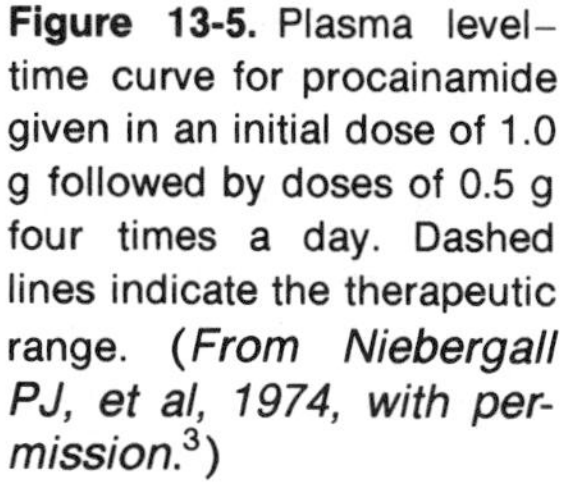

Figure 13-5. Plasma level–time curve for procainamide given in an initial dose of 1.0 g followed by doses of 0.5 g four times a day. Dashed lines indicate the therapeutic range. (*From Niebergall PJ, et al, 1974, with permission.*[3])

DETERMINATION OF BIOAVAILABILITY AND BIOEQUIVALENCY IN A MULTIPLE-DOSE REGIMEN

A number of drugs are given in a multiple-dose regimen for prophylactic treatment of a chronic disease. Examples of such drugs include anticonvulsants, cardiotonics, hypoglycemics, and others which patients use to prevent a sudden acute attack of the given illness. To evaluate the bioequivalence of a drug in these patients with only a single dose could be dangerous. Furthermore, repeated administration of drugs may cause a change in body clearance through an alteration in hepatic metabolism and/or renal excretion. The extent of bioavailability, measured by assuming the $[\mathrm{AUC}]_0^\infty$, is dependent on clearance:

$$[\mathrm{AUC}]_0^\infty = \frac{FD_0}{\mathrm{Cl_T}} \qquad (13.34)$$

Determination of bioavailability using multiple doses reveals changes that are normally not detected in a single-dose study. With some drugs a drug-induced malabsorption syndrome can also alter the percentage of drug absorbed. Thus, drug bioavailability may decrease after repeated doses if the fraction of the dose absorbed (F) decreases or if the total body clearance (KV_d) increases.

In evaluating drug bioavailability information, one must consider the experimental design used to obtain the data. Otherwise, differences due to artifact might be mistaken for real differences in bioavailability. Estimation of the absorption rate constant during multiple dosing is difficult, since the residual drug from the previous dose superimposes on the dose that follows. However, the data obtained in multiple doses is useful in calculating a steady-state plasma level.

Bioavailability may be determined during a multiple-dose regimen only after a steady-state plasma drug level has been reached. As discussed, the time needed to reach the steady-state plasma level is related to the elimination $t_{1/2}$ of the drug. As observed in Table 13-2, it takes approximately 6.6 half-lives to reach 99% of the C_{av}^∞.

The parameters for bioavailability of a drug using plasma level data from a multiple-dose regimen are similar to those obtained with a single-dose regimen. In the former case the first plasma samples are taken just prior to the second dose of the drug. Thereafter, plasma samples are taken periodically after the dose is administered to adequately describe the entire plasma level–time curve (Fig. 13-1). Parameters including AUC, time for peak drug concentration, and peak drug concentration are then used to describe the bioavailability of the drug.

In a bioequivalence study the first step is to determine the bioavailability of a standard or well-known drug product (Fig. 13-6, drug product A). Once this is accomplished, the patient begins to take equal oral doses of an alternate drug product. Again, time must be allowed for the theoretical attainment of C_{av}^∞ with the second drug product. When steady state is reached, the plasma level–time curve for a dosage interval with the second drug product is described (Fig. 13-6, drug product B). Using the same plasma parameters as before, the bioequivalence or lack of bioequivalence may be determined.

There are a number of advantages to using this method for the determination of bioequivalence: (1) the patient acts as his or her own control; (2) the patient maintains a minimum plasma drug concentration; and (3) the plasma samples after

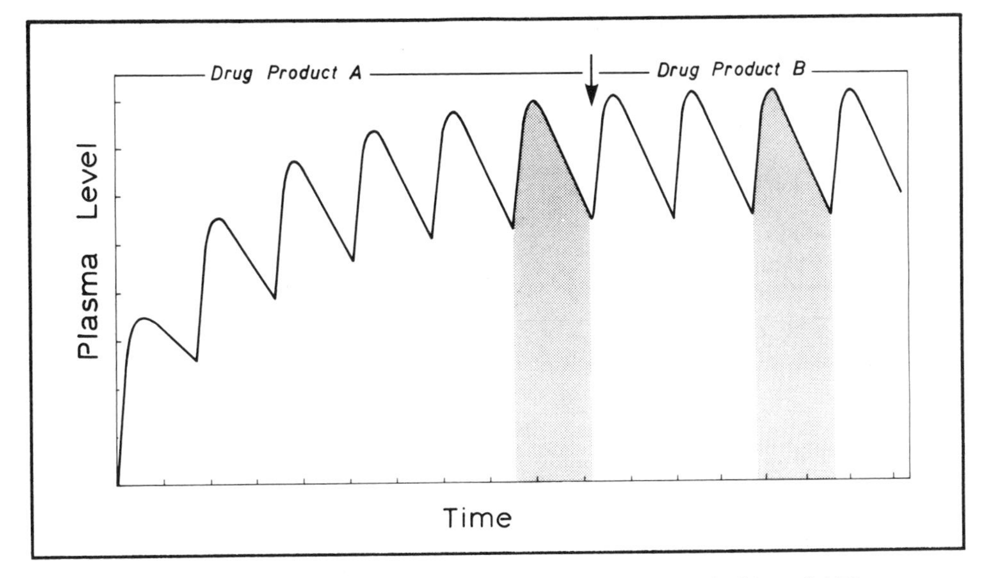

Figure 13-6. Multiple-dose bioequivalency study comparing the bioavailability of drug product *B* to the bioavailability of drug product *A*. Blood levels for such studies must be taken after C_{av}^{∞} is reached. The arrow represents the start of therapy with drug product *B*.

multiple doses contain more drug and can be assayed more accurately. The disadvantages for using this method include the following: (1) the study takes more time to perform, since steady-state conditions must be reached, and (2) sometimes more plasma samples must be obtained from the patient to ascertain that steady state is reached and to describe the plasma level–time curve accurately.

Since the C_{av}^{∞} depends primarily on the dose of the drug and the time interval between doses, the extent of drug systemically available is more important than the rate of drug availability. If there is wide variation in the rate of a drug's availability, then it is possible that initial high blood levels may lead to toxicity.

If the blood level–time curve of the second drug product is comparable to that of the reference drug product, the second product is considered to be bioequivalent. If the second drug has less bioavailability (assuming that only the extent of drug absorption is less than that of the reference drug), the resulting C_{av}^{∞} will be smaller than that obtained with the first drug. Usually the drug manufacturer will perform dissolution tests prior to performing a bioequivalence study. These in vitro dissolution tests will help to ensure that the C_{av}^{∞} obtained from each drug product in vivo will not be largely different from each other. In contrast, if the extent of drug availability is greater in the second drug product, the C_{av}^{∞} will be higher.

PRACTICE PROBLEMS

1. Patient C.S. is a 35-year-old male weighing 76.6 kg. The patient is to be given multiple intravenous bolus injections of an antibiotic every 6 hr. The effective concentration of this drug is 15 μg/ml. After the patient is given a

single IV dose, the elimination half-life for the drug is determined to be 3.0 hr and the apparent V_d is 196 ml/kg.

a. Determine a multiple IV dose regimen for this drug (assume drug is given every 6 hr).

Solution

$$C_{av}^{\infty} = \frac{FD_0}{V_d K \tau}$$

For IV dose $F = 1$,

$$D_0 = (15\ \mu g/ml)\left(\frac{0.693}{3\ hr}\right)(196\ ml/kg)(6\ hr)$$
$$= 4.07\ mg/kg \text{ every } 6\ hr$$

Since patient C.S. weighs 76.6 kg, the dose should be

$$D_0 = (4.07\ mg/kg)(76.6\ kg)$$
$$= 312\ mg \text{ every } 6\ hr$$

Solution

After the condition of this patient has stabilized, the patient is to be given the drug orally for convenience of drug administration. It is desirable to design an oral dosage regimen which will produce the same steady-state blood level as the multiple IV doses. The drug dose will depend on the bioavailability of the drug from the drug product, the desired therapeutic drug level, and the dosage interval chosen. Assume that the antibiotic is 90% bioavailable and the physician would like to continue oral medication every 6 hr.

The average or steady-state plasma drug level is given by

$$C_{av}^{\infty} = \frac{FD_0}{V_d K \tau}$$

Since $K = 0.693/t_{1/2}$,

$$C_{av}^{\infty} = \frac{FD_0 1.44 t_{1/2}}{V_d \tau}$$

Since the literature may give the total body clearance Cl_T for the drug, the above equation is equivalent to

$$C_{av}^{\infty} = \frac{FD_0}{Cl_T \tau}$$

Where $Cl_T = KV_d$ for a one-compartment model, or $Cl_T = bV_p$ for a two-compartment model.

$$D_0 = \frac{(15\ \mu g/ml)(196\ ml/kg)(6\ hr)}{(0.9)(1.44)(3\ hr)}$$

$$= 4.54\ mg/kg$$

Since patient C.S. weighs 76.6 kg, he should be given the following dose.

$$D_0 = (4.54\ mg/kg)(76.6\ kg)$$

$$= 348\ mg\ \text{every 6 hr}$$

For drugs with equal absorption but slower absorption rates (F is the same but K_a is smaller), the initial dosing period may show a lower blood level; however, the steady-state blood level will be unchanged.

2. In practice, drug products are usually commercially available in certain specified strengths. Using the information provided in the preceding problem, assume that the antibiotic is available in 125-, 250-, and 500-mg tablets. Therefore, the pharmacist or prescriber must now decide which tablets are to be given to the patient. In this case it may be possible to give the patient 375 mg (i.e., one 125-mg tablet and one 250-mg tablet) every 6 hr. However, the C_{av}^{∞} should be calculated to determine if the plasma level is approaching a toxic value. Alternatively, a new dosage interval might be appropriate for the patient. It is very important to design the dosage interval and dose to be as simple as possible so that the patient will not be confused and will be able to comply with the medication program properly.

a. What is the new C_{av}^{∞} if the patient is given 375 mg every 6 hr?

Solution

$$C_{av}^{\infty} = \frac{(0.9)(375{,}000)(1.44)(3)}{(196)(76.6)(6)}$$

$$= 16.2\ \mu g/ml$$

Since the therapeutic objective was to achieve a minimum effective concentration (MEC) of 15 $\mu g/ml$, a value of 16.2 $\mu g/ml$ is reasonable.

b. The patient has difficulty in distinguishing tablets of different strengths. Can the patient take a 500-mg dose (i.e., two 250-mg tablets)?

Solution

The dosage interval, τ, for the 500-mg tablet would have to be calculated as follows.

$$\tau = \frac{(0.9)(500{,}000)(1.44)(3)}{(196)(76.6)(15)}$$

$$= 8.63\ hr$$

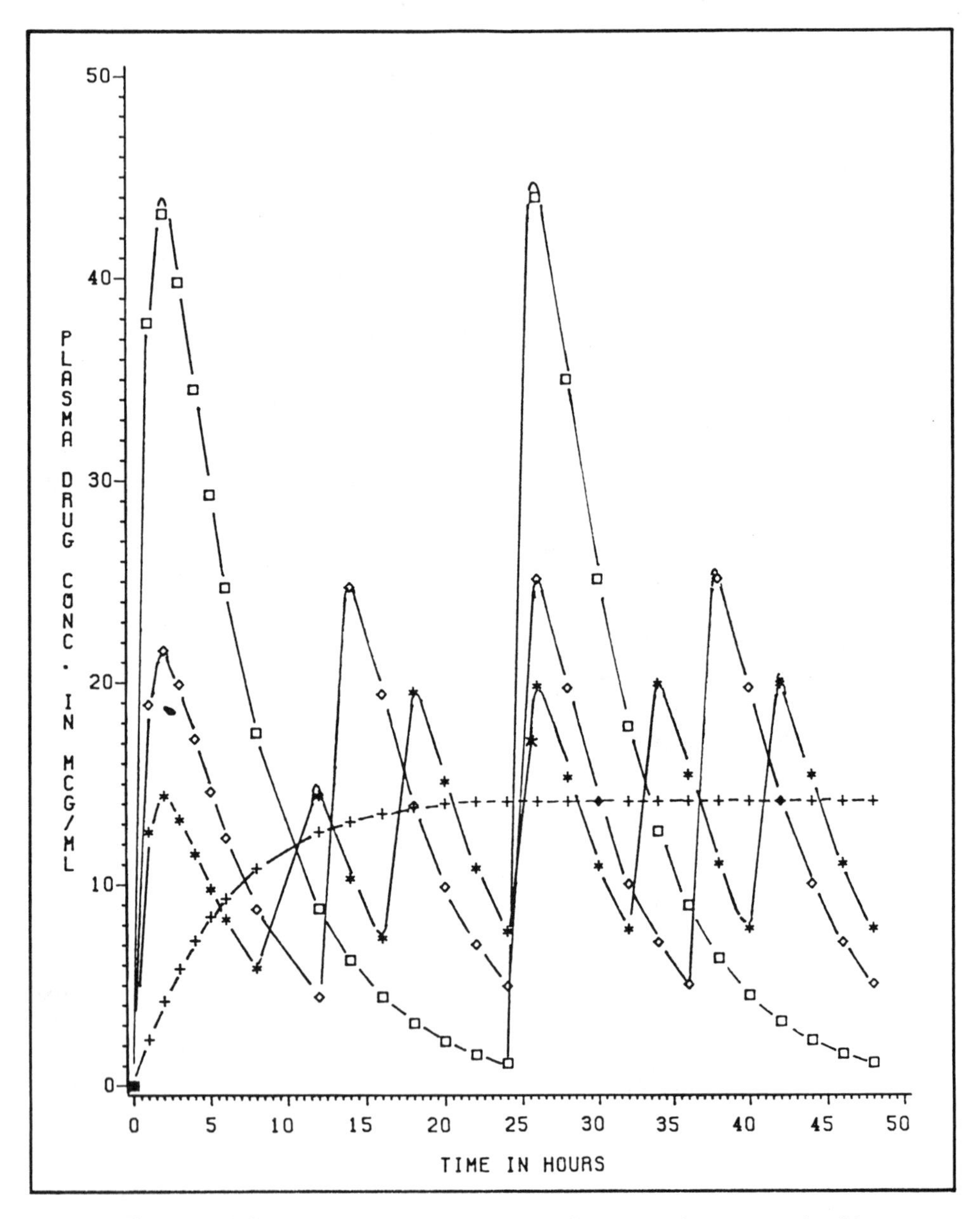

Figure 13-7. Simulated plasma drug concentration versus time curves after IV infusion and oral multiple doses for a drug with an elimination half-life of 4 hours and apparent V_d of 10 L. X, IV infusion given at a rate of 25 mg / hr, oral multiple doses are 200 mg every 8 hr, 300 mg every 12 hr, and 600 mg every 24 hr.

c. A dosage interval of 8.63 hr is difficult to remember. Is a dosage regimen of 500 mg every 8 hr reasonable?

Solution

$$C_{av}^{\infty} = \frac{(0.9)(500{,}000)(1.44)(3)}{(196)(76.6)(8)}$$

$$= 16.2\ \mu g/ml$$

Notice that a larger dose is necessary if the drug is given at longer intervals.

In designing a dosage regimen, one should consider a regimen that is practical and convenient for the patient. For example, the dosage interval should be spaced conveniently for the patient for improved compliance. In addition, one should consider the dosage of the drug that is commercially available.

The use of Equation 13.17 to initially estimate a dosage regimen has wide utility. The C_{av}^{∞} is equal to the dosing rate divided by the total body clearance of the drug in the patient:

$$C_{av}^{\infty} = \frac{FD_0}{\tau}\frac{1}{Cl_T} \qquad (13.35)$$

where FD_0/τ is equal to the dosing rate, R and $1/Cl_T$ is equal to $1/KV_d$.

In designing dosage regimens, the dosing rate, D_0/τ is adjusted for the patient's drug clearance to obtain the desired C_{av}^{∞}. For an IV infusion the zero-order rate of infusion, R, is used to obtain the desired steady-state plasma drug concentration, C_{ss}. If R is substituted for FD_0/τ in Equation 13.35, then the following equation for estimating the C_{ss} after an IV infusion

TABLE 13-4. EFFECT OF DOSING SCHEDULE ON PREDICTED STEADY-STATE PLASMA DRUG CONCENTRATIONS*

Dosing Schedule			Steady-State Drug Concentration ($\mu g/ml$)		
Dose (mg)	τ (hr)	Dosing Rate, D_0/τ (mg/hr)	C_{max}^{∞}	C_{av}^{∞}	C_{min}^{∞}
—	—	25†	14.5	14.5	14.5
100	4	25	16.2	14.5	11.6
200	8	25	20.2	14.5	7.81
300	12	25	25.3	14.5	5.03
600	24	25	44.1	14.5	1.12
400	8	50	40.4	28.9	15.6
600	8	75	60.6	43.4	23.4

*Drug has an elimination half-life of 4 hr and an apparent V_d of 10 L.
†Drug given by IV infusion. The first-order absorption rate constant K_a is 1.2 hr^{-1} and the drug follows a one-compartment open model.

is obtained:

$$C_{ss} = R\frac{1}{Cl_T} \tag{13.36}$$

From Equations 13.35 and 13.36 all dosage schedules having the same dosing rate, D_0/τ, or R will have the same C_{av}^{∞} or C_{ss}, whether the drug is given by multiple doses or by IV infusion. For example, dosage schedules of 100 mg every 4 hr, 200 mg every 8 hr, 300 mg every 12 hr, and 600 mg every 24 hr will yield the same C_{av}^{∞} in the patient. An IV infusion rate of 25 mg/hr in the same patient will given a C_{ss} equal to the C_{av}^{∞} obtained with the multiple-dose schedule (Fig. 13-7; Table 13-4).

QUESTIONS

1. Gentamycin has an average elimination half-life of approximately 2 hr and an apparent volume of distribution of 20% of body weight. It is necessary to give gentamycin, 1 mg/kg every 8 hr by multiple IV injections, to a 50-kg woman with normal renal function. Calculate (a) C_{max}, (b) C_{min}, and (c) C_{av}^{∞}.
2. A physician wants to give theophylline to a young male asthmatic patient (age 29, 80 kg). According to the literature, the elimination half-life for theophylline is 5 hr and the apparent V_d is equal to 50% of body weight. The plasma level of theophylline required to provide adequate airway ventilation is approximately 10 μg/ml.
   a. The physician wants the patient to take medication every 6 hr around the clock. What dose of theophylline would you recommend (assume theophylline is 100% bioavailable)?
   b. If you were to find that theophylline is available to you only in 225-mg capsules, what dosage regimen would you recommend?
3. What pharmacokinetic parameter is most important in determining the time at which the steady-state plasma drug level (C_{av}^{∞}) is reached?
4. Name two ways in which the fluctuations of plasma concentrations (between C_{max}^{∞} and C_{min}^{∞}) can be minimized for a person on a multiple-dose drug regimen without altering the C_{av}^{∞}.
5. What is the purpose of giving a loading dose?
6. What is the loading dose for an antibiotic ($K = 0.23\ hr^{-1}$) with a maintenance dose of 200 mg every 3 hr?
7. What is the main advantage of giving a potent drug by IV infusion as opposed to multiple IV injections?

REFERENCES

1. van Rossum JM, Tomey AHM: Rate of accumulation and plateau concentration of drugs after chronic medication. J Pharm Pharmacol 20:390–2, 1968
2. Kruger-Thiemer E: Pharmacokinetics and dose-concentration relationships. In Ariens EJ (ed), Physico-Chemical Aspects of Drug Action. New York, Pergamon Press, 1968, p. 97

3. Niebergall PJ, Sugita ET, Schnaare RC: Potential dangers of common drug dosing regimens. Am J Hosp Pharm 31:53–58, 1974

BIBLIOGRAPHY

Gibaldi M, Perrier D: Pharmacokinetics, 2nd ed. New York, Marcel Dekker, 1962, pp. 451–57

Levy G: Kinetics of pharmacologic effect. Clin Pharmacol Ther 7:362, 1966

van Rossum JM: Pharmacokinetics of accumulation. J Pharm Sci 75:2162–64, 1968

Wagner JG: Kinetics of pharmacological response, I: Proposed relationship between response and drug concentration in the intact animal and man. J Theor Biol 20:173, 1968

Wagner JG: Relations between drug concentrations and response. J Mond Pharm 14:279–310, 1971

CHAPTER FOURTEEN

Nonlinear Pharmacokinetics

In the previous chapters linear pharmacokinetic models using simple first-order kinetics were introduced to describe the course of drug action. These linear models assumed that the pharmacokinetic parameters for a drug would not change when different doses or multiple doses of a drug were given. With some drugs increased doses or chronic medication can cause deviations from the linear pharmacokinetic profile observed with single low doses of the same drug. This nonlinear pharmacokinetic behavior is also termed dose-dependent pharmacokinetics.

Many of the processes of drug absorption, distribution, biotransformation, and excretion involve enzymes or carrier-mediated systems. For some drugs given at therapeutic levels, one of these specialized processes may become saturated. As shown in Table 14-1, various causes of nonlinear pharmacokinetic behavior are theoretically possible. Besides saturation of a carrier-mediated system, drugs may demonstrate nonlinear pharmacokinetics due to a pathologic alteration in drug absorption, distribution, and elimination. For example, aminoglycosides may cause renal nephrotoxicity, thereby altering renal drug excretion. In addition, an obstruction of the bile duct due to the formation of gallstones will alter biliary drug excretion. In all cases, the main pharmacokinetic observation is a change in the apparent elimination rate constant.

There are a number of drugs for which saturation or capacity-limited metabolism in man has been demonstrated. These drug processes include glycine conjugation of salicylate, sulfate conjugation of salicylamide, acetylation of *p*-aminobenzoic acid, and the elimination of phenytoin.[1] Drugs which demonstrate saturation kinetics usually show the following characteristics.

1. Elimination of drug does not follow simple first-order kinetics–i.e., elimination kinetics are nonlinear.
2. The elimination half-life becomes greater as dose is increased.
3. The AUC is not proportional to the amount of bioavailable drug.

TABLE 14-1. EXAMPLES OF CAUSES OF DRUGS SHOWING DOSE- AND TIME-DEPENDENT KINETICS

Cause*	Drug
Absorption	
Saturable transport in gut wall	Riboflavin
Drug comparatively insoluble	Griseofulvin
Saturable gut wall or hepatic metabolism on first pass	Propranolol, salicylamide
Pharmacologic effect on GI motility	Metoclopramide, chloroquine
Saturable gastric or GI decomposition	Some penicillins
Distribution	
Saturable plasma protein binding	Phenylbutazone, salicylate
Saturable tissue binding	—
Saturable transport into or out of tissues	Methotrexate
Renal Elimination	
Active secretion	Penicillin G
Active reabsorption	Ascorbic acid
Change in urine pH	Salicylic acid
Saturable plasma protein binding	Salicylic acid
Nephrotoxic effect at higher doses	Aminoglycosides
Diuretic effect	Theophylline, alcohol
Extrarenal Elimination	
Capacity-limited metabolism; enzyme saturation or cofactor limitation	Phenytoin, theophylline Salicylic acid, alcohol
Saturable biliary excretion	—
Enzyme induction	Carbamazepine
Hepatotoxic at higher doses	Acetaminophen
Saturable plasma protein binding	Phenylbutazone
Altered hepatic blood flow	Propranolol
Metabolite inhibition	Diazepam

*Hypothermia, metabolic acidosis, altered cardiovascular function, and coma are additional causes of dose and time dependencies in drug overdose.
From Tozer TN, et al, 1981, with permission.[1]

4. The saturation of capacity-limited processes may be affected by other drugs that require the same enzyme or carrier-mediated system.
5. The composition of the metabolites of a drug may be affected by a change in the dose.

Since these drugs have a changing apparent elimination constant with larger doses, prediction of drug concentration in the blood based on a small dose is difficult. Drug concentration in the blood can increase rapidly once an elimination process is saturated. In general, metabolism (biotransformation) and active tubular secretion of drugs by the kidney are the processes most usually saturated. Figure 14-1 shows plasma level–time curves for a drug that exhibits saturable kinetics. When a large dose is given, a curve is obtained with an initial slow elimination phase followed by a much more rapid elimination at lower blood concentrations (Fig. 14-1, curve *A*). With a small dose of the drug apparent first-order kinetics are observed,

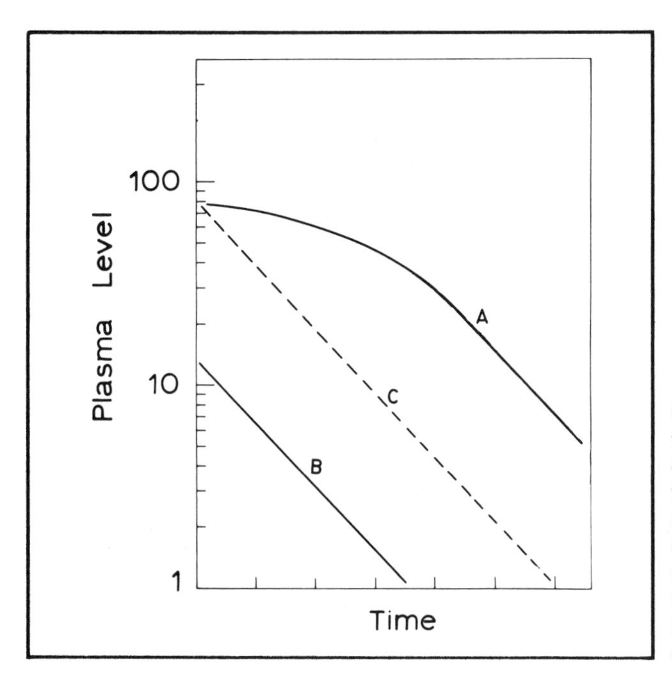

Figure 14-1. Plasma level–time curves for a drug which exhibits a saturable elimination process. Curves *A* and *B* represent high and low doses of drug, respectively, given in a single IV bolus. Curve *C* represents the normal first-order elimination of a different drug.

since no saturation kinetics occur (Fig. 14-1, curve *B*). If the pharmacokinetic data were estimated only from the blood levels described by curve *B*, then a twofold increase in the dose would give the blood profile presented in curve *C* (Fig. 14-1), which considerably underestimates the drug concentration as well as the duration of action. In order to determine whether a drug is following dose-dependent kinetics, the drug is given at various dosage levels and a plasma level–time curve is obtained for each dose. The curves should exhibit parallel slopes if the drug follows dose-independent kinetics. Alternatively, a plot of the areas under the plasma level–time curves at various doses should be linear (Fig. 14-2).

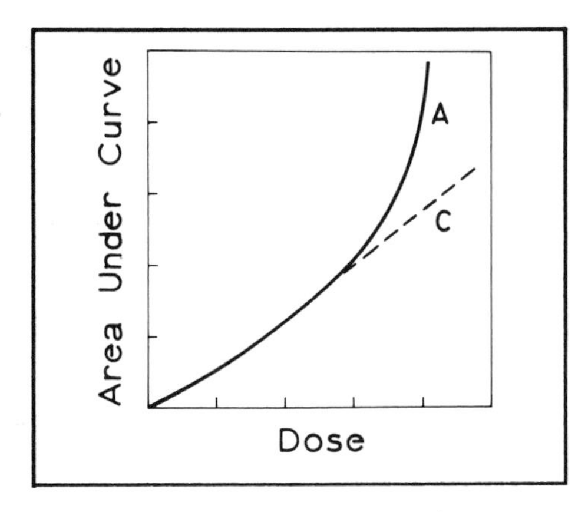

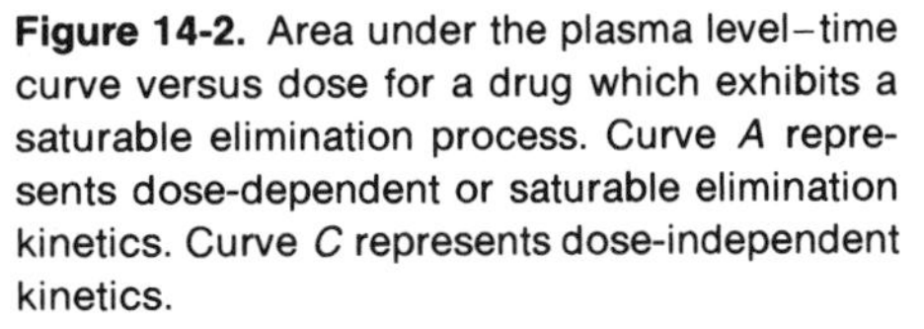
Figure 14-2. Area under the plasma level–time curve versus dose for a drug which exhibits a saturable elimination process. Curve *A* represents dose-dependent or saturable elimination kinetics. Curve *C* represents dose-independent kinetics.

SATURABLE ENZYMATIC ELIMINATION PROCESSES

The elimination of drug by a saturable enzymatic process is described by *Michaelis–Menten* kinetics. If C_p is the concentration of drug in the plasma, then

$$\text{Elimination rate} = -\frac{dC_p}{dt} = \frac{V_m C_p}{K_m + C_p} \tag{14.1}$$

where V_m is the maximum elimination rate and K_m is the Michaelis constant. The values for K_m and V_m are dependent on the nature of the drug and the enzymatic process involved.

The elimination rate of a hypothetical drug with a K_m of 0.1 μg/ml and a V_m of 0.5 μg/ml hr is calculated in Table 14-2 by means of Equation 14.1. Since the ratio of elimination rate to drug concentration changes as the drug concentration changes, the rate of drug elimination is not a first-order or linear process. A first-order elimination process would yield a constant elimination rate: drug concentration value known as the rate constant. At drug concentrations of 0.4–10 μg/ml, the enzyme system is not saturated and the rate of elimination is a *mixed* or *nonlinear* process. At higher drug concentrations, 11.2 μg/ml and above, the elimination rate approaches the maximum velocity (V_m) of approximately 0.5 μg/ml hr.

Equation 14.1 describes a nonlinear enzyme process that encompasses a broad range of drug concentrations. When the drug concentration, C_p, is large in relation to the K_m, saturation of the enzymes occurs and the rate of elimination proceeds at a

TABLE 14-2. EFFECT OF DRUG CONCENTRATION ON THE ELIMINATION RATE AND RATE CONSTANT*

Drug Concentration (μg/ml)	Elimination Rate (μg/ml hr)	Elimination Rate / Concentration† (hr^{-1})
0.4	0.400	1.000
0.8	0.444	0.556
1.2	0.462	0.385
1.6	0.472	0.294
2.0	0.476	0.238
2.4	0.480	0.200
2.8	0.483	0.172
3.2	0.485	0.152
10.0	0.495	0.0495
10.4	0.495	0.0476
10.8	0.495	0.0459
11.2	0.496	0.0442
11.6	0.496	0.0427

*K_m = 0.1 μg/ml, V_m = 0.5 μg/ml hr.
†The ratio of the elimination rate to the concentration is equal to the rate constant.

fixed or constant rate equal to V_m. Thus, elimination of drug becomes a zero-order process.

$$-\frac{dC_p}{dt} = \frac{V_m C_p}{C_p} = V_m \qquad (14.2)$$

PRACTICE PROBLEMS

1. Using the hypothetical drug considered in Table 14-2 ($V_m = 0.5$ μg/ml hr, $K_m = 0.1$ μg/ml), how long would it take for the plasma drug concentration to decrease from 20 to 12 μg/ml?

Solution

Since 20 μg/ml is above the saturable level, as indicated in the table, elimination occurs at a zero-order rate of 0.5 μg/hr.

$$\text{Time needed for the drug to decrease to 12 } \mu\text{g/ml} = \frac{20 - 12\ \mu\text{g}}{0.5\mu\text{g/hr}} = 16\ \text{hr}$$

Based on data generated from Equation 14.1, Table 14-3 shows how enzymatic drug elimination can change from a nonlinear to a linear process over a restricted concentration range.

When the drug concentration, C_p, is small in relation to the K_m ($C_p \leq 0.05$ μg/ml, Table 14-3), the rate of drug elimination becomes a first-order process. This is evident since the rate constant (or elimination rate–drug concentration) values are constant. At drug concentrations below 0.05 μg/ml, the ratio of elimination rate to drug concentration has a

TABLE 14-3. EFFECT OF DRUG CONCENTRATION ON THE ELIMINATION RATE AND RATE CONSTANT*

Drug Concentration (C_p) (μg/ml)	Elimination Rate (μg/ml hr)	Elimination Rate Concentration† (hr^{-1})
0.01	0.011	1.1
0.02	0.022	1.1
0.03	0.033	1.1
0.04	0.043	1.1
0.05	0.053	1.1
0.06	0.063	1.0
0.07	0.072	1.0
0.08	0.082	1.0
0.09	0.091	1.0

*$K_m = 0.8$ μg/ml, $V_m = 0.9$ μg/ml hr.
† The ratio of the elimination rate to the concentration is equal to the rate constant.

constant value of 1.1 hr^{-1}. Mathematically, when C_p is much smaller than K_m, C_p in the denominator is negligible.

$$-\frac{dC_p}{dt} = \frac{V_m C_p}{C_p + K_m} = \frac{V_m}{K_m} C_p$$

$$-\frac{dC_p}{dt} = K'C_p \qquad (14.3)$$

The first-order rate constant, K', can be calculated from Equation 14.3:

$$K' = \frac{V_m}{K_m} = \frac{0.9}{0.8} = \sim 1.1 \text{ hr}^{-1}$$

This calculation confirms the data in Table 14-3, since enzymatic drug elimination at drug concentrations below 0.05 μg/ml is a first-order rate process with a rate constant of 1.1 hr^{-1}. Therefore, the $t_{1/2}$ due to enzymatic elimination can be calculated:

$$t_{1/2} = \frac{0.693}{1.1} = 0.63 \text{ hr}$$

2. How long would it take for the plasma concentration of the drug in Table 14-3 to decline from 0.05 to 0.005 μg/ml?

Solution

Since drug elimination is a first-order process for the specified concentrations,

$$C_p = C_p^0 e^{-Kt}$$

$$\log C_p = \log C_p^0 - \frac{Kt}{2.3}$$

$$t = 2.3 \frac{\log C_p - \log C_p^0}{K}$$

Since $C_p^0 = 0.05$ μg/ml, $K = 1.1 \text{ hr}^{-1}$, and $C_p = 0.005$ μg/ml,

$$t = \frac{2.3(\log 0.05 - \log 0.005)}{1.1} = \frac{2.3(-1.30 + 2.3)}{1.1} = \frac{2.3}{1.1} = 2.09 \text{ hr}$$

When given in therapeutic doses, most drugs produce plasma drug concentrations well below the K_m for all carrier-mediated enzyme systems affecting the pharmacokinetics of the drug. Therefore, most drugs at normal therapeutic concentrations follow first-order rate processes. Only a few drugs, such as salicylate and phenytoin, tend to saturate the hepatic mixed-function oxidases at higher therapeutic doses. With these drugs, elimination kinetics are first-order with very small doses and *mixed* at higher doses and may approach zero-order with very high therapeutic doses.

DRUG ELIMINATION BY CAPACITY-LIMITED PHARMACOKINETICS: ONE-COMPARTMENT MODEL, IV BOLUS INJECTION

The rate of elimination of a drug that follows capacity-limited pharmacokinetics is governed by the V_m and K_m of the drug. Equation 14.1 describes the elimination of a drug that distributes in the body as a single compartment and is eliminated by Michaelis–Menten or capacity-limited pharmacokinetics. If a single IV bolus injection of drug, D_0, is given at $t = 0$, the drug concentration, C_t, in the plasma at any time t may be calculated by an integrated form of Equation 14.1 described by

$$\frac{C_0 - C_t}{t} = V_m - \frac{K_m}{t} \ln \frac{C_0}{C_t} \qquad (14.4)$$

Alternatively, the amount of drug in the body after an IV bolus injection may be calculated by the following relationship. Equation 14.5 may be used to simulate the decline of drug in the body after various size doses are given provided the K_m and V_m of drug are known.

$$\frac{D_0 - D_t}{t} = V_m - \frac{K_m}{t} \ln \frac{D_0}{D_t} \qquad (14.5)$$

where D_0 is the amount of drug in the body at $t = 0$. In order to calculate the time for the dose of the drug to decline to a certain amount of drug in the body, Equation 14.5 must be rearranged and solved for time t:

$$t = \frac{1}{V_m}\left(D_0 - D_t + K_m \ln \frac{D_0}{D_t} \right) \qquad (14.6)$$

The relationship of K_m and V_m on the time for an IV bolus injection of drug to decline to a given amount of drug in the body is illustrated in Figures 14-3 and 14-4. Using Equation 14.6, the time for a single 400-mg dose given by IV bolus injection to decline to 20 mg was calculated for a drug with a K_m of 38 mg and a V_m that is varied from 200 to 100 mg/hr (Table 14-4). With a V_m of 200 mg/hr the time for the 400-mg dose to decline to 20 mg in the body is 2.46 hr; whereas when the V_m is decreased to 100 mg/hr, the time for the 400-mg dose to decrease to 20 mg is increased to 4.93 hr. Thus, there is an inverse relationship between the time for the dose to decline to a certain amount of drug in the body and the V_m as shown in Equation 14.6.

Using a similar example, the effect of the K_m on the time for a single 400-mg dose given by IV bolus injection to decline to 20 mg in the body is described in Table 14-5 and Figure 14-4. Assuming the V_m is 200 mg/hr, the time for the drug to decline from 400 to 20 mg is 2.46 hr when the K_m is 38 mg; whereas when the K_m is 76 mg, the time for the drug dose to decline to 20 mg is 3.03 hr. Thus, an increase in the K_m (with no change in the V_m) will increase the time for the drug to be eliminated from the body. It is important to note that the K_m is not an elimination constant. The K_m is actually a hybrid rate constant in enzyme kinetics representing both the forward and backward reaction rates and is equal to the drug concentration or amount of drug in the body at $\frac{1}{2}V_m$.

The one-compartment open model with capacity-limited elimination pharmacokinetics adequately describes the plasma drug concentration–time profiles for

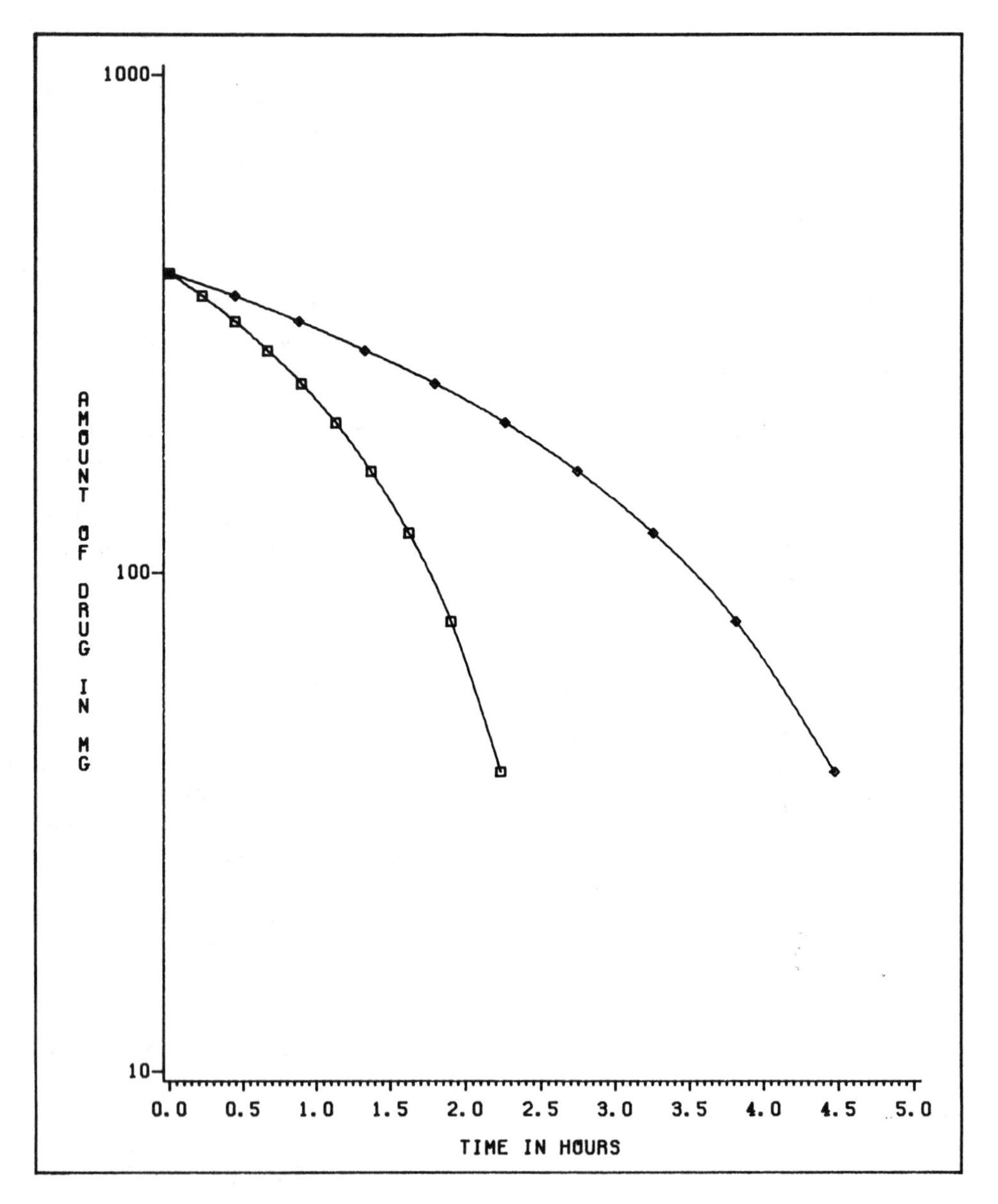

Figure 14-3. Amount of drug in the body versus time for a capacity-limited drug following an intravenous dose. The data are generated using V_m of 100 mg/hr (◆) and V_m of 200 mg/hr (□). K_m is kept constant.

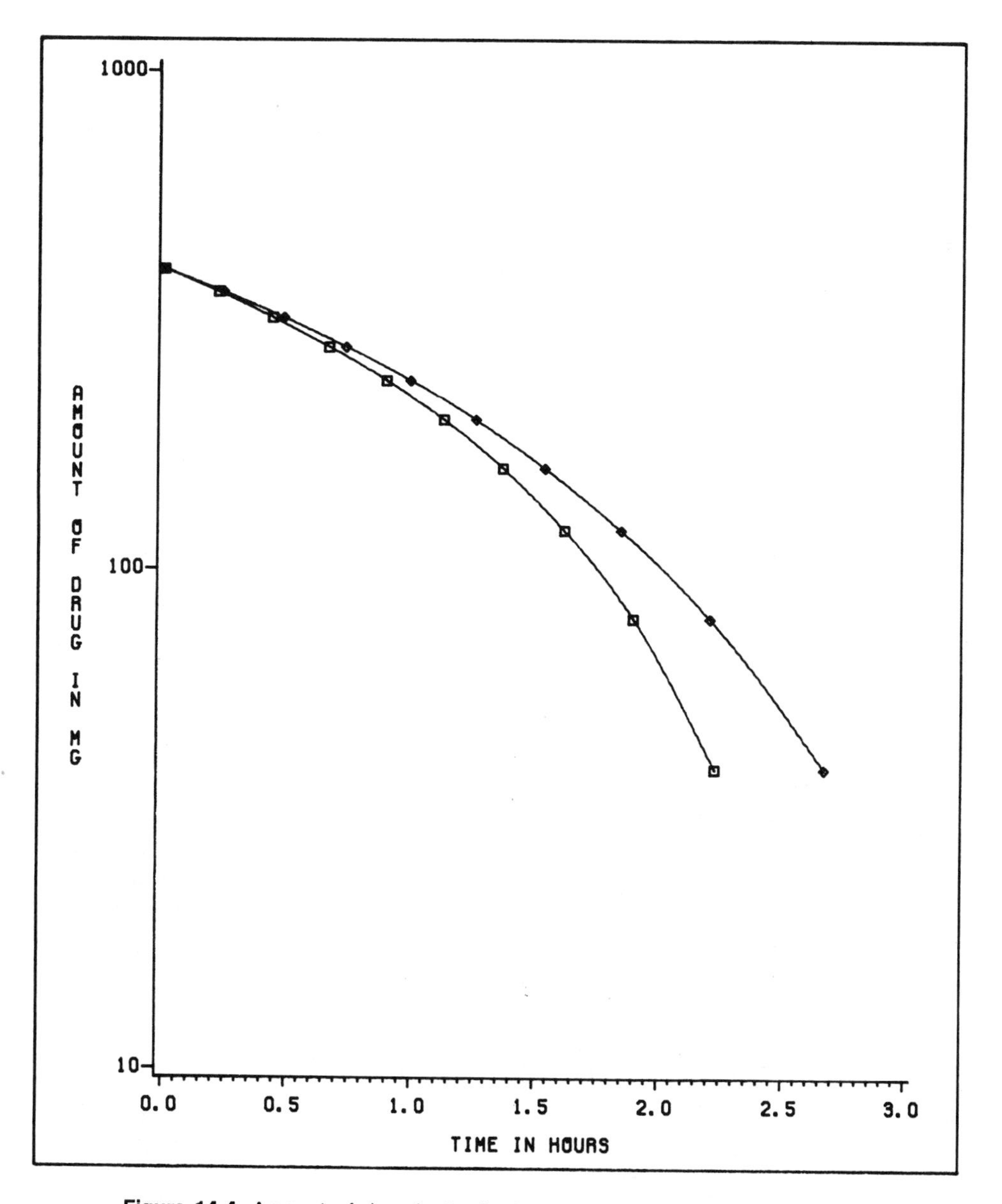

Figure 14-4. Amount of drug in the body versus time for a capacity-limited drug following an intravenous dose. The data are generated using K_m of 38 mg (□) and K_m of 76 mg (◆). V_m is kept constant.

TABLE 14-4. CAPACITY-LIMITED PHARMACOKINETICS: EFFECT OF V_m. ON THE ELIMINATION OF DRUG*

Amount of Drug in Body (mg)	Time for Drug Elimination (hr)	
	$V_m = 200\ mg/hr$	$V_m = 100\ mg/hr$
400	0	0
380	0.109	0.219
360	0.220	0.440
340	0.330	0.661
320	0.442	0.884
300	0.554	1.10
280	0.667	1.33
260	0.781	1.56
240	0.897	1.79
220	1.01	2.02
200	1.13	2.26
180	1.25	2.50
160	1.37	2.74
140	1.49	2.99
120	1.62	3.25
100	1.76	3.52
80	1.90	3.81
60	2.06	4.12
40	2.23	4.47
20	2.46	4.93

*A single 400-mg dose is given by IV bolus injection. The drug is distributed into a single compartment and is eliminated by capacity-limited pharmacokinetics. K_m is 38 mg. The time for drug to decline from 400 to 20 mg is calculated from Equation 14.6 assuming the drug has a $V_m = 200$ mg/hr or $V_m = 100$ mg/hr.

some drugs. The mathematics needed to describe nonlinear pharmacokinetic behavior of drugs that follow two-compartment models and/or have both combined capacity-limited and first-order kinetic profiles are very complex and have little practical applications for dosage calculations and therapeutic drug monitoring.

PRACTICE PROBLEMS

1. A drug eliminated from the body by capacity-limited pharmacokinetics has a K_m of 100 mg and a V_m of 50 mg/hr. If 400 mg of the drug is given to a patient by IV bolus injection, calculate the time for the drug to be 50% eliminated. If 320 mg of the drug is to be given by IV bolus injection, calculate the time for 50% of the dose to be eliminated. Explain why there is a difference in the time for 50% elimination of a 400-mg dose compared to a 320-mg dose.

Solution

Use Equation 14.6 to calculate the time for the dose to decline to a given amount of drug in the body. For this problem D_t is equal to 50% of the dose D_0.

TABLE 14-5. CAPACITY-LIMITED PHARMACOKINETICS: EFFECTS OF K_m ON THE ELIMINATION OF DRUG*

Amount of Drug in Body (mg)	Time for Drug Elimination (hr)	
	$K_m = 38$ *mg*	$K_m = 76$ *mg*
400	0	0
380	0.109	0.119
360	0.220	0.240
340	0.330	0.361
320	0.442	0.484
300	0.554	0.609
280	0.667	0.735
260	0.781	0.863
240	0.897	0.994
220	1.01	1.12
200	1.13	1.26
180	1.25	1.40
160	1.37	1.54
140	1.49	1.69
120	1.62	1.85
100	1.76	2.02
80	1.90	2.21
60	2.06	2.42
40	2.23	2.67
20	2.46	3.03

*A single 400-mg dose is given by IV bolus injection. The drug is distributed into a single compartment and is eliminated by capacity-limited pharmacokinetics. V_m is 200 mg/hr. The time for drug to decline from 400 to 20 mg is calculated from Equation 14.6 assuming the drug has a $K_m = 38$ mg or $K_m = 76$ mg.

If the dose is 400 mg,

$$t = \frac{1}{50}\left(400 - 200 + 100 \ln \frac{400}{200}\right) = 5.39 \text{ hr}$$

If the dose is 320 mg,

$$t = \frac{1}{50}\left(320 - 160 + 100 \ln \frac{320}{160}\right) = 4.59 \text{ hr}$$

For capacity-limited elimination, the elimination half-life is dose dependent since the drug elimination process is partially saturated. Therefore, small changes in the dose will produce large differences in the time for 50% drug elimination. The parameters K_m and V_m determine when the dose is saturated.

2. Using the same drug as in Problem 1, calculate the time for 50% elimination of the dose when the dose is 10 and 5 mg, respectively. Explain why the times for 50% drug elimination are similar even though the dose is reduced by one-half.

Solution

As in practice problem 1, use Equation 14.6 to calculate the time for the amount of drug in the body at zero time (D_0) to decline 50%.

TABLE 14-6. INFORMATION NECESSARY FOR GRAPHIC DETERMINATION OF V_m AND K_m.

OBS	C (μM/ml)	V (μM/ml min)	$1/V$ (ml min/μM)	$1/C$ (ml/μM)
1	1	0.500	2.000	1.000
2	6	1.636	0.611	0.166
3	11	2.062	0.484	0.090
4	16	2.285	0.437	0.062
5	21	2.423	0.412	0.047
6	26	2.516	0.397	0.038
7	31	2.583	0.337	0.032
8	36	2.504	0.379	0.027
9	41	2.673	0.373	0.024
10	46	2.705	0.369	0.021

If the dose is 10 mg,

$$t = \frac{1}{50}\left(10 - 5 + 100\ln\frac{10}{5}\right) = 1.49 \text{ hr}$$

If the dose is 5 mg,

$$t = \frac{1}{50}\left(5 - 2.5 + 100\ln\frac{5}{2.5}\right) = 1.44 \text{ hr}$$

Whether the patient is given a 10- or a 5-mg dose by IV bolus injection, the times for the amount of drug to decline 50% are approximately the same. At 10- and 5-mg doses the amount of drug in the body is much less than the K_m of 100 mg. Therefore, the amount of drug in the body is well below saturation of the elimination process and the drug declines at a first-order rate.

Determination of K_m and V_m

Equation 14.1 relates the rate of drug biotransformation to the concentration of the drug in the body. The same equation may be applied to determine the rate of enzymatic reaction of a drug in vitro (Eq. 14.7). When an experiment is performed with solutions of various concentration of the drug C, a series of reaction rates (V) may be measured for each concentration. Special plots may then be used to determine K_m and V_m.

It can be seen that Equation 14.7 may be rearranged into Equation 14.8:

$$V = \frac{V_m C}{K_m + C} \tag{14.7}$$

$$\frac{1}{V} = \frac{K_m}{V_m}\frac{1}{C} + \frac{1}{V_m} \tag{14.8}$$

Equation 14.8 is a linear equation when $1/V$ is plotted against $1/C$. The intercept for the line is $-1/K_m$ and the slope is K_m/V_m. An example of a drug reacting enzymatically with rate (V) at various concentrations C is shown in Table 14-6 and Figure 14-5. A plot of the $1/V$ versus $1/C$ is shown in Figure 14-6. A plot of $1/V$ versus $1/C$ is linear with an intercept of 0.33 μmol. Therefore,

$$\frac{1}{V_m} = 0.33 \text{ min ml}/\mu\text{mol}$$

$$V_m = 3\ \mu\text{mol/ml min}$$

since slope $= 1.65 = K_m/V_m = K_m/3$ or $K_m = 3 \times 1.65\ \mu\text{mol/ml} = 5\ \mu\text{mol/ml}$. Alternatively, K_m may be found from the x intercept where $-1/K_m$ is equal to the x

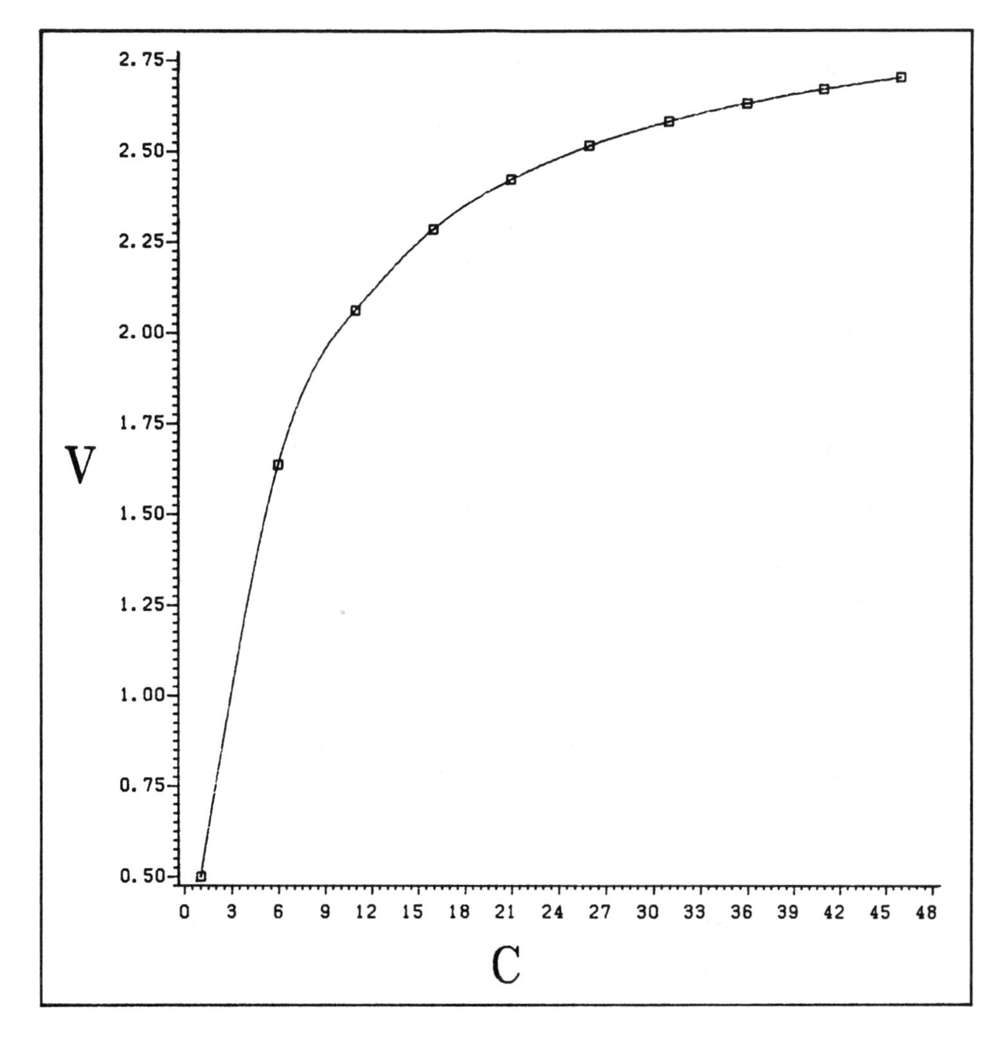

Figure 14-5. Plot of rate of drug metabolism at various drug concentrations. $K_m = 5.0\ \mu\text{mol/ml}$; $V_m = 3\ \mu\text{mol/ml min}$.

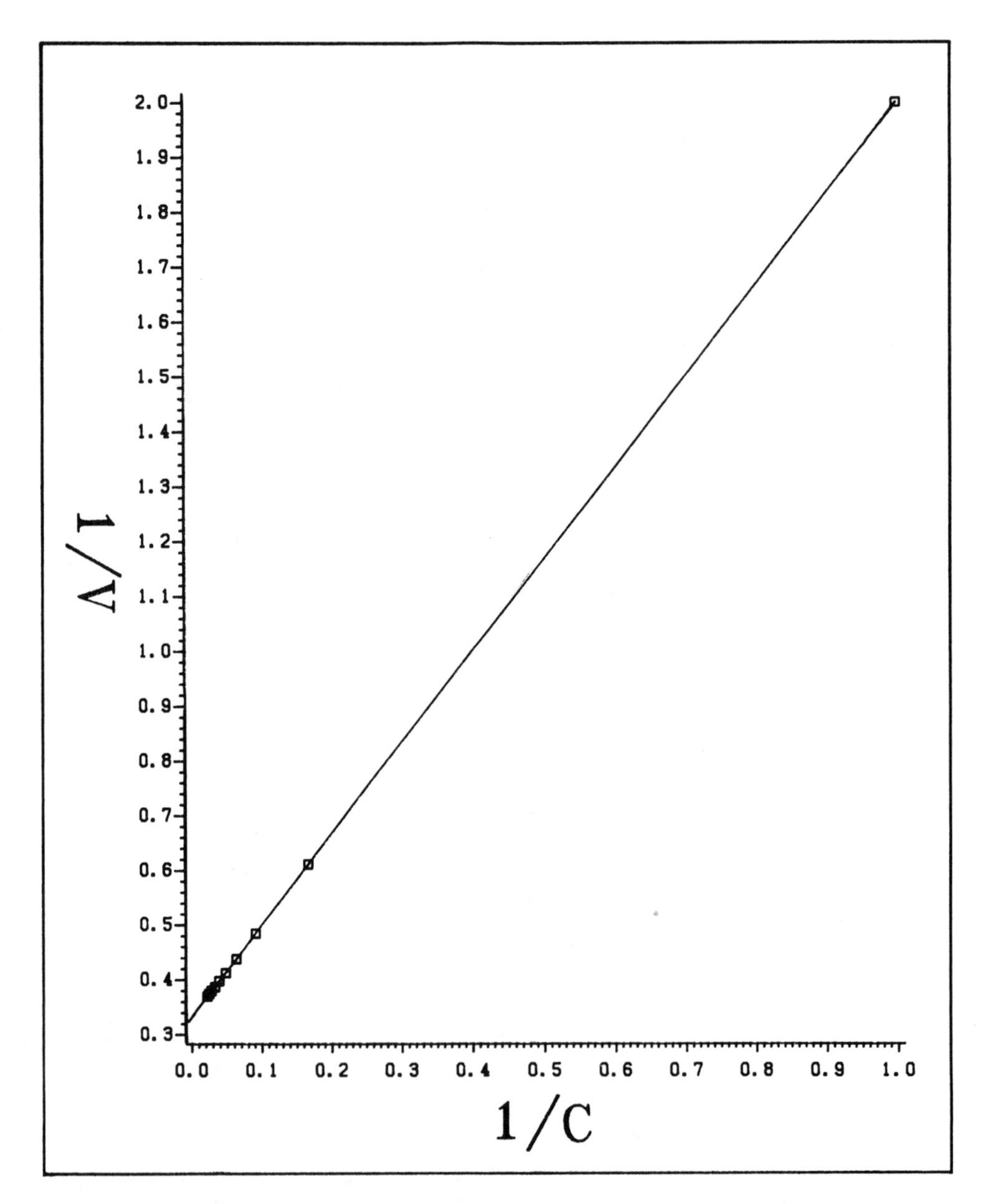

Figure 14-6. Plot of $1/V$ versus $1/C$ for determining K_m and V_m.

TABLE 14-7. CALCULATIONS NECESSARY FOR GRAPHIC DETERMINATION OF K_m AND V_m

C (μM/ml)	V (μM/ml min)	C/V (min)	V/C (1/min)
1	0.500	2.000	0.500
6	1.636	3.666	0.272
11	2.062	5.333	0.187
16	2.285	7.000	0.142
21	2.423	8.666	0.115
26	2.516	10.333	0.096
31	2.583	12.000	0.083
36	2.634	13.666	0.073
41	2.673	15.333	0.065
46	2.705	17.000	0.058

intercept (may be seen by extending the graph to intercept the x axis at the negative region).

With this plot (Fig. 14-6) the points are clustered. Other methods are available which may spread the points more evenly. These methods are derived from rearranging Equation 14.8 into Equations 14.10 and 14.11:

$$\frac{C}{V} = \frac{1}{V_m} C + \frac{K_m}{V_m} \tag{14.9}$$

$$V = -K_m \frac{V}{C} + V_m \tag{14.10}$$

A plot of C/V versus C would yield a straight line with $1/V_m$ as slope and K_m/V_m as intercept (Eq. 14.9). A plot of V versus V/C would yield a slope of $-K_m$ and an intercept of V_m (Eq. 14.10).

The necessary calculations needed for making the above plots are shown in Table 14-7. The plots are shown in Figures 14-7 and 14-8. It should be noted that the data are spread out better by the two latter plots. Calculations from the slope shows that the same K_m and V_m are obtained as in Figure 14-6. When the data are more scattered, one method may be more accurate than the other; a simple approach is to graph the data and examine the linearity of the graphs. The same basic type of plots are used in the clinical literature to determine K_m and V_m for individual patients for drugs that undergo capacity-limited kinetics.

Determination of K_m and V_m in Patients

Equation 14.7 shows that the rate of drug metabolism (V) is dependent on the concentration of the drug (C) in the beaker. The same basic concept may be applied to the rate of drug metabolism of a capacity-limited drug in the body. The body may be regarded as a single compartment with drug dissolved in it. The rate of drug

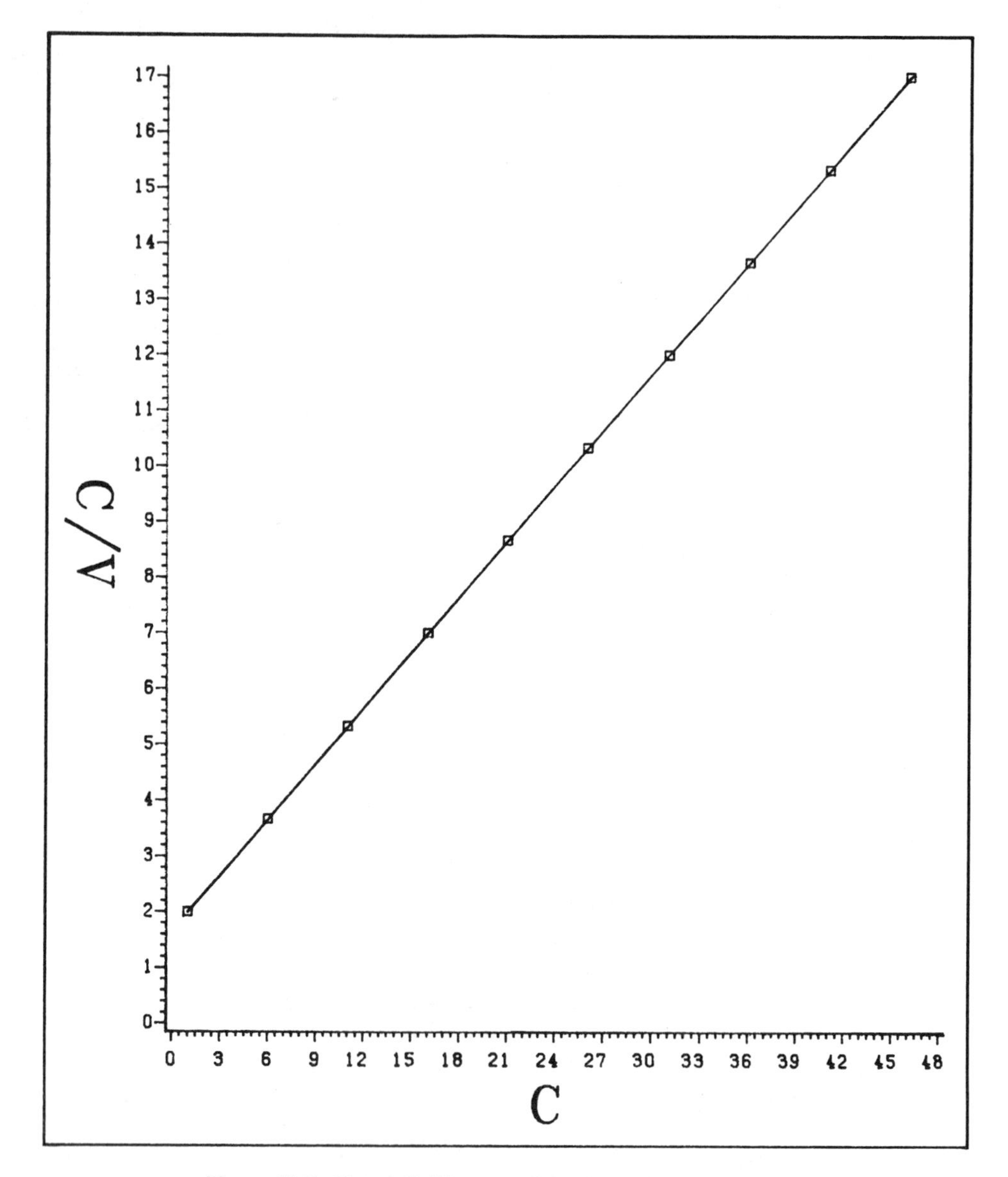

Figure 14-7. Plot of C/V versus C for determining K_m and V_m.

metabolism will vary depending on the concentration of drug C_p as well as the metabolic rate constants K_m and V_m of the drug in the individual.

An example for the determination of K_m and V_m is given for the drug phenytoin. Phenytoin undergoes capacity-limited kinetics in the body. To determine K_m and V_m, two doses are given at different times, until steady state is reached. The steady state drug concentrations are then measured by assay. At steady state the rate

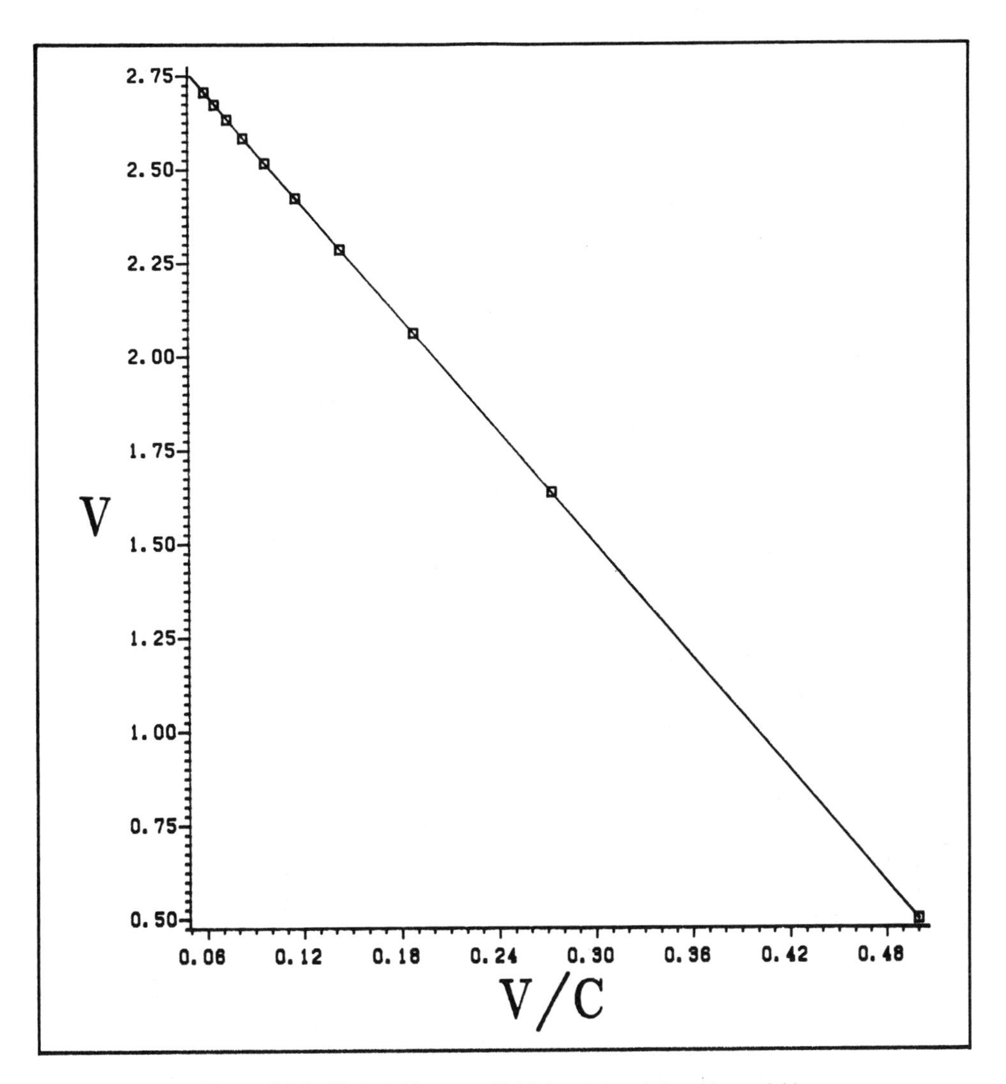

Figure 14-8. Plot of V versus V/C for determining K_m and V_m.

of drug metabolism (V) is assumed to be the same as the rate of drug input R (dose/day). Therefore Equation 14.11 may be written for drug metabolism in the body similar to the way drugs are metabolized in vitro (Eq. 14.7).

$$R = \frac{V_m C_{ss}}{K_m + C_{ss}} \tag{14.11}$$

R = dose/day or dosing rate; C_{ss} = steady-state plasma drug concentration; V_m = maximum metabolic rate constant in the body; K_m = *Michaelis-Menten* constant of the drug in the body.

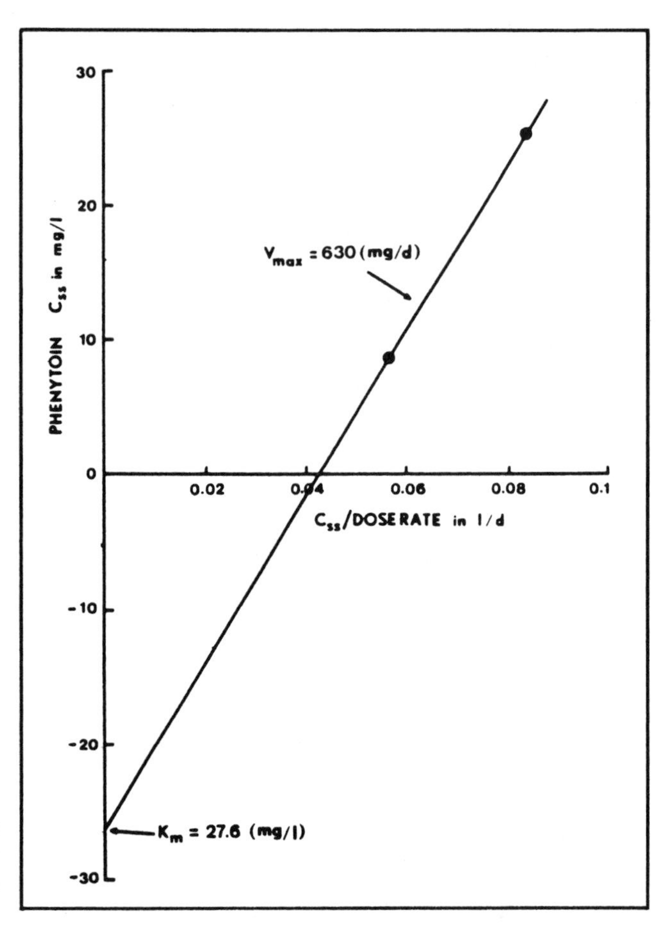

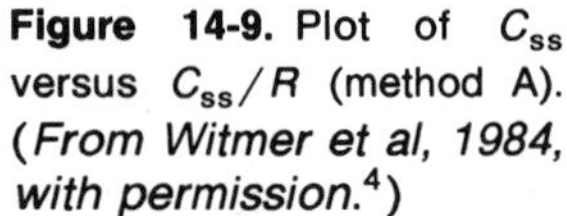
Figure 14-9. Plot of C_{ss} versus C_{ss}/R (method A). (*From Witmer et al, 1984, with permission.*[4])

EXAMPLE

The drug phenytoin was administered to a patient at dosing rates of 150 mg/day and 300 mg/day, respectively. The steady-state plasma concentration found was 8.6 mg/L and 25.1 mg/L, respectively. Find the K_m and V_m of this patient. What would be the dose needed to achieve a steady-state concentration of 11.3 mg/L?

Solution

There are three methods for solving this problem, all based on the same basic equation (Eq. 14.11).

Method A

Inverting Equation 14.11 on both side yields

$$\frac{1}{R} = \frac{K_m}{V_m}\frac{1}{C_{ss}} + \frac{1}{K_m} \qquad (14.12)$$

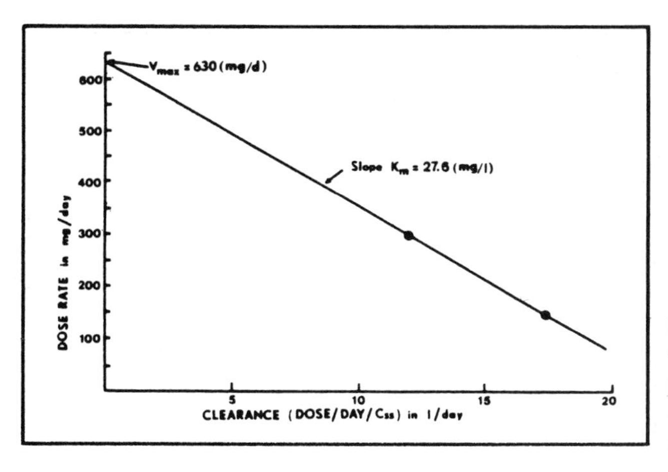

Figure 14-10. Plot of R versus R/C_{ss} or clearance (method B). (*From Witmer et al, 1984, with permission.*[4])

Multiply both sides by $[C_{ss}V_m]$

$$\frac{V_m C_{ss}}{R} = K_m + C_{ss}$$

Rearrange:

$$C_{ss} = \frac{V_m C_{ss}}{R} - K_m \tag{14.13}$$

A plot of C_{ss} versus C_{ss}/R is shown in Figure 14-9. V_m is equal to the slope, 630 mg/day, and K_m is equal to the y-intercept, 27.6 mg/L.

Method B

From Eq. 14.11:

$$RK_m + RC_{ss} = V_m C_{ss}$$

Divide both side by C_{ss} yields

$$R = V_m - \frac{K_m R}{C_{ss}} \tag{14.14}$$

A plot of R versus R/C_{ss} is shown in Figure 14-10. The K_m and V_m found are similar to those by the previous method (Figure 14-9).

Method C

A plot of R versus C_{ss} is shown in Figure 14-11. To determine K_m and V_m:

1. Mark points for R of 300 mg/day and C_{ss} of 25.1 mg/L as shown. Connect with a straight line.
2. Mark points for R of 150 mg/day and C_{ss} of 8.6 mg/L as shown. Connect with a straight line.
3. Where lines from first two steps cross is called point A.

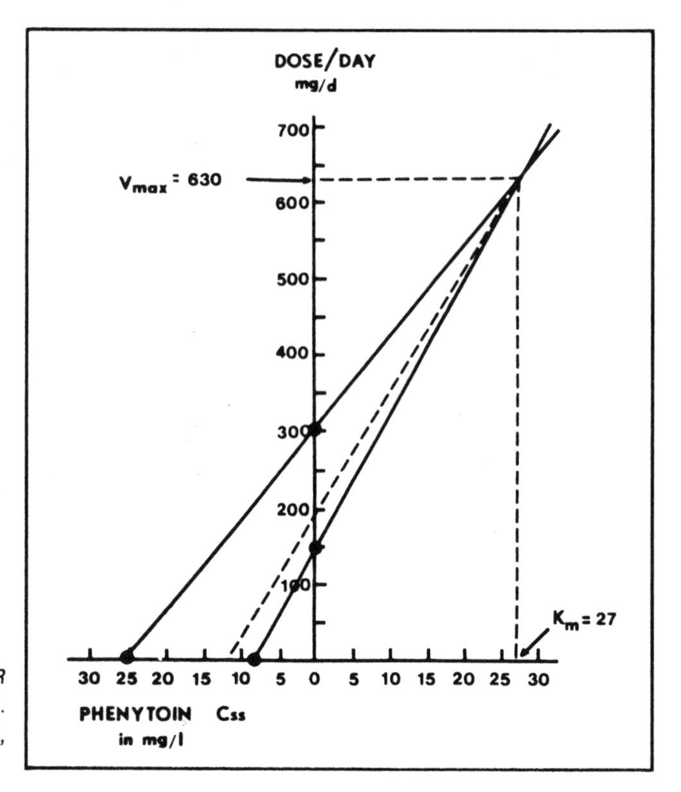

Figure 14-11. Plot of R versus C_{ss} (method C). (*From Witmer et al, 1984, with permission.*[4])

4. From point A, read V_m on y axis, and K_m on x-axis. (Again V_m of 630 mg/day and K_m of 27 mg/L is found.)

This V_m and K_m can be used in Eq. 14.11 to find R. Alternatively, join point A on the graph to meet 11.3 mg/L on the x axis; R can be read where this line meets y axis (190 mg/day).

To calculate the dose needed to keep steady state phenytoin concentration of 11.3 mg/L in this patient, use Eq. 14.11:

$$R = \frac{(630 \text{ mg/day})(11.3 \text{ mg/L})}{27 \text{ mg/day} + 11.3 \text{ mg/L}} = \frac{7119 \text{ mg/day}}{38.3} = 186 \text{ mg/day}$$

This compares very closely with the value obtained by the graphic method. All three methods have been used clinically. Vozeh et al[5] recently introduced a method that allows for an estimation of phenytoin dose based on steady-state concentration resulting from one dose. This method is based on the statistically compiled Nomogram that makes it possible to project a most likely dose for the patient.

Determination of K_m and V_m by Direct Method

When steady-state concentrations of phenytoin are known only at two dose levels, there is no advantage in using the graphic method. K_m and V_m may be calculated by solving two simultaneous equations formed by substituting C_{ss} and R (Eq. 14.11) with C_1, R_1, C_2, and R_2. The equations contain two unknowns, K_m and V_m, and may be solved easily:

$$R_1 = \frac{V_m C_1}{K_m + C_1}$$

$$R_2 = \frac{V_m C_2}{K_m + C_2}$$

Combining the two equations yields Equation 14.15:

$$K_m = \frac{R_2 - R_1}{\dfrac{R_1}{C_1} - \dfrac{R_2}{C_2}} \tag{14.15}$$

where C_1 is steady-state plasma drug concentration after dose 1; C_2 is steady-state plasma drug concentration after dose 2; R_1 is the first dosing rate; and R_2 is the second dosing rate. To calculate K_m and V_m, use Equation 14.15 with the values $C_1 = 8.6$ mg/L; $C_2 = 25.1$ mg/L; $R_1 = 150$ mg/day; and $R_2 = 300$ mg/day. The results are

$$K_m = \frac{300 - 150}{\dfrac{150}{8.6} - \dfrac{300}{25.1}} = 27.3 \text{ mg/L}$$

Substitute K_m into either of the two simultaneous equations to solve for V_m:

$$150 = \frac{V_m(8.6)}{27.3 + 8.6}$$

$$V_m = 626 \text{ mg/day}$$

NONLINEAR PHARMACOKINETICS DUE TO DRUG–PROTEIN BINDING

Protein binding may prolong the elimination half-life of a drug. Drugs that are protein bound must dissociate into the free or nonbound form to be eliminated by glomerular filtration. The nature and extent of drug–protein binding affects the magnitude of the deviation from normal linear or first-order elimination rate process.

For example, consider the plasma level–time curves of two hypothetical drugs given intravenously in equal doses (Fig. 14-12). One drug is 90% protein bound whereas the other drug does not bind plasma protein. Both drugs are eliminated solely by glomerular filtration through the kidney.

The plasma curves in Figure 14-12 demonstrate that the protein-bound drug is more concentrated in the plasma than a drug that is not protein bound, and the protein-bound drug is eliminated at a slower, nonlinear rate. Since the two drugs are eliminated by identical mechanisms, the characteristically slower elimination rate for the protein-bound drug is due to the fact that less free drug is available for glomerular filtration in the course of renal excretion.

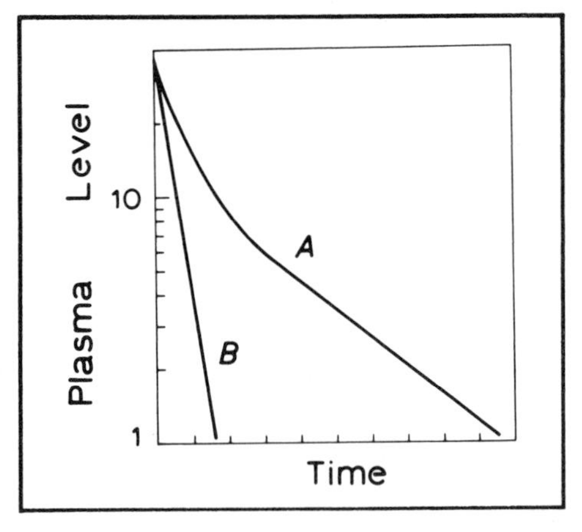

Figure 14-12. Plasma curve comparing the elimination of two drugs given in equal IV doses. Curve *A* represents a drug 90% bound to plasma protein. Curve *B* represents a drug not bound to plasma protein.

The concentration of free drug, C_f, can be calculated at any time, as follows.

$$C_f = C_p(1 - \text{fraction bound}) \tag{14.16}$$

For any protein-bound drug the free drug concentration, C_f, will always be less than the total drug concentration, C_p.

A careful examination of Figure 14-12 shows that the slope of the bound drug decreases gradually as the drug concentration decreases. This indicates that the percent of drug bound is not constant. In vivo, the percent of drug bound usually increases as the plasma drug concentration decreases (see Chap. 11). Since protein binding of drug can cause nonlinear elimination rates, pharmacokinetic fitting of protein-bound drug data to a simple one-compartment model without accounting for binding results in erroneous estimates of the volume of distribution and elimination half-life. Sometimes plasma drug data for drugs that are highly protein bound have been fitted inappropriately to two-compartment models.

ONE-COMPARTMENT MODEL DRUG WITH PROTEIN BINDING

The process of elimination of a drug distributed in a single compartment with protein binding is illustrated in Figure 14-13. The one compartment contains both free drug and bound drug, which are dynamically interconverted with rate constants K_1 and K_2. Elimination of drug occurs only with the free drug at a first-order rate. The bound drug is not eliminated. Assuming a saturable and instantly reversible drug-binding process: P = protein concentration in plasma; C_f = plasma concentration of free drug; $K_d = K_2/K_1$ = dissociation constant of the protein drug complex; C_p = total plasma drug concentration; and C_b = plasma concentration of bound drug.

$$\frac{C_b}{P} = \frac{\frac{1}{K_d} C_f}{1 + \left(\frac{1}{K_d}\right) C_f} \tag{14.17}$$

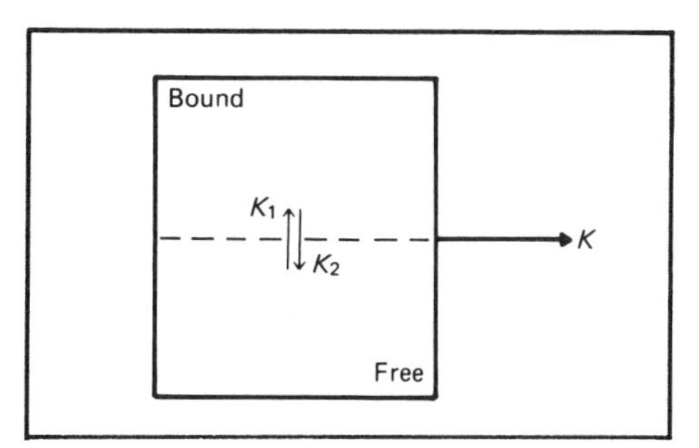

Figure 14-13. One-compartment model with drug–protein binding.

This equation can be rearranged as follows:

$$C_b = \frac{PC_f}{K_d + C_f} = C_p - C_f \tag{14.18}$$

Solving for C_f,

$$C_f = \tfrac{1}{2}\left[-(P + K_d - C_p) + \sqrt{(P + K_d - C_p)^2 + 4K_dC_p}\right] \tag{14.19}$$

Since the rate of drug elimination is dC_p/dt,

$$\frac{dC_p}{dt} = -KC_f$$

$$\frac{dC_p}{dt} = -\frac{K}{2}\left[-(P + K_d - C_p) + \sqrt{(P + K_d - C_p)^2 + 4K_dC_p}\right] \tag{14.20}$$

This differential equation describes the relationship of changing plasma drug concentrations during elimination. This equation is not easily integrated but could be solved by means of a numerical method. Figure 14-14 shows the plasma drug concentration curves for a one-compartment protein-bound drug having a volume of distribution of 50 ml/kg and an elimination half-life of 30 min. The protein concentration is 4.4% and the molecular weight of the protein is 67,000. At various doses the pharmacokinetics of elimination of the drug as shown by the plasma curves range from linear to nonlinear, depending on the total plasma drug concentration.

Nonlinear elimination pharmacokinetics occur more dramatically at higher doses, since more free drug is then available and initial drug elimination occurs more rapidly. For drugs demonstrating nonlinear pharmacokinetics, the free drug concentration may increase slowly at first, but when the dose of drug is raised beyond the protein-bound saturation point, free plasma drug concentrations may rise abruptly. Therefore, the concentration of free drug should always be calculated in order to make sure the patient receives a proper dose.

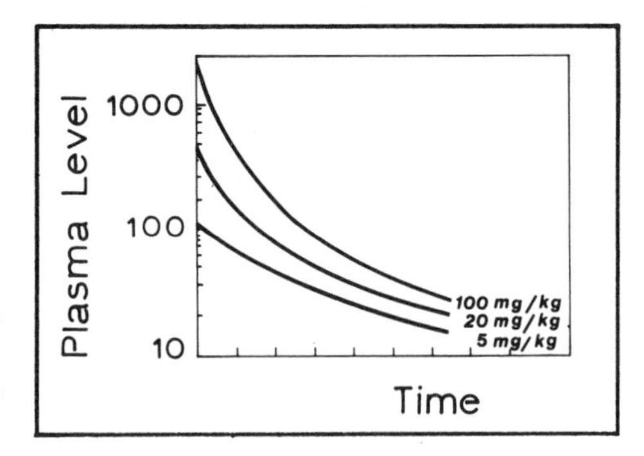

Figure 14-14. Plasma drug concentrations for various doses of a one-compartment model drug with protein binding. (*Adapted from Coffey J, et al, 1971, with permission.*[3])

QUESTIONS

1. What processes of drug absorption, distribution, and elimination may be considered "capacity limited," "saturated," or "dose dependent?"
2. Drugs such as phenytoin and salicylates have been reported to follow dose-dependent elimination kinetics. What changes in pharmacokinetic parameters, including $t_{1/2}$, V_d, AUC, and C_p, could be predicted if the amounts of these drugs administered were increased from low pharmacologic doses to high therapeutic doses?
3. A given drug is metabolized by capacity-limited pharmacokinetics. Assume K_m is 50 μg/ml, V_m is 20 μg/ml hr, and the apparent V_d is 20 L/kg.
   a. What is the reaction order for the metabolism of this drug when given in a single intravenous dose of 10 mg/kg?
   b. How much time is necessary for the drug to be 50% metabolized?
4. How would induction or inhibition of the hepatic enzymes involved in drug biotransformation theoretically affect the pharmacokinetics of a drug which demonstrates nonlinear pharmacokinetics due to saturation of its hepatic elimination pathway?
5. Assume that both the active parent drug and its inactive metabolites are excreted by active tubular secretion. What might be the consequences of increasing the dosage of the drug on its elimination half-life?
6. The drug isoniazid was reported to interfere with the metabolism of phenytoin. Patients taking both drugs together would result in a higher phenytoin level in the body. Using the basic principles in this chapter, do you expect K_m to increase or decrease in patients taking both drugs? (Hint: See Fig. 14-4.)
7. Explain why K_m are often seen to have units of μM/ml and sometimes mg/L.

REFERENCES

1. Tozer TN, et al: In Breimer DD, Speiser P (eds), Topics in Pharmaceutical Sciences. New York, Elsevier, 1981, p. 4

2. Gibaldi M: Pharmacokinetic aspects of drug metabolism. Ann NY State Acad Sci 179:19, 1971
3. Coffey J, Bullock FJ, Schoenemann PT: Numerical solution of nonlinear pharmacokinetic equations: Effect of plasma protein binding on drug distribution and elimination. J Pharm Sci 60:1623, 1971
4. Witmer DR, Ritschel WA: Phenytoin isoniazid interaction: A kinetic approach to management. Drug Intell Pharmacokinet 18:483–86, 1984
5. Vozeh S, Muir KT, Sheiner LB: Predicting phenytoin dosage. J Pharm Biopharm 9:131–46, 1981

BIBLIOGRAPHY

Amsel LP, Levy G: Drug biotransformation interactions in man, II: A pharmacokinetic study of the simultaneous conjugation of benzoic and salicylic acids with glycine. J Pharm Sci 58:321–26, 1969

Kruger-Theimer E: Nonlinear dose concentration relationships. II Farmaco 23:718–56, 1968

Levy G: Pharmacokinetics of salicylate in man. Drugs Metab Rev 9:3–19, 1979

Levy G, Tsuchiya T: Salicylate accumulation kinetics in man. N Eng J Med 287:430–32, 1972

Ludden TM, Hawkins DW, Allen JP, Hoffman SF: Optimum phenytoin dosage regimen. Lancet 1:307–08, 1979

Mullen, PW: Optimal phenytoin therapy: A new technique for individualizing dosage. Clin Pharm Ther 23:228–32, 1978

Mullen PW, Foster RW: Comparative evaluation of six techniques for determining the Michaelis–Menten parameters relating phenytoin dose and steady state serum concentrations. J Pharm Pharmacol 31:100–04, 1979

Wagner J: Properties of the Michaelis–Menten equation and its integrated form which are useful in pharmacokinetics. J Pharm Biopharm 1:103, 1973

CHAPTER FIFTEEN

Application of Pharmacokinetics in Clinical Situations

The success of drug therapy is highly dependent on the dosage regimen design. A properly designed dosage regimen tries to achieve an optimum concentration of the drug at a receptor site to produce an optimal therapeutic response with minimum adverse effects. Individual variation in pharmacokinetics and pharmacodynamics makes the design of dosage regimens difficult. Therefore, the application of pharmacokinetics to dosage regimen design must be coordinated with proper clinical evaluation and monitoring.

THERAPEUTIC DRUG MONITORING

In administering potent drugs to patients the physician must maintain the plasma drug level within a narrow range of therapeutic concentrations. Various pharmacokinetic methods may be used to calculate the initial dose or dosage regimen. Usually, the initial dosage regimen is calculated empirically or estimated after a careful consideration of the known pharmacokinetics for the drug, the pathophysiologic condition of the patient, and the patient's drug history.

Due to interpatient variability in drug absorption, distribution, and elimination as well as changing pathophysiologic conditions in the patient, therapeutic drug-monitoring (TDM) services have been established in many hospitals to evaluate the response of the patient to the recommended dosage regimen. The functions of a TDM service are listed below.

- Select drug.
- Design dosage regimen.
- Evaluate patient's response.
- Determine need for measuring serum drug concentrations.

- Assay for drug.
- Perform pharmacokinetic evaluation of drug levels.
- Readjust dosage regimen.
- Monitor serum drug concentrations.
- Recommend special requirements.

Drug Selection

The choice of drug and drug therapy is usually made by the physician. However, many practitioners consult with the clinical pharmacist in drug product selection and dosage regimen design.

The choice of drug therapy is usually made on the basis of physical diagnosis of the patient, presence of any pathophysiologic problems in the patient, previous medical history in the patient, concurrent drug therapy, known allergies or drug sensitivities, and pharmacodynamic actions of the drug.

Dosage Regimen Design

Once the proper drug is selected for the patient, there are a number of factors that must be considered when designing a therapeutic dosage regimen. First, the usual pharmacokinetics of the drug including its absorption, distribution, and elimination profile are considered in the patient. Second, the physiology of the patient, such as age, weight, gender, and nutritional status, are considered. Third, any pathophysiologic conditions such as renal dysfunction, hepatic disease, and congestive heart failure, are considered since these could affect the normal pharmacokinetic profile of the drug. Fourth, one should consider the exposure of the patient to other medication or environmental factors (such as smoking) that also might alter the usual pharmacokinetics. Finally, the dosage regimen design should consider the target drug concentration at the receptor site for the patient including any change in receptor sensitivity to drug. Mathematical approaches to dosage regimen design will be given in a later section.

Evaluation of Patient's Response

After a drug product is chosen and the patient is receiving the initial dosage regimen, the practitioner should clinically evaluate the patient's response. If the patient is not responding to drug therapy as expected, then the drug and dosage regimen should be reviewed. The dosage regimen should be reviewed for adequacy, accuracy, and patient compliance to the drug therapy. The practitioner should then determine whether or not serum drug concentrations should be measured in the patient. In many situations sound clinical judgment may preclude the need for measuring serum drug concentrations.

Measurement of Serum Drug Concentrations

Before blood samples are taken from the patient, the practitioner should establish if there is need to measure the serum drug concentration. In some cases the patient's response may not be related to the serum drug concentration. For example, allergy or mild nausea may not be dose related.

A major assumption made by the practitioner is that serum drug concentrations relate to the therapeutic and/or toxic effects of the drug. For many drugs clinical studies have demonstrated that there is a therapeutically effective range of serum concentrations. Therefore, knowledge of the serum drug concentration may clarify why a patient is not responding to the drug therapy or why the patient is having an adverse effect. In addition, the practitioner may want to clarify the accuracy of the dosage regimen.

When ordering serum drug concentrations to be measured, a single serum drug concentration may not yield useful information unless other factors are considered. For example, the dosage regimen of the drug, including size of dose and dosage interval, route of drug administration, and time of sampling (peak, trough, or steady-state), should be known.

In many cases a singular blood sample is insufficient and several blood samples are needed to clarify the adequacy of the dosage regimen. In practice, trough serum concentrations are easier to obtain than peak or C_{av}^{∞} samples during a multiple-dose regimen. In addition, there may be limitations in terms of the number of blood samples which may be taken, the total volume of blood needed for the assay, and the time to perform the drug analysis. The practitioner who orders the measurement of serum concentrations should also consider the cost of the assays, the risks and discomfort for the patient, and the utility of the information gained.

Assay for Drug

Drug analyses are usually performed by either a clinical chemistry laboratory or a clinical pharmacokinetics laboratory. A variety of analytic techniques are available for drug measurement including high-pressure liquid chromatography, gas chromatography, spectrophotometry, fluorometry, immunoassay, and radioisotopic methods. The method used by the analytic laboratory may depend on such factors as the physicochemical characteristics of the drug, the target concentration for measurement, the amount and nature of the biological specimen (serum, urine), the available instrumentation, cost for each assay, and the analytical skills of the laboratory personnel. The laboratory should have a standard operating procedure for each drug analysis technique and follow good laboratory practices. Moreover, analytic method used for the assay of drugs in serum should be validated with respect to the following:

- Specificity
- Linearity
- Sensitivity
- Precision
- Accuracy
- Stability

Specificity. Specificity should be established by the demonstration via chromatographic evidence that the method is specific for the drug. The method should demonstrate that there is no interference between the drug, metabolites of the drug, and endogenous or exogenous substances. In addition, the internal standard should be resolved completely and also demonstrate no interference with other compounds. Colorimetric and spectrophotometric assays are usually less specific. Interference from other material may erroneously inflate the results.

Sensitivity. Sensitivity is the minimum detectable level or concentration of drug in serum which may be approximated as that lowest drug concentration which is 2–3 times the background noise. A minimum quantifiable level (MQL) is a statistical method for the determination of the precision of the lower level.

Linearity. The assay must demonstrate suitable linearity by using processed standard concentrations covering the range of the predicted unknown concentration. Linearity refers to a proportional relationship between the drug concentration and the instrument response (or signal) used to measure the drug.

Precision. Precision relates to the variation or reproducibility of the data. Precision measurements should be obtained by replication of various drug concentrations and by replication of standard concentration curves prepared separately on different days. A suitable statistical measurement of the dispersion of the data, such as standard deviation or coefficient of variation, is then performed.

Accuracy. Accuracy refers to the difference between the average assay values and the true or known drug concentrations. Control (known) drug serum concentrations should be prepared by an independent technician using such techniques to minimize any error in their preparation. These samples, including a "zero" drug concentration, are assayed by the technician assigned to the study along with a suitable standard drug concentration curve.

Stability. Standard drug concentrations should be maintained under the same storage conditions as the unknown serum samples and assayed periodically.

The stability study should continue for at least the same length of time as that for which the study samples are to be stored.

Serum samples obtained from subjects on a drug study should be assayed along with a minimum of three standard processed serum samples containing known standard drug concentrations and a minimum of three control serum samples whose concentrations are unknown to the analyst. These control serum samples should be randomly distributed in each day's run. Control samples should be replicated in duplicate to evaluate within day precision and between day precision. The concentration of drug in each serum sample is based on each day's processed standard curve.

Since each method for drug assay may have differences in sensitivity, precision, and specificity, the pharmacokineticist should be aware of which drug assay method the laboratory used.

Pharmacokinetic Evaluation

After the serum drug concentrations are measured, the pharmacokineticist must properly evaluate the data. Most laboratories report total drug (free plus bound drug) concentrations in the serum. The pharmacokineticist should be aware of the usual therapeutic range of serum concentrations from the literature. However, the literature may not indicate if the values were trough or peak serum levels. Moreover, the assay used in reporting the methodology might be different in terms of specificity and precision.

The assay results from the laboratory might show that the patient's serum drug levels are higher, lower, or equivalent to the expected serum levels. The pharmacokineticist should carefully evaluate these results while considering the patient and the patient's pathophysiologic condition. Table 15-1 gives a number of factors for the pharmacokineticist to consider when interpreting the drug serum concentration. Often, other data such as a high serum creatinine and high blood urea nitrogen (BUN) might help verify the reason that the observed high serum drug concentration in the patient was due to slow renal drug clearance due to compromised kidney function. In addition, a complaint by the patient of overstimulation and insomnia might also collaborate the laboratory's finding of higher than anticipated serum concentrations of theophylline. Therefore, the clinician or pharmacokineticist should evaluate the data using sound medical judgment and observation. The therapeutic decision should not be based solely on serum drug concentrations.

TABLE 15-1. PHARMACOKINETIC EVALUATION OF SERUM DRUG CONCENTRATIONS

Serum Concentrations Lower than Anticipated
Patient compliance
Error in dosage regimen
Wrong drug product (controlled release instead of immediate release)
Poor bioavailability
Rapid elimination
Enlarged apparent volume of distribution
Steady state not reached
Timing of blood sample
Serum Concentrations Higher than Anticipated
Patient compliance
Error in dosage regimen
Wrong drug product (immediate release instead of controlled release)
Rapid bioavailability
Smaller than anticipated apparent volume of distribution
Slow elimination
Serum Concentration Correct but Patient does not Respond to Therapy
Altered receptor sensitivity (e.g., tolerance)
Drug interaction at receptor site

Dosage Adjustment

From the serum drug concentration data and patient observations the clinician or pharmacokineticist might recommend an adjustment in the dosage regimen. Ideally, the new dosage regimen should be calculated using the pharmacokinetic parameters derived from the patient's serum drug concentrations. Although there might not be enough data for a complete pharmacokinetic profile, the pharmacokineticist should still be able to derive a new dosage regimen based on the available data and the pharmacokinetic parameters in the literature that are based on average population data.

Monitor Serum Drug Concentrations

In many cases the patient's pathophysiology might be unstable, either improving or further deteriorating. For example, proper therapy for congestive heart failure will improve cardiac output and renal perfusion, thereby increasing renal drug clearance. Therefore, continuous monitoring of serum drug concentrations are necessary to ensure proper drug therapy for the patient. For some drugs an acute pharmacologic response can be monitored in lieu of actual serum drug concentration. For example, prothrombin clotting time might be useful for monitoring anticoagulant therapy and blood pressure monitoring for hypotensive agents.

Special Recommendations

At times the patient might not be responding to drug therapy due to other factors. For example, the patient is not following the instructions for taking the medication (patient compliance). The patient may be taking the drug after a meal instead of before. The patient is not adhering to a special diet (e.g., low salt). Therefore, the patient might need special instructions which are simple and easy to follow.

DESIGN OF DOSAGE REGIMENS

There are a variety of methods that may be used to design a dosage regimen. Generally, the initial dosage of the drug is estimated using average population pharmacokinetic parameters obtained from the literature. The patient is then monitored for the therapeutic response by physical diagnosis and if necessary by measurement of serum drug levels. After evaluation of the patient a readjustment of the dosage regimen might be indicated with further therapeutic drug monitoring.

Individualized Dosage Regimens

The most accurate approach to dosage regimen design would be the calculation of the dose based on the pharmacokinetics of the drug in the patient. This approach is not feasible for the calculation of the initial dose. However, once the patient has been medicated, the readjustment of the dose may be calculated using pharmacokinetic parameters derived from measurement of the serum drug levels after the initial dose.

Dosage Regimens Based on Population Averages

The method most often used to calculate a dosage regimen is based on average pharmacokinetic parameters obtained from clinical studies which have been published in the drug literature. This method may be based on a fixed or adaptive model.[1,2]

In the fixed model it is assumed that the population average pharmacokinetic parameters may be used directly to calculate a dosage regimen for the patient without any alteration. Usually pharmacokinetic parameters, such as absorption rate constant K_a, bioavailability factor F, apparent volume of distribution V_d, and elimination rate constant K, are assumed to remain constant. Most often the drug is assumed to follow the pharmacokinetics of a one-compartment model. When a multiple-dosage regimen is designed, then the multiple-dosage equations based on principle of superposition (Chapter 13) are used to evaluate the dose. The practitioner may use the usual dosage suggested by the literature and also make a small adjustment of the dosage based on the patient's weight and/or age.

When using the adaptive model to calculate a dosage regimen, the pharmacokineticist makes use of patient variables such as weight, age, sex, and body surface area and known patient pathophysiology such as renal disease, as well as the known population average pharmacokinetic parameters of the drug. In this case the calculation of dosage regimen takes into consideration any changing pathophysiology of the patient and attempts to adapt or modify the dosage regimen according to the needs of the patient.

Dosage Regimen Based on Partial Pharmacokinetic Parameters

For many drugs the entire pharmacokinetic profile for the drug is unfortunately unknown or unavailable. Therefore, the pharmacokineticist might have to make some assumptions in order to calculate the dosage regimen. For example, a common assumption is to let the bioavailability factor F equal to 1 or 100%. Thus, if the drug is less than fully absorbed systemically, then the patient would be undermedicated rather than overmedicated. Obviously, some of these assumptions will be dependent on the nature of the drug and its therapeutic range.

Adaptive Dosage Regimen with Feedback

A more accurate method for calculating a dosage regimen uses the available pharmacokinetic parameters for the drug and the patient characteristics to decide the initial dosage regimen. Then the patient is monitored using an acute pharmacologic response and/or serum drug concentrations as a means of readjusting the dosage regimen accordingly. As an adjunct to dosage regimen design, computer simulations of the predicted serum drug concentrations are compared with observed serum drug concentrations from the patient. This method has one advantage of matching more closely the dosage regimen to the patient's needs. In addition, there is a learning situation from which the practitioner may improve the initial dosage regimen calculation for another patient who has a similar syndrome.

Empirical Dosage Regimens

In many cases the physician selects a dosage regimen for the patient without using any pharmacokinetic variables. In this situation the physician makes the decision based on empirical clinical data, personal experience, and observations. The physician characterizes the patient as representative of a similar well-studied clinical population that has used the drug successfully.

CONVERSION FROM INTRAVENOUS INFUSION TO ORAL DOSING

After the patient's condition is controlled by intravenous infusion, it is often desirable to continue to medicate the patient with the same drug using the oral route of administration. As discussed in Chapter 12, once the intravenous infusion is stopped, then the serum drug concentration decreases according to first-order elimination kinetics. For immediate-release oral drug products the time to reach steady state is dependent on the first-order elimination rate constant for the drug. Therefore, if the patient starts the dosage regimen with the oral drug product at the same time when the intravenous infusion is stopped, then the exponential decline of serum levels from the intravenous infusion should just match the exponential increase in serum drug levels from the oral drug product.

The conversion from intravenous infusion to a sustained-release oral medication given once or twice daily has become more common with the availability of sustained-released-drug products such as theophylline[6] and quinidine. Computer simulation for the conversion of intravenous theophylline (aminophylline) therapy to oral sustained-release theophylline demonstrated that oral therapy should be started at the same time as intravenous infusion is stopped.[3] With this method there is minimal fluctuations between the peak and trough serum theophylline levels. Moreover, giving the first oral dose may make it easier for the nursing staff or patient to comply with the dosage regimen.

The following methods may be used to calculate an appropriate oral dosage regimen for a patient whose condition has been stabilized by an intravenous drug infusion. Both methods assume that the patient's plasma drug concentration is at steady state.

Method 1

This method assumes that the steady-state plasma drug concentration, C_{ss}, after IV infusion is identical to the desired C_{av}^{∞} after multiple oral doses of the drug. Therefore, the following equation may be used:

$$C_{av}^{\infty} = \frac{SFD_0}{KV_d\tau} \quad (15.1)$$

solving for dosing rate, $D_0/\tau = C_{av}^{\infty}KV_d/SF$ where S is the salt form of the drug.

(15.2)

EXAMPLE

An adult male asthmatic patient (age 55, 78 kg) has been maintained on an intravenous infusion of aminophylline at a rate of 34 mg/hr. The steady-state theophylline drug concentration was 12 μg/ml and total body clearance was calculated as 3.0 L/hr. Calculate an appropriate oral dosage regimen of theophylline for this patient.

Solution

Aminophylline is a soluble salt of theophylline and contains 85% of theophylline ($S = 0.85$). Theophylline is 100% bioavailable ($F = 1$) after an oral dose. Since total body clearance $Cl_T = KV_d$, Equation 15.2 may be expressed as

$$\frac{D_0}{\tau} = \frac{C_{av}^{\infty}Cl_T}{SF} \quad (15.3)$$

The dose rate, D_0/T, (34 mg/hr) was calculated on the basis of aminophylline. The patient, however, will be given theophylline orally. To convert to oral theophylline, S and F should be considered:

$$\begin{matrix}\text{Theophylline} \\ \text{dose rate}\end{matrix} = \frac{SFD_0}{T} = \frac{(0.85)(1)(34)}{1} = 28.9 \text{ mg/hr}$$

The theophylline dose rate of 28.9 mg/hr must be converted to a reasonable schedule for the patient with a consideration of the various commercially available theophylline drug products. Therefore, the total daily dose is 28.9 mg/hr × 24 hr or 693.6 mg/day. Possible theophylline dosage schedules could be 700 mg/day, 350 mg every 12 hr or 175 mg every 6 hr. Each of these dosage regimens would achieve the same C_{av}^{∞} but different C_{max}^{∞} and C_{min}^{∞}, which should be calculated. The dose of 350 mg every 12 hr should be given in sustained-release form to avoid any excessive high drug concentration in the body.

Method 2

This method assumes that the rate of intravenous infusion (mg/hr) is the same desired rate of oral dosage. Using the example in method 1, the following calculations may be used.

Solution

The aminophylline is given by IV infusion at a rate of 34 mg/hr. The total daily dose of aminophylline would be 34 mg/hr. Then 24 hr = 816 mg. The equivalent daily dose in terms of theophylline would be 816 × 0.85 = 693.6 mg. Thus, the patient should receive approximately 700 mg of theophylline per day.

DETERMINATION OF DOSE

The dose of a drug is estimated with the objective of delivering a desirable therapeutic level of the drug to the body. For many drugs the desirable therapeutic drug levels and pharmacokinetic parameters are available in the clinical literature. However, the literature in some cases may not yield complete drug information, or the information available may be partly equivocal. Therefore, the pharmacokineticist must make certain necessary assumptions in accordance with the best pharmacokinetic information available.

For a drug that is administered for an extended period of time, the dose is usually calculated so that the average steady-state blood level is within the therapeutic range. The dose can be calculated with Equation 15.4, which expresses the C_{av}^{∞} in terms of dose (D), dosing interval (τ), volume of distribution (V_d), and the elimination half-life of the drug. F is the fraction of drug absorbed and is equal to 1 for drugs administered intravenously.

$$C_{av}^{\infty} = \frac{1.44 D t_{1/2} F}{V_d \tau} \qquad (15.4)$$

PRACTICE PROBLEMS

1. The pharmacokinetic data of clindamycin were reported by DeHann et al[4] (1972) as follows:

$$K = 0.247 \text{ hr}^{-1}$$

$$t_{1/2} = 2.81 \text{ hr}$$

$$V_d = 43.9 \text{ L}/1.73 \text{ m}^2$$

What is the steady-state concentration of the drug after 150 mg of the drug have been given orally every 6 hr for a week (assume the drug is 100% absorbed)?

Solution

$$C_{av}^{\infty} = \frac{1.44 D_0 t_{1/2} F}{V_d \tau}$$

$$= \frac{1.44 \times 150{,}000 \times 2.81 \times 1}{43{,}900 \times 6} \ \mu g/ml$$

$$= 2.3 \ \mu g/ml$$

2. The elimination half-life of tobramycin was reported by Regamey et al[5] to be 2.15 hr; the volume of distribution was reported to be 33.5% of body weight.

a. What is the dose for an 80-kg individual if a steady-state level of 2.5 μg/ml is desired? Assume that the drug is given intravenously every 8 hr.

Solution

Assuming the drug is 100% bioavailable due to IV injection,

$$C_{av}^{\infty} = \frac{1.44 D_0 t_{1/2} F}{V_d \tau}$$

$$2.5 = \frac{1.44 \times 2.15 \times 1 \times D_0}{80 \times 0.335 \times 1000 \times 8}$$

$$D_0 = \frac{2.5 \times 80 \times 0.335 \times 1000 \times 8}{1.44 \times 2.15} \ \mu g$$

$$= 173 \ mg$$

The dose should be 173 mg every 8 hr.

b. The manufacturer has suggested that in normal cases tobramycin should be given at a rate of 1 mg/kg every 8 hr. With this dosage regimen, what would the average steady-state level be?

Solution

$$C_{av}^{\infty} = \frac{1.44 \times 1 \times 1000 \times 2.15}{0.335 \times 1000 \times 8}$$

$$= 1.16 \ \mu g/ml$$

Since the bacteriocidal concentration of an antibiotic varies with the organism involved in the infection, the dose prescribed may change. The average plasma concentration of a drug is used to indicate whether optimum drug level has been reached. With certain antibiotics, however, the steady-state peak and trough levels are sometimes used as therapeutic indicators, largely as a matter of convenience. For example, the effective concentration of tobramycin was reported to be around 4–5 μg/ml for peak level and around 2 μg/ml for trough level when administered intramuscularly every 12 hr. Although peak and trough levels are frequently reported in clinical journals, these drug levels are only transitory in the body. Peak and trough drug levels are less useful pharmacokinetically, since the information cannot be applied directly to a different dosing schedule. Moreover, peak and trough levels fluctuate more and are usually reported less accurately than average plasma drug concentrations. When the average plasma drug concentration is used as a therapeutic indicator, an optimum dosing interval must be chosen. The dosing interval is usually set at approximately 1–2 elimination half-lives of the drug, unless the drug has a very narrow therapeutic index. In this case the drug must be given in small doses more frequently or by infusion.

EFFECT OF CHANGING DOSE AND DOSING INTERVAL ON C^{∞}_{max}, C^{∞}_{min}, AND C^{∞}_{av}

The C^{∞}_{av} is used most often in dosage calculation. However, when monitoring serum drug concentrations, C^{∞}_{av} cannot be measured directly but may be obtained by the AUC/τ during multiple-dosage regimens. As discussed in Chapter 13, the C^{∞}_{av} is not the arithmetic average of C^{∞}_{max} and C^{∞}_{min} since serum concentrations decline exponentially. In contrast, the C_{ss} may be used to monitor the steady-state serum concentrations after intravenous infusion. When considering therapeutic drug monitoring of serum concentrations after the initiation of a multiple-dosage regimen, the trough serum drug concentrations or C^{∞}_{min} may be used to validate the dosage regimen. The blood sample withdrawn just prior to the administration of the next dose represents C^{∞}_{min}. To obtain the C^{∞}_{max}, the blood sample must be withdrawn exactly at the time for peak absorption, or closely spaced blood samples must be taken and the plasma drug concentrations graphed. In practice, an approximate time for maximum drug absorption is estimated and a blood sample is withdrawn. Due to differences in rates of drug absorption, the C^{∞}_{max} measured in this manner is only an approximation of the true C^{∞}_{max}.

The advantage of using C^{∞}_{av} as an indicator for deciding therapeutic blood level is that C^{∞}_{av} is determined on a set of points and is generally less fluctuating than either C^{∞}_{max} or C^{∞}_{min}. Moreover, when the dosing interval is changed, the dose may be proportionally increased to keep C^{∞}_{av} constant. This approach works well for some drugs. For example, if the drug diazepam is given either 10 mg tid or 15 mg bid, the same C^{∞}_{av} is obtained as shown by Equation 15.1. In fact, if the daily dose is the same, the C^{∞}_{av} should be the same.

The dosing interval must be set with the elimination half-life of the drug; otherwise the patient may suffer either toxic effect of a high C^{∞}_{max} even if the C^{∞}_{av} is kept constant. For example, using the same example of diazepam, the same C^{∞}_{av} is achieved at 10 mg tid or 60 mg every other day. Obviously, the C^{∞}_{max} of the latter dose regimen would produce C^{∞}_{max} which is several times larger than that achieved with 10 mg tid dose regimen. In general, if a drug has a relatively wide therapeutic index and a relatively long elimination half-life, then there is good flexibility in changing the dose or dosing interval using C_{av}^{∞} as an indicator. When the drug has a narrow therapeutic index, C_{max}^{∞} and C_{min}^{∞} must be monitored to ensure safety and efficacy.

As the size of the dose or dosage intervals change proportionately, the C_{av}^{∞} may be the same but the steady-state peak, C_{max}^{∞}, and trough, C_{min}^{∞}, drug levels will change. The C_{max}^{∞} is influenced by the size of the dose and dosage interval. An increase in the size of the dose given at a longer dosage interval will cause an increase in C_{max}^{∞} and a decrease in C_{min}^{∞}. In this case the C_{max}^{∞} may be very close or above the minimum toxic drug concentration (MTC). However, the C_{min}^{∞} may be lower than the minimum effective drug concentration (MEC). In this latter case the low C_{min}^{∞} may be subtherapeutic and dangerous for the patient depending on the nature of the drug.

DETERMINATION OF FREQUENCY OF DRUG ADMINISTRATION

The size of a drug dose is often related to the frequency of drug administration. The more frequently a drug is administered, the smaller the dose must be. Thus, a dose of 250 mg every 3 hr could be changed to 500 mg every 6 hr without affecting the average steady-state plasma concentration of the drug. However, as the dosing interval get longer, the size of the dose required to maintain the average plasma drug concentration gets correspondingly larger. When an excessively long dosing interval is chosen, the large dose may result in peak plasma levels that are above toxic drug concentration, although the C_{av}^{∞} will remain the same. In general, the dosing interval for most drugs is determined by the elimination half-life. Drugs like penicillins, which have relatively low toxicity, may be given at intervals much longer than their elimination half-lives without any toxicity problems. Drugs having a narrow therapeutic index, such as digoxin and phenytoin, must be given relatively frequently to minimize excessive "peak and trough" fluctuations in blood levels. For example, the common maintenance schedule for digoxin is 0.25 mg/day and the elimination half-life of digoxin is 1.7 days. In contrast, penicillin G is given at 250 mg every 6 hr, while the elimination half-life of penicillin G is 0.75 hr. Penicillin is given at a dosage interval equal to 8 times its elimination half-life, whereas digoxin is given at a dosing interval only 0.59 times its elimination half-life. The toxic plasma concentration of penicillin G is over 100 times greater than its effective concentration, whereas digoxin has an effective concentration of 1–2 ng/ml and a toxicity level of 3 ng/ml. The toxic concentration of digoxin is only 1.5 times the effective concentration. Therefore, a drug with a large therapeutic index can be given in large doses and at relatively long dosing intervals.

DETERMINATION OF BOTH DOSE AND DOSAGE INTERVAL

Both the dose and dosage interval should be considered in the dosage regimen calculations. Ideally, the calculated dosage regimen should maintain the serum drug concentrations between the C_{max}^{∞} and C_{min}^{∞}. For intravenous multiple-dosage regimens the ratio of $C_{max}^{\infty}/C_{min}^{\infty}$ may be expressed by

$$\frac{C_{max}^{\infty}}{C_{min}^{\infty}} = \frac{C_p^0/(1 - e^{-k\tau})}{C_p^0 e^{-kT}/(1 - e^{-k\tau})} \tag{15.5}$$

which can be simplified to

$$\frac{C_{max}^{\infty}}{C_{min}^{\infty}} = \frac{1}{e^{-k\tau}} \tag{15.6}$$

From Equation 15.6 a maximum dosage interval, τ, may be calculated which will maintain the serum concentration between the C_{min}^{∞} and C_{max}^{∞}. After the dosage interval is calculated, then a dose may be calculated.

PRACTICE PROBLEM

1. The elimination half-life of an antibiotic is 3 hr with an apparent volume of distribution equivalent to 20% of body weight. The usual therapeutic range for this antibiotic is between 5 and 15 μg/ml. Adverse toxicity for this drug is often observed at serum concentrations greater than 20 μg/ml. Calculate a dosage regimen (multiple IV doses) which will just maintain the serum drug concentrations between 5 and 15 μg/ml.

Solution

From Equation 15.6 determine the dosage interval τ:

$$\frac{15}{5} = \frac{1}{e^{-(0.693/3)\tau}}$$

$$e^{-0.231\tau} = 0.333$$

Take the natural logarithm (ln) on both sides of the equation:

$$-0.231\tau = -1.10$$

$$\tau = 4.76 \text{ hr}$$

Then determine the dose from Equation 15.7 after substitution of $C_p^0 = D_0/V_d$:

$$C_{max}^{\infty} = \frac{D_0/V_d}{1 - e^{-K\tau}} \tag{15.7}$$

Solve for dose, D_0, letting $V_d = 200$ ml/kg (20% body weight):

$$15 = \frac{D_0/200}{1 - e^{-(0.231)(4.76)}}$$

$$D_0 = 2 \text{ mg/kg}$$

To check this dose for therapeutic effectiveness, calculate C_{min}^{∞}, and C_{av}^{∞}:

$$C_{min}^{\infty} = \frac{(D_0/V_d)e^{-K\tau}}{1 - e^{-K\tau}} = \frac{(2000/200)e^{0.231(4.76)}}{1 - e^{-(0.231)(4.76)}}$$

$$C_{min}^{\infty} = 4.99\ \mu\text{g/ml}$$

As a further check on the dosage regimen, the C_{av}^{∞} is calculated:

$$C_{av}^{\infty} = \frac{D_0}{V_d K \tau} = \frac{2000}{(200)(0.231)(4.76)}$$

$$C_{av}^{\infty} = 9.09\ \mu g/ml$$

By calculation, the dose of this antibiotic should be 2 mg/kg every 4.76 hr to maintain the serum drug concentrations between 5 and 15 μg/ml.

In practice, rather than a dosage interval of 4.76 hr the dosage regimen and the dosage interval should be made as convenient as possible for the patient and the size of the dose should take into account the commercially available drug formulation. Therefore, the dosage regimen should be recalculated to have a convenient value (4–6 hr) and the size of the dose adjusted accordingly.

NOMOGRAMS IN DESIGNING DOSAGE REGIMENS

For ease of calculation of dosage regimens many clinicians rely on nomograms to calculate the proper dosage regimen for their patients. The use of a nomogram may give a quick approximation of the dosage regimen for initial drug therapy. However, as with any method of calculation, there are a number of limitations of which the clinician should be aware. For example, the nomogram may be based on empirical clinical observations in various patients who were given the drug. The nomogram may have dosage regimen adjustments for patients with various characteristics such as obesity, smoker, age, etc. In addition, the nomogram may be based on population-average pharmacokinetic parameters and the assumption that the drug follows a specific pharmacokinetic model. In order to keep the dosage regimen calculation simple, complicated equations are often solved diagramatically to produce a simple dose recommendation based on a specially designed nomogram. The dosage regimen may give a constant dose but change the dosage interval or keep a constant dosage interval but change the size of the dose. A few nomograms do make use of certain pharmacologic or physiologic parameters such as serum creatinine concentration to help modify the dosage regimen accordingly. Lastly, the nomograms based on small population averages may not take into consideration the predicted pharmacokinetic behavior of the drug in the individual patient.

DETERMINATION OF ROUTE OF ADMINISTRATION

The selection of the proper route of administration is an important consideration in drug therapy. The rate of drug absorption and the duration of action are influenced by the route of drug administration. Moreover, there are physiologic considerations that often preclude the use of certain routes of administration. Drugs which are unstable in the gastrointestinal tract or drugs which undergo extensive first-pass effect are not suitable for oral administration. For example, insulin is destroyed in the stomach, and drugs like xylocaine and nitroglycerin are not suitable for oral administration because of rapid removal of the drug due to the first-pass effect.

Furthermore, certain drugs are not suitable for administration intramuscularly due to erratic drug release, pain, or local irritation. Even though the drug is injected into the muscle mass, the drug must reach the circulatory system or other body fluid to become bioavailable. The anatomic site of the intramuscular injection will affect the rate of drug absorption. A drug injected into the deltoid muscle is more rapidly absorbed than a drug similarly injected into the gluteus maximus due to better blood flow in the former. In general, the method of drug administration which is most consistent and which provides greatest bioavailability should be given to ensure maximum therapeutic effect. The various methods of drug administration can be classified as either extravascular or intravascular (Table 15-2).

Intravenous administration is the fastest and most reliable way of delivering the drug into the circulatory system. Drugs administered intravenously are removed more rapidly because the entire dose is subject to elimination immediately. Consequently, more frequent drug administration is required. Drugs administered extravascularly must be absorbed into the bloodstream and the total absorbed dose is eliminated more slowly. The frequency of administration can be lessened by using routes of administration which give a sustained rate of drug absorption. Intramuscular injection generally provides more rapid absorption than does oral administration of preparations that are not very soluble. However, precipitation of the drug at the injection site may result in slower absorption and a delayed response. For example, a dose of 50 mg of chlordiazepoxide (Librium) is more quickly absorbed after oral administration than after intramuscular injection.

TABLE 15-2. COMMON ROUTES OF DRUG ADMINISTRATION

Intramuscular
- Intravenous infusion (IV drip)
- Intravenous injection (IV bolus)
- Intra-arterial injection

Extravascular
- Enteral
  - Oral
  - Sublingual
  - Buccal
  - Rectal
- Parental
  - Intramuscular injection
  - Subcutaneous injection
  - Intradermal injection
  - Intrathecal injection
- Inhalation
- Transdermal

DOSING OF DRUGS IN INFANTS

Dosing of drugs in infants requires a thorough consideration of the differences between the infant and the adult as concerns the pharmacokinetics and pharmacology of the drug. The variation in body composition and the maturity of liver and kidney function are potential sources of differences in pharmacokinetics with respect to age. For convenience, "infants" are here arbitrarily defined as children 0–2 years of age. Within this group, special consideration is necessary for infants less than 4 weeks old because their ability to handle drugs often differs from more mature infants.

In general, hepatic function is not attained until the third week of life. Oxidative processes are fairly well developed in infants, but there is a deficiency of conjugative enzymes. In addition, many drugs exhibit reduced binding to plasma albumin in infants.

Newborns show only 30–50% the renal activity of adults on an activity per unit of body weight basis (Table 15-3). Drugs that are heavily dependent on renal excretion will have a sharply increased elimination half-life. For example, the penicillins are excreted for the most part through the kidney. The elimination half-lives of such drugs are much reduced in infants, as shown in Table 15-4.

PRACTICE PROBLEMS

The elimination half-life of penicillin G is 0.5 hr in adults and 3.2 hr in neonates (0–7 days old). Assuming that the normal adult dose of penicillin G is 4 mg/kg every 4 hr, calculate the dose of penicillin G for an 11-lb infant.

TABLE 15-3. COMPARISON OF NEWBORN AND ADULT RENAL CLEARANCES.*

	Average Infant	Average Adult
Body weight (kg)	3.5	70
Body water		
(%)	77	58
(L)	2.7	41
Inulin clearance		
(ml/min)	Approx. 3	130
$k(\text{min}^{-1})$	3/2700 = 0.0011	130/41,000 = 0.0032
$t_{1/2}$(min)	630	220
PAH clearance		
(ml/min)	Approx. 12	650
$k(\text{min}^{-1})$	12/2800 = 0.0043	650/41,000 = 0.016
$t_{1/2}$(min)	160	43

*Computations are for a drug distributed in the whole body water, but any other V_d would give the same relative values.

Data for average infant from West et al. By permission of Charles C. Thomas and Cambridge University Press.[11]

TABLE 15-4. ELIMINATION HALF-LIVES OF DRUGS IN INFANTS AND ADULTS

Drug	Half-Life in Neonates* (hr)	Half-Life in Adults (hr)
Penicillin G	3.2	0.5
Ampicillin	4	1 to 1.5
Methicillin	3.3/1.3	0.5
Carbenicillin	5 to 6	1 to 1.5
Kanamycin	5 to 5.7	3 to 5
Gentamicin	5	2 to 3

*0–7 days old

Solution

$$\frac{\tau_1}{\tau_2} = \frac{(t_{1/2})_1}{(t_{1/2})_2}$$

$$t_{1/2} = 0.5 \text{ hr}$$

$$\tau_2 = \frac{4 \times 3.2}{0.5} = 25.6 \text{ hr}$$

Therefore, this infant may be given the following dose:

$$\text{Dose} = 4 \text{ mg/kg} \times \frac{11 \text{ lb}}{2.2 \text{ lb/kg}} = 20 \text{ mg every 24 hr}$$

Alternatively, 10 mg every 12 hr would achieve the same C_{av}^{∞}.

The dosages of drugs given to infants should be based on pharmacokinetic considerations. A number of empirical rules are available for calculation of the dosages of drugs for infants. For example, *Clark's rule* states

$$\text{Child dose} = \frac{\text{weight in lb} \times \text{adult dose}}{150}$$

Using the previous example for penicillin G and an adult dose of 300 mg (for a 75-kg adult), the dose for an 11-lb infant should be

$$\text{Child dose} = \frac{11}{150} \times 300 = 22 \text{ mg}$$

Although the dose calculated in this case is similar to the dose calculated using a pharmacokinetic approach, the dosage interval is not determined for drugs where the elimination half-life is different in the infants. In the case of penicillin the drug may be handled rather differently in the infant. The other rules (such as Young's rule* and Clark's rule) for dose adjustment are, at best, crude approximations that

*Young's rule (for a patient 2 years of age or older):

$$\text{Child dose} = \frac{\text{age (yr)}}{\text{age (yr)} + 12} \times \text{adult dose}$$

assume that only body age and size change with growth and do not consider the rate of drug elimination. Another dose adjustment method is based on *body surface area*. This approach has the advantage of avoiding bias due to obesity or unusual body weight since the height and weight of the patient are both considered. Again, the body surface area method gives only a rough estimation of the proper dose, since the pharmacokinetic differences of specific drugs are not considered.

DOSING OF DRUGS IN THE ELDERLY

The physiologic changes due to aging may necessitate special considerations in administering drugs to the elderly. The body composition of the elderly patient is modified in many ways. Fatty tissues are increased and metabolic processes are slowed. For example, fat-soluble drugs may have an altered volume of distribution due to the increased amount of fatty tissues. Free drug concentration in the body may be increased because of reduced drug plasma–protein binding. The cardiac output of the elderly patient is only slightly modified. However, perfusion of blood to the intestinal region is reported to be greatly reduced, potentially affecting the absorption of drugs from the gastrointestinal tract. The glomerular filtration rate in elderly patients is significantly reduced, creating longer elimination half-lives for renally excreted drugs and potential drug accumulation in the body. Finally, the receptor sensitivity or response to drugs in the elderly patient may be also modified. Indeed, a number of drugs were reported to elicit an increased incidence of side effects when administered to elderly patients. The correction of the dose in the elderly for drugs excreted by glomerular filtration is calculated from creatinine clearance by means of the Jellife equation or the nomogram in Chapter 16. The reduction in creatinine clearance in the elderly is quantitated to calculate a reduced dose. If other pharmacokinetic parameters are available for elderly patients, the dose can be modified accordingly.

PRACTICE PROBLEMS

1. Kanamycin has a normal elimination half-life of 107 min in young adults. In patients 70–90 years old the elimination half-life of kanamycin is 282 min. The normal dose of kanamycin is 15 mg/kg day divided into two doses. What is the dose for a 75-year-old patient, assuming that the volume of distribution per body weight is not changed by the patient's age?

Solution

The longer elimination half-life of kanamycin in the elderly is due to a decrease in renal function. A good inverse correlation has been obtained of elimination half-life to kanamycin and creatinine clearance. To maintain the same average concentration of kanamycin in the elderly as in young adults, the dose may be reduced.

$$C_{av}^{\infty} = \frac{1.44 D_N (t_{1/2})_N}{\tau_N V_N} = \frac{1.44 D_0 (t_{1/2})_0}{\tau_0 V_0}$$

$$\frac{D_N (t_{1/2})_N}{\tau_N} = \frac{D_0 (t_{1/2})_0}{\tau_0}$$

Keeping the dose constant,

$$D_N = D_0$$

where D_N is the new dose

$$\frac{\tau_0}{\tau_N} = \frac{(t_{1/2})_0}{(t_{1/2})_N}$$

$$\tau_0 = 12 \times \frac{282}{107} = 31.6 \text{ hr}$$

Therefore, the same dose of kanamycin may be administered every 32 hr without affecting the average steady-state level of kanamycin.

2. The clearance of lithium was determined to be 41.5 ml/min in a group of patients with an average age of 25 years. In a group of elderly patients with an average age of 63 years, the clearance of lithium was 7.7 ml/min. What percentage of the normal dose of lithium should be given to a 65-year-old patient?

Solution

The dose should be proportional to clearance; therefore,

$$\text{Dose reduction } (\%) = \frac{7.7 \times 100}{41.5} = 18.5\%$$

The dose of lithium may be reduced to about 20% of the regular dose in the 65-year-old patient without affecting the steady-state blood level.

DOSING OF DRUGS IN THE OBESE PATIENT

The obese patient has a greater accumulation of fat tissue than necessary for normal body functions. The patient is considered obese if the actual body weight exceeds the ideal or desirable body weight by 20%, according to the Metropolitan Life Insurance data. In contrast, atheletes who have a greater body weight due to greater muscle mass are not considered obese. Adipose (fat) tissue has a smaller proportion of water compared to muscle tissue. Thus, the obese patient has a smaller proportion of total body water to total body weight compared to the patient with ideal body weight, which could affect the apparent volume of distribution of the drug. For example, Abernethy et al[8] have shown a significant difference in the apparent volume of distribution of antipyrine in obese patients (0.46 L/kg) compared to the ideal body weight patient (0.62 L/kg) based on actual total body weight.

In addition to the differences in total body water per kilogram body weight in the obese patient, the greatest proportion of body fat in this patient could lead to the distributional changes in the drug's pharmacokinetics due to partitioning of the drug between lipid and aqueous environments. Drugs such as digoxin and gentamycin are very polar and tend to distribute into water rather than into fat tissue. Other pharmacokinetic parameters may be altered in the obese patient due to possible physiologic alterations such as fatty infilteration of the liver affecting biotransformation and cardiovascular changes which might affect renal blood flow and renal excretion.[9]

QUESTIONS

1. Penicillin G has a volume of distribution of 42 L/1.73 m^2 and an elimination rate constant of 1.034 hr^{-1}. Calculate the maximum peak concentration that would be produced if the drug were given intravenously at a rate of 250 mg every 6 hr for a week.
2. Dicloxacillin has an elimination half-life of 42 min and a volume of distribution of 20 L. Dicloxacillin is 97% protein bound. What would be the steady-state free concentration of dicloxacillin if the drug were given intravenously at a rate of 250 mg every 6 hr?
3. The normal elimination half-life of cefamandole is 1.49 hr and the apparent volume of distribution (V_d) is 39.2% of body weight. The elimination half-life for a patient with a creatinine clearance of 15 ml/min was reported by Czerwinski and Pederson[10] to be 6.03 hr, and creatinine's V_d is 23.75% of body weight. What doses of cefamandole should be given the normal and the uremic patient (respectively) if the drug is administered intravenously every 6 hr and the desired objective is to maintain an average steady concentration of 2 μg/ml?
4. The maintenance dose of digoxin was reported to be 0.5 mg/day for a 60-kg patient with normal renal function. The half-life of digoxin is 0.95 days and the volume of distribution is 306 L. The bioavailability of the digoxin tablet is 0.56.
   a. Calculate the steady-state concentration of digoxin.
   b. Determine whether the patient is adequately dosed (effective serum digoxin concentration is 1–2 ng/ml).
   c. What is the steady-state concentration if the patient is dosed with the elixir instead of the tablet (assume the elixir to be 100% bioavailable).
5. An antibiotic has an elimination half-life of 2 hr and an apparent volume of distribution of 200 ml/kg. The minimum effective serum concentration is 2 μg/ml and the minimum toxic serum concentration is 16 μg/ml. A physician ordered a dosage regimen of this antibiotic to be given 250 mg every 8 hr by repetitive intravenous bolus injections.

a. Comment on the appropriateness of this dosage regimen for an adult male patient (23 years, 80 kg) whose creatinine clearance is 122 ml/min.
b. Would you suggest an alternate dosage regimen for this patient? Give your reasons and suggest an alternative dosage regimen.

6. Gentamycin (Garamycin, Schering) is a highly water soluble drug. The dosage of this drug in obese patients should be based on an estimate of the lean body mass or "ideal body weight." *Why*?
7. Why is the calculation for the loading dose, D_L, for a drug based on the apparent volume of distribution; whereas, the calculation of the maintenance dose is based on the elimination rate constant?
8. A potent drug with a narrow therapeutic index is ordered for a patient. After making rounds, the attending physician observes that the patient is not responding to drug therapy and orders a single plasma level measurement. Comment briefly on the value of measuring the drug concentration in a single blood sample and on the usefulness of the information which might be gained.
9. Calculate an oral dosage regimen for a cardiotonic drug for an adult male (68 kg, 63 years old) with normal renal function. The elimination half-life for this drug is 30 hr and its apparent volume of distribution is 4 L/kg. The drug is 80% bioavailable when given orally and the suggested therapeutic serum concentrations for this drug are from 0.001–0.002 μg/ml.
   a. This cardiotonic drug is commercially supplied as 0.075 mg, 0.15 mg, and 0.30 mg white, scored, compressed tablets. Using these readily available tablets, what dose would you now recommend for this patient?
   b. Are there any advantages for this patient to give smaller doses more frequently compared to a higher dosage less frequently? Any disadvantages?
   c. Would you suggest a loading dose for this drug? Why? What loading dose would you recommend?
   d. Is there a rationale for preparing a controlled-release product of this drug?
10. The dose of sulfisoxazole (Gantrisin, Roche Labs) recommended for an adult female patient (age 26, 63 kg) with a urinary tract infection was 1.5 g every 4 hr. The drug is 85% bound to serum proteins. The elimination half-life of this drug is 6 hr and the apparent volume of distribution is 1.3 L/kg. Sulfisoxazole is 100% bioavailable.
    a. Calculate the steady-state plasma concentration of sulfisoxazole in this patient.
    b. Calculate an appropriate loading dose of sulfisoxazole for this patient.
    c. Gantrisin (sulfisoxazole) is supplied in tablets containing 0.5 g of drug. How many tablets would you recommend for the loading dose?
    d. If no loading dose were given, how long would it take to achieve 95–99% of steady state?
11. The desired plasma level for an antiarrythmic agent is 5 μg/ml. The drug has an apparent volume of distribution of 173 ml/kg and an elimination half-life of 2.0 hr. The kinetics of the drug follow the kinetics of a one-compartment open model.

a. An adult male patient (75 kg, 56 years of age) is to be given an IV injection of this drug. What loading dose (D_L) and infusion rate (R) would you suggest?

b. The patient did not respond very well to drug therapy. Plasma levels of drug were measured and found to be 2 μg/ml. How would you readjust the infusion rate to increase the plasma drug level to the desired 5 μg/ml?

c. How long would it take to achieve 95% of steady-state plasma drug levels in this patient assuming no loading dose was given and the apparent V_d was unaltered?

12. An antibiotic is to be given to an adult male patient (75 kg, 58 years of age) by intravenous infusion. The elimination half-life for this drug is 8 hr and the apparent volume of distribution is 1.5 L/kg. The drug is supplied in 30-ml ampules at a concentration of 15 mg/ml. The desired steady-state serum concentration for this antibiotic is 20 μg/ml.

a. What infusion rate (R) would you suggest for this patient?

b. What loading dose would you suggest for this patient?

c. If the manufacturer suggests a starting infusion rate of 0.2 ml/hr kg body weight, what is the expected steady-state serum concentration in this patient?

d. You would like to verify that this patient received the proper infusion rate; at what time after the start of the IV infusion would you take a blood sample to monitor the serum antibiotic concentration? Why?

e. Assume that the measured serum antibiotic concentration was measured and found to be higher than anticipated; what reasons based on sound pharmacokinetic principles would account for this situation?

13. Nomograms are frequently used in lieu of pharmacokinetics calculations to determine an appropriate drug dosage regimen for a patient. Discuss the advantages and disadvantages for using nomograms to calculate a drug dosage regimen.

REFERENCES

1. Mawer GE: Computer assisted prescribing of drugs. Clin Pharmacokin 1:67–78, 1976
2. Greenblatt DJ: Predicting steady state serum concentrations of drugs. Ann Rev Pharmacol Toxicol 19:347–56, 1979
3. Iafrate RP, Glotz VP, Robinson JD, Lupkiewicz SM: Computer simulated conversion from intravenous to sustained-release oral theophylline drug. Intel Clin Phar 16:19–25, 1982
4. DeHaan RM, Metzler CM, Schellenberg D, et al: Pharmacokinetic study of clindamycin hydrochloride in humans. Int J Clin Pharmacol Biopharm 6:105–19, 1972
5. Regamey C, Gordon RC, Kirby WMM: Comparative pharmacokinetics of tobramysin and gentamicin. Clin Pharmacol Ther 14:396–403, 1973
6. Stein GE, Haughey DB, Ross RJ, Vakoutis J: Conversion from intravenous to oral dosing using sustained release theophylline tablets. Clin Pharm 1:772–73, 1982
7. Shirkey HC: Dosage (Dosology). In Shirkey HC (ed), Pediatric Therapy. St. Louis, Mosby, 1975, pp. 19–33

8. Abernethy DR, Greenblatt DJ, Divoll M, et al: Alterations in drug distribution and clearance due to obesity. J Pharmacol Exptl Therap 217:681–85, 1981
9. Abernethy DR, Greenblatt DJ: Pharmacokinetics of drugs in obesity. Clin Pharmacokin 7:108–24, 1982
10. Czerwinski AW, Pederson JA: Pharmacokinetics of cefamandole in patients with renal impairment. Antimicrob Agents Chemother 15:161–64, 1979
11. West JR, Smith HW, Chasis H: Glomerular filtration rate, effective blood flow and maximal tubular excretory capacity in infancy. J Pediat 32:10, 1948

BIBLIOGRAPHY

Benet LZ (ed): The Effect of Disease States on Drug Pharmacokinetics. Washington, D.C., American Pharmaceutical Association, 1976

Benowitz NL, Meister W: Pharmacokinetics in patients with cardiac failure. Clin Pharmacokinet 1:389–405, 1976

Clinical symposium on drugs and the unborn child. Clin Pharmacol Ther 14(2):621–770, 1973

Crooks J, O'Malley K, Stevenson IH: Pharmacokinetics in the elderly. Clin Pharmacokinet 1:280–96, 1976

DeVane CL, Jusko WJ: Dosage regimen design. Pharmac Ther 17:143–63, 1982

Dimascio A, Shader RI: Drug administration schedules. Am J Psychiatry 126:6, 1969

Evans WE, Schentag JJ, Jusko WJ: Applied Pharmacokinetics. Principles of Therapeutic Drug Monitoring. San Francisco, Applied Therapeutics, 1980

Friis-Hansen B: Body-water compartments in children: Changes during growth and related changes in body composition. Pediatrics 28:169–81, 1961

Giacoia GP, Gorodisher R: Pharmacologic principles in neonatal drug therapy. Clin Perinatol 2:125–38, 1975

Holloway DA: Drug problems in the geriatric patient. Drug Intelligence Clin Pharm 8:632–42, 1974

Jusko WJ: Pharmacokinetic principles in pediatric pharmacology. Pediatr Clin North Am 19:81–100, 1972

Krasner J, Giacoia GP, Yaffe SJ: Drug–protein binding in the newborn infant. Ann NY State Acad Sci 226:102–14, 1973

Kristensen M, Hansen JM, Kampmann J, et al: Drug elimination and renal function. Int J Clin Pharmacol Biopharm 14:307–8, 1974

Latini R, Bonati M, Tognoni G: Clinical role of blood levels. Ther Drug Monit 2:3–9, 1980

Lehmann K, Merten K: Die Elimination von Lithium in Alhangigkeit vom Lebensalten bei Gesunden und Nieweminsuffizienten. Int J Clin Pharmacol Biopharm 10:292–98, 1974

Levy G (ed): Clinical Pharmacokinetics: A Symposium. Washington, D.C., American Pharmaceutical Assoc., 1974

Morselli PL: Clinical pharmacokinetics in neonates. Clin Pharmacokinet 1:81–98, 1976

Mungall DR: Applied Clinical Pharmacokinetics. New York, Raven Press, 1983

Niebergall PJ, Sugita ET, Schnaare RL: Potential dangers of common drug dosing regimens. Am J Hosp Pharm 31:53–58, 1974

Rane A, Sjoquist F: Drug metabolism in the human fetus and newborn infant. Pediatr Clin North Am 19:37–49, 1972

Rane A, Wilson JT: Clinical pharmacokinetics in infants and children. Clin Pharmacokinet 1:2–24, 1976

Richey DP, Bender DA: Pharmacokinetic consequences of aging. Annu Rev Pharmacol Toxicol 17:49–65, 1977

Rowland M, Tozer TN: Clinical Pharmacokinetics Concepts and Applications. Philadelphia, Lea & Febiger, 1980

Schumacher GE, Griener JC: Using Pharmacokinetics in drug therapy II. Rapid estimates of dosage regimens and blood levels without knowledge of pharmacokinetic variables. Am J Hosp Pharm 35:454–59, 1978

Thompson PD, Melmon KL, Richardson JA, et al: Lidocaine pharmacokinetics in advanced heart failure, liver disease, and renal failure in humans. Ann Intern Med 78:499–508, 1973

Vestel RE: Drug use in the elderly: A review of problems and special considerations. Drugs 16:358–82, 1978

Winter ME: Basic Clinical Pharmacokinetics. San Francisco, Applied Therapeutics, 1980

CHAPTER SIXTEEN

Dosage Adjustment in Renal Disease

The kidney is an important organ in regulating body fluid levels, electrolyte balance, and metabolic waste and drug removal from the body. Impairment or degeneration of the kidney functions will have an impact on the pharmacokinetics of drugs. Some of the more common causes of kidney failure include disease, injury, and drug intoxication. Table 16-1 lists some of the conditions that may lead to chronic or acute renal failure. The condition in which glomerular filtration is impaired or reduced, leading to accumulation of excessive fluid and blood nitrogenous products in the body, is commonly described as *uremia*. Uremia can also be caused by acute diseases or trauma to the kidney. However, the influence of uremia on drug elimination is pharmacokinetically the same, generally producing a reduction of glomerular filtration and/or active secretion which leads to a longer elimination half-life of the administered drug.

The disturbance in electrolytes and fluids in the body due to renal failure may cause change in the volume of distribution of the drug. In addition, drug–protein binding may be altered, which also affects the volume of distribution. During uremia, binding of most weak acid drugs is decreased whereas binding of weak bases is less affected. The decrease in drug–protein binding results in an increase in the volume of distribution and may also facilitate biotransformation and excretion of drugs in the body. In practice, however, the net elimination half-life of drugs rarely increases due to the dominant effect of reduced glomerular filtration.

As a result of a decreased elimination rate constant, total body drug clearance is also reduced, since total body clearance, Cl_T, is the product of volume of distribution and the elimination rate constant of the drug.

Total body clearance is a useful parameter in deciding the appropriate dose of drug. The dose for a uremic patient is calculated from the dosing interval, the uremic clearance of the drug, and the desired average plasma concentration of the drug.

In clinical practice calculation of drug clearance for uremic patients is often impossible due to the lack of initial plasma drug concentrations for analysis. Moreover, the patient's condition may be changing too rapidly to allow pharmacokinetic analysis. The dose adjustment for such patients is often based on change in

TABLE 16-1. COMMON CAUSES OF KIDNEY FAILURE

Pyelonephritis	Inflammation and deterioration of the pyelonephrons due to infection, antigens, or other idiopathic causes.
Hypertension	Chronic overloading of the kidney with fluid and electrolytes may lead to kidney insufficiency.
Diabetes mellitus	The disturbance of sugar metabolism and acid–base balance may lead to or predispose a patient to degenerative renal disease.
Nephrotoxic drugs/ metals	Certain drugs taken chronically may cause irreversible kidney damage—e.g., the aminoglycosides, phenacetin, and heavy metals such as mercury and lead.
Hypovolemia	Any condition which causes a reduction in renal blood flow will eventually lead to renal ischemia and damage.
Neophroallergens	Certain compounds may produce an immune type of sensitivity reaction with nephritic syndrome—e.g., quartan malaria nephrotoxic serum.

the elimination constant, neglecting the change in the volume of distribution. The usefulness of such an approach differs with the drug and according to the condition of the patient. The limitations and assumptions involved must be carefully assessed by the clinician before this approach is taken.

DOSE ADJUSTMENT BASED ON DRUG CLEARANCE

This method tries to maintain the desired C_{av}^{∞} after multiple oral doses or multiple IV bolus injections as total body clearance, Cl_T, changes. The calculation for C_{av} is

$$C_{av}^{\infty} = \frac{FD_0}{Cl_T \tau} \tag{16.1}$$

For patients with a uremic condition or renal impairment, total body clearance will change to a new value, Cl_T^u. Therefore, to maintain the same desired C_{av}^{∞}, the dose must change to $D_0^{u\prime}$ or the dosage interval must change to τ^u as shown in the following equation:

$$C_{av}^{\infty} = \underset{\text{(normal)}}{\frac{D_0^N}{Cl_T^N \tau^N}} = \underset{\text{(uremic)}}{\frac{D_0^u}{Cl_T^u \tau^u}} \tag{16.2}$$

where the superscripts N and u represent normal and uremic conditions, respectively.

Rearranging Equation 16.2 and solving for D_0,

$$D_0^u = \frac{D_0^N Cl_T^u \tau^u}{Cl_T^N \tau} \tag{16.3}$$

If the dosage interval τ is kept constant, then the uremic dose D_0^u is equal to a fraction (Cl_T^u/Cl_T^N) of the normal dose, as shown in the equation

$$D_0^u = \frac{D_0^N Cl_T^u}{Cl_T^N} \tag{16.4}$$

For IV infusions the same desired C_{ss} is maintained both for patients with normal function and for patients with renal impairment. Therefore, the rate of infusion, R, must be changed to a new value of R^u for the uremic patient as described by the equation

$$C_{ss} = \underset{\text{(normal)}}{\frac{R}{Cl_T^N}} = \underset{\text{(uremic)}}{\frac{R^u}{Cl_T^u}} \tag{16.5}$$

METHOD BASED ON CHANGES IN THE ELIMINATION RATE CONSTANT

The overall elimination rate constant for many drugs is reduced in the uremic patient. A dosage regimen may be designed for the uremic patient either by reducing the normal dose of the drug and keeping the frequency of dosing (dosage interval) constant or by decreasing the frequency of dosing (prolong the dosage interval) and keeping the dose constant. Doses of drugs with a narrow therapeutic window should be reduced particularly if the drug has accumulated in the patient prior to deterioration of kidney function.

The usual approach to estimating a multiple-dosage regimen in the normal patient is to maintain a desired C_{av}^{∞} as shown in Equation 16.2. Assuming the V_d is the same in both normal and uremic patients and τ is constant, then the uremic dose, D_0^u is a fraction (K^u/K^N) of the normal dose:

$$D_0^u = \frac{D_0^N K^u}{K^N} \tag{16.6}$$

When the elimination rate constant for a drug in the uremic patient cannot be determined directly, indirect methods are available to calculate the predicted elimination rate constant based on the renal function of the patient. The assumptions on which these dosage regimens are calculated include:

1. The elimination rate constant decreases proportionately as renal function decreases.
2. The nonrenal routes of elimination (primarily, the rate constant for metabolism) remains unchanged.
3. Changes in the renal clearance of the drug is reflected by changes in the creatinine clearance.

The overall elimination rate constant is the sum total of all the routes of elimination in the body including the renal rate and the nonrenal rate constants:

$$K^u = K_{NR} + K_R^u \tag{16.7}$$

where K_{NR} is the nonrenal elimination rate constant and K_R is the renal excretion rate constant.

Renal clearance is the product of the apparent volume of distribution and the rate constant for renal excretion:

$$Cl_R^u = K_R^u V_d^u \tag{16.8}$$

Rearrangement of Equation 16.8 gives

$$K_R^u = \frac{1}{V_d^u} Cl_R^u \tag{16.9}$$

Assuming that the apparent volume of distribution and nonrenal routes of elimination do not change in uremia, the $K_{NR}^u = K_{NR}^u$ and $V_d^u = V_d^N$.

Substitution of Equation 16.9 into Equation 16.7 gives

$$K^u = K_{NR} + \frac{1}{V_d} Cl_R^u \tag{16.10}$$

From Equation 16.10 a change in the renal clearance, Cl_R^u, due to renal impairment will be reflected by a change in the overall elimination rate constant K^u. Since changes in the renal drug clearance cannot be assessed directly in the uremic patient, Cl_R^u is usually related to a measurement of kidney function as the glomerular filtration rate (GFR) which, in turn, is estimated by changes in the patient's clearance creatinine.

GENERAL APPROACHES FOR DOSE ADJUSTMENT IN RENAL DISEASE

There are several methods for estimating the appropriate dosage regimen for a patient with renal impairment. Most of these methods assume that the required therapeutic plasma drug concentration in uremic patients is similar to that required in patients with normal renal function. Uremic patients are maintained on the same C_{av}^{∞} after multiple oral doses or multiple IV bolus injections. For IV infusions the same C_{ss} is maintained. (C_{ss} is the same as C_{av}^{∞} after the plasma drug concentration reaches steady-state.)

The design of dosage regimens for the uremic patient is based on the pharmacokinetic changes that have occurred due to the uremic condition. Generally, drugs in patients with uremia or kidney impairment have prolonged elimination half-lives and a change in the apparent volume of distribution. In less severe uremic conditions there may not be edema nor a significant change in the apparent volume of distribution. Consequently, the methods for dose adjustment in uremic patients are based on an accurate estimation of the drug clearance in these patients.

Several specific clinical approaches for the calculation of drug clearance based on monitoring kidney function are presented later in this chapter. Two general pharmacokinetic approaches for dose adjustment include methods based on drug clearance and methods based on the elimination half-life.

MEASUREMENT OF GLOMERULAR FILTRATION RATE

Several drugs and endogenous substances have been used as markers to measure GFR. These markers are carried to the kidney by the blood via the renal artery and are filtered at the glomerulus.

Several criteria are necessary for using a drug to measure GFR:

1. The drug must be freely filtered at the glomerulus.
2. The drug must not be reabsorbed nor actively secreted by the renal tubules.
3. The drug should not be metabolized.
4. The drug should not bind significantly to plasma proteins.
5. The drug should not have an effect on the filtration rate nor alter renal function.
6. The drug should be nontoxic.
7. The drug may be infused in a sufficient dose which permits simple and accurate quantitation in plasma and in urine.

Therefore, the rate at which these markers are filtered from the blood into the urine per unit of time reflects the filtration rate of the kidney. Changes in GFR reflect changes in kidney function which may be diminished in uremic conditions.

Inulin, a fructose polysaccharide, fulfills most of the criteria listed above and is therefore used as a standard reference for the measurement of GFR. In practice, however, the use of inulin involves a time-consuming procedure in which inulin is given by intravenous infusion until a constant steady-state plasma level is obtained. Clearance of inulin may then be measured by the rate of intravenous infusion divided by the steady-state plasma inulin concentration. While this procedure gives an accurate value for GFR, inulin clearance is not used frequently in clinical practice.

The clearance of creatinine is used most extensively as a measurement of GFR. Creatinine is an endogenous substance formed during muscle metabolism from creatine phosphate. Creatinine production varies with the age, weight, and sex of the individual. In humans creatinine is mainly filtered at the glomerulus with no reabsorption. However, a small amount may be actively secreted by the renal tubules, and the values for GFR obtained by the creatinine clearance tend to be higher than GFR measured by inulin clearance.

SERUM CREATININE CONCENTRATION AND CREATININE CLEARANCE

Under normal circumstances creatinine production is roughly equal to creatinine excretion, so that the serum creatinine level remains constant. In a patient with reduced glomerular filtration, serum creatinine will accumulate in accordance with the degree of loss of glomerular filtration in the kidney. The serum creatinine concentration is frequently used to determine creatinine clearance, which is a rapid and convenient way of monitoring kidney function. Pharmacokinetically, *creatinine clearance* may be defined as the rate of urinary excretion of creatinine/serum creatinine. Creatinine clearance can be calculated directly by determining the patient's serum creatinine concentration and the rate of urinary excretion of creatinine. The approach is similar to that used in the determination of drug clearance. In practice, the rate of urinary excretion of creatinine is measured for the entire day to obtain a reliable excretion rate. The serum creatinine concentration is determined at the midpoint of the urinary collection period. Creatinine clearance is clinically expressed in ml/min and serum creatinine concentration in mg%. The following equation is used to calculate creatinine clearance in ml/min when the serum creatinine concentration is known:

$$Cl_{Cr} = \frac{\text{rate of urinary excretion of creatinine}}{\text{serum concentration of creatinine}}$$

$$Cl_{Cr} = \frac{C_u V 100}{C_{Cr} 1440} \tag{16.11}$$

where C_{Cr} = creatinine concentration (mg%) of the serum taken at the 12th hour or at the midpoint of the urine collection period; V = volume of urine excreted (ml) in 24 hr; C_u = concentration of creatinine in urine (mg/ml); and Cl_{Cr} = creatinine clearance in ml/min.

Creatinine clearance has been normalized both to body surface area using 1.73 m^2 as the average and to body weight for a 70-kg adult male. Creatinine distributes into total body water, and when clearance is normalized to a standard V_d, similar drug half-lives in adults and children correspond with identical clearances. One approach by Hallynck et al[1] is to normalize clearance to the lean body mass (LBM) of 50 kg in an average male. A measurement of LBM may be obtained from a skinfold technique or by the following equations.

Males:

$$\text{LBM} = 1.10 \times (\text{weight}) - 128 \times (\text{weight}^2/\text{height}^2) \tag{16.12}$$

Females:

$$\text{LBM} = 1.07 \times (\text{weight}) - 148 \times (\text{weight}^2/\text{height}^2) \tag{16.13}$$

where weight is in kilograms and height is in centimeters. Creatinine clearance is expressed as ml/min per 50-kg LBM.

Several other equations have been used to estimate lean body mass in the obese patients. In a few cases the actual body weight may be the same or lower than the lean body weight. In this case the actual body weight should be used in the calculation.

Calculation of Creatinine Clearance from Serum Creatinine Concentration

Several methods are available for the calculation of creatinine clearance from the serum creatinine concentration. In general, these methods should only be used in patients with intact liver function and no abnormal muscle disease, such as muscle hypertrophy or dystrophy. In obese patients Cl_{Cr} should be calculated with the lean body weight formula. The first method presented here is a general approach to calculating the Cl_{Cr} when the age and weight of the patient are unavailable. This method[2] is not as accurate as the Jellife[11] or Nomogram[4] method.

For the male

$$Cl_{Cr} = \frac{100}{C_{Cr}} - 12 \tag{16.14}$$

For the female

$$Cl_{Cr} = \frac{80}{C_{Cr}} - 7 \tag{16.15}$$

where the Cl_{Cr} is given in ml/min 1.73 m^2.

Adults. The following method by Jellife[11] is more accurate than the previous method. This method takes into account the patient's age and is generally applicable for adult patients age 20–80 years. With this method the older the patient, the smaller the creatinine clearance for the same serum creatinine concentration.

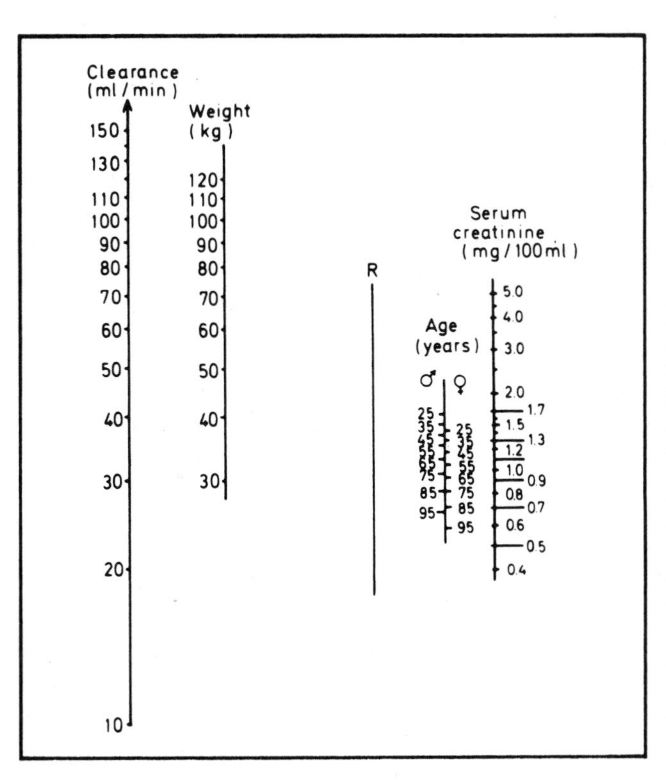

Figure 16-1. Nomogram for evaluation of endogenous creatinine clearance. To use the nomogram, connect with a ruler the patient's weight on the second line from the left with the patient's age on the fourth line. Note the point of intersection on *R* and keep the ruler there. Turn the right part of the ruler to the appropriate serum creatinine value and the left side will indicate the clearance in ml/min. (*From Kampmann J, Siersback-Nielsen, JM, 1974, with permission.*[4])

The Jellife method is as follows. For female patients, one would use 90% of the Cl_{Cr} obtained for males.

$$Cl_{Cr} = \frac{98 - 0.8\,(\text{age} - 20)}{C_{Cr}} \tag{16.16}$$

The method by Cockcroft and Gault[3] (Eq. 16.17) is also used to estimate creatinine clearance from serum creatinine concentration. This method does include both age and weight of the patient.

Males:

$$Cl_{Cr} = \frac{[140 - \text{age (yr)}] \times \text{body weight (kg)}}{72(C_{Cr})} \tag{16.17}$$

Females:

For female patients use 85% of the Cl_{Cr} value obtained in males.

The lean body weight (LBW) may be used in the Cockcroft and Gault (1976) method.

The nomogram method estimates creatinine clearance on the basis of age, weight, and serum creatinine concentration, as shown in Figure 16-1.

The lean body weight (LBW) formula is as follows.

$$\text{Male LBW} = 0.3281W + 0.33929H - 29.5336$$

$$\text{Female LBW} = 0.29569W + 0.41813H - 43.2933$$

where W is weight in kilograms and H is height in centimeters.

A more recent nomogram (Fig. 16-2) by Bjornsson et al[5] has also been used to estimate creatinine clearance from the serum creatinine concentration with knowledge of the patient's age and weight. This nomogram was tested in 50 hospitalized patients of both sexes ranging in age from 24 to 88 years. In patients with low creatinine clearance the nomogram tends to overestimate the creatinine clearance.

Children. There are a number of methods for calculation of creatinine clearance in children based on body length and serum creatinine concentration. Equation 16.18 is a method by Schwartz et al:[6]

$$Cl_{Cr} = \frac{0.55\ \text{body length (cm)}}{C_{Cr}} \tag{16.18}$$

where Cl_{Cr} is given in ml/min 1.73 m^2.

Another method for the calculation of creatinine clearance in children uses the nomogram by Traub and Johnson[7] shown in Figure 16-3. This nomogram was based on observations of 81 children ages 6–12 years and requires the patient's height and serum creatinine concentration.

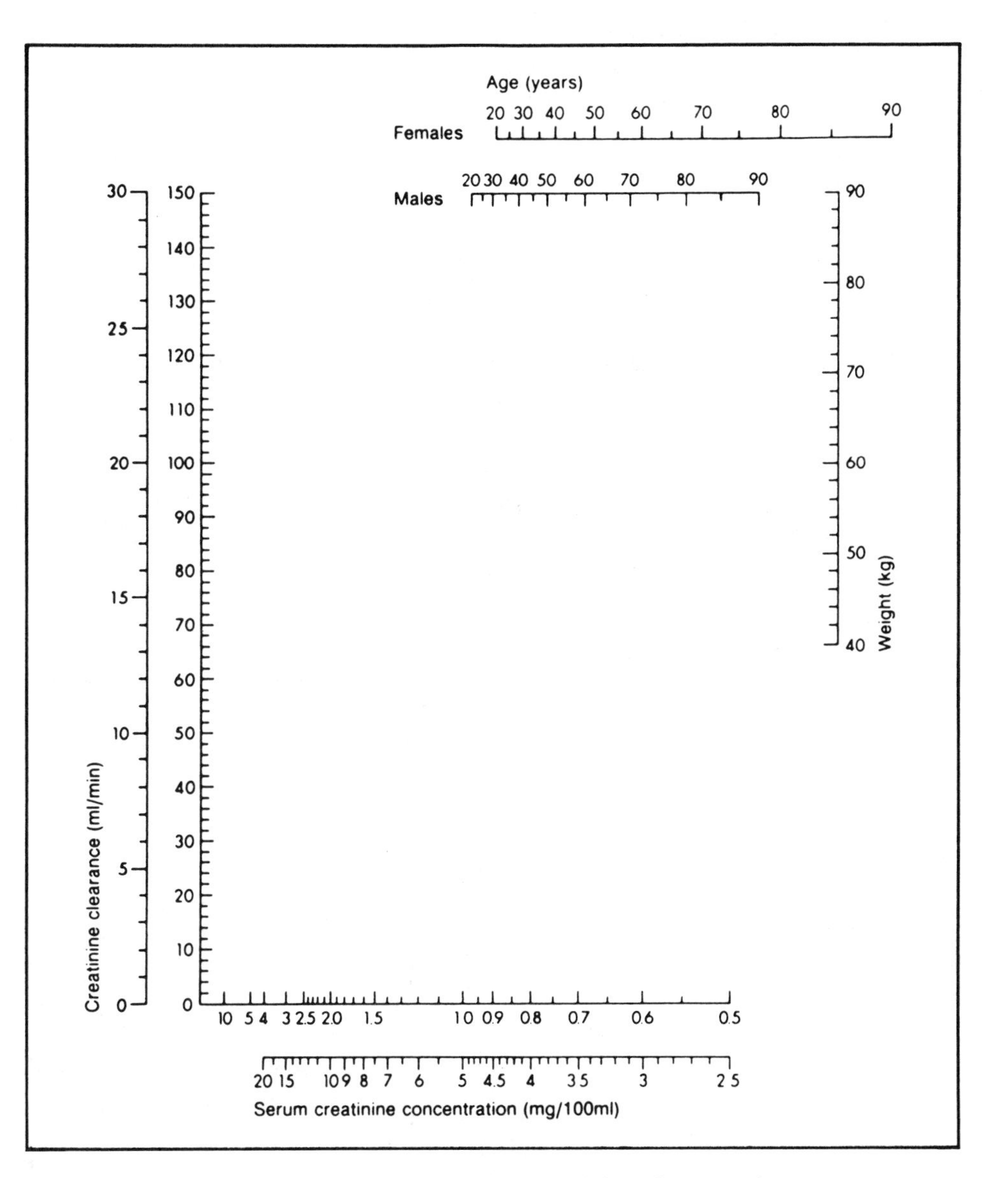

Figure 16-2. Nomogram for estimating creatinine clearance from serum creatinine concentrations in adults. Step 1: Define a point where lines perpendicular to the axes for the individual patient's age (sex) and bodyweight cross. Step 2: Draw a line connecting this point and the origin. Step 3: For any given serum creatinine concentration, a corresponding creatinine clearance is determined by this line. Use the outer scales for serum creatinine concentrations higher than 2.5 mg/100 ml. (*From Bjornsson TD, et al, 1983, with permission.*[5])

PRACTICE PROBLEMS

1. What is the creatinine clearance for an adult male patient having a serum creatinine concentration of 1 mg%?

Solution

Using Equation 16.2,

$$\mathrm{Cl}_{\mathrm{Cr}} = \frac{100}{C_{\mathrm{Cr}}} - 12 = \frac{100}{1} - 12 = 88 \text{ ml/min } 1.73 \text{ m}^2$$

2. What is the creatinine clearance for a 25-year-old male patient with a C_{Cr} of 1 mg% and a body weight of 80 kg?

Solution

Using the Jellife equation (Eq. 16.4),

$$\mathrm{Cl}_{\mathrm{Cr}} = \frac{98 - 0.8(25 - 20)}{1\%} = 94 \text{ ml/min } 1.73 \text{ m}^2$$

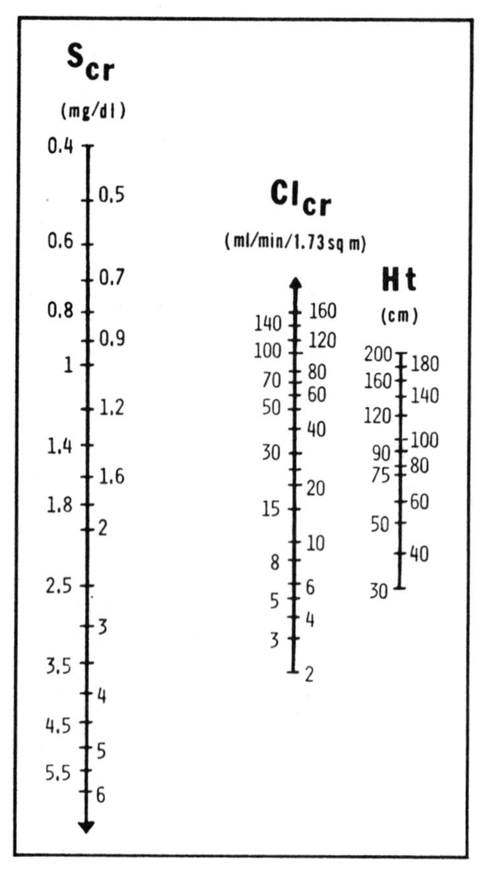

Figure 16-3. Nomogram for rapid evaluation of endogenous creatinine clearance ($\mathrm{Cl}_{\mathrm{Cr}}$) in pediatric patients (aged 6–12 years). To predict $\mathrm{Cl}_{\mathrm{Cr}}$, connect the child's S_{Cr} (serum creatinine) and Ht (height) with a ruler and read the $\mathrm{Cl}_{\mathrm{Cr}}$ where the ruler intersects the center line. (*From Traub SL, Johnson CE, 1980, with permission.*[7])

Using the nomogram (Fig. 16-1), join the points at 25 years (male) and 80 kg with a ruler—let the line intersect line R. Connect the intersection point at line R with the creatinine concentration point of 1 mg%—extend the line to intersect the "clearance line." The extended line will intersect the clearance line at 110 ml/min, giving the creatinine clearance for the patient.

3. What is the creatinine clearance for a 25-year-old male patient with a C_{Cr} of 1 mg%. The patient is 152 cm in height and weighs 103 kg.

Solution

The patient is obese and the Cl_{Cr} calculation should be based on lean body weight (LBW) using the equation

$$\begin{aligned} \text{LBW} &= 0.3281(103) + 0.33929(152) - 29.5336 \\ &= 55.83 \text{ kg} \end{aligned}$$

Using the Cockcroft and Gault method (Eq. 16.17), the Cl_{Cr} can be calculated:

$$Cl_{Cr} = \frac{(140 - 25)(55.83)}{72(1)} = 89.2 \text{ ml/min}$$

The practice problems show that, depending on the formula used, the calculated Cl_{Cr} can vary considerably. Consequently, unless a significant change in the creatinine clearance occurs, use of these methods will result in a rather large margin of error. Therefore, dosage adjustment on the basis of these methods alone is not justified.

The serum creatinine methods for the estimation of the creatinine clearance assume stabilized kidney function and a steady-state serum creatinine concentration. In acute renal failure and in other situations in which kidney function is changing, the serum creatinine may not represent steady-state conditions. If C_{Cr} is measured daily and the C_{Cr} value is constant, then the serum creatinine concentration is probably at steady state. If the C_{Cr} values are changing daily, then kidney function is changing and the serum creatinine is not at steady state.

DOSAGE ADJUSTMENT FOR UREMIC PATIENTS

The Nomogram Method

The method of Welling and Craig[8] provides a convenient way of estimating the ratio of the uremic elimination rate constant K_u to the normal elimination rate constant K_N on the basis of creatinine clearance.

In this method the nomogram plots K_u/K_N for various drugs as a function of Cl_{Cr} (Fig. 16-4). The K_u/K_N ratio of a drug will decrease as the creatinine clearance decreases, depending on the percentage of drug normally removed by the kidney. For example, drug L in Figure 16-4 is completely excreted by the kidney. Therefore, at end-state renal failure ($Cl_{Cr} = 0$), $K_u/K_N = 0$. As the kidney function increases, the K_u/K_N ratio will increase sharply. With drug A, which is exclusively metabolized, kidney function does not significantly affect the K_u/K_N ratio and therefore no change in K_u/K_N will occur as Cl_{Cr} changes. With drug D, which is probably representative of most drugs (i.e., eliminated by both hepatic metabolism and renal excretion), the K_u/K_N decreases gradually as Cl_{Cr} decreases. The intercept represents the nonrenal rate constant, expressed as a percentage of the normal elimination rate constant. It is interesting to note that at a Cl_{Cr} of 100 ml/min, all the three drugs in Figure 16-4 converged at a single point (i.e., $K_u/K_N = 100\%$), indicating that 100 ml/min is regarded as the normal clearance with this process.

To use the nomogram method, follow the steps below:

1. Locate the group to which the drug belongs in Table 16-2.
2. Find K_u/K_N at the point corresponding to the Cl_{Cr} of the patient (Fig. 16-4).
3. Determine K_u for the patient.
4. Make the dose adjustment in accordance with pharmacokinetic principles.

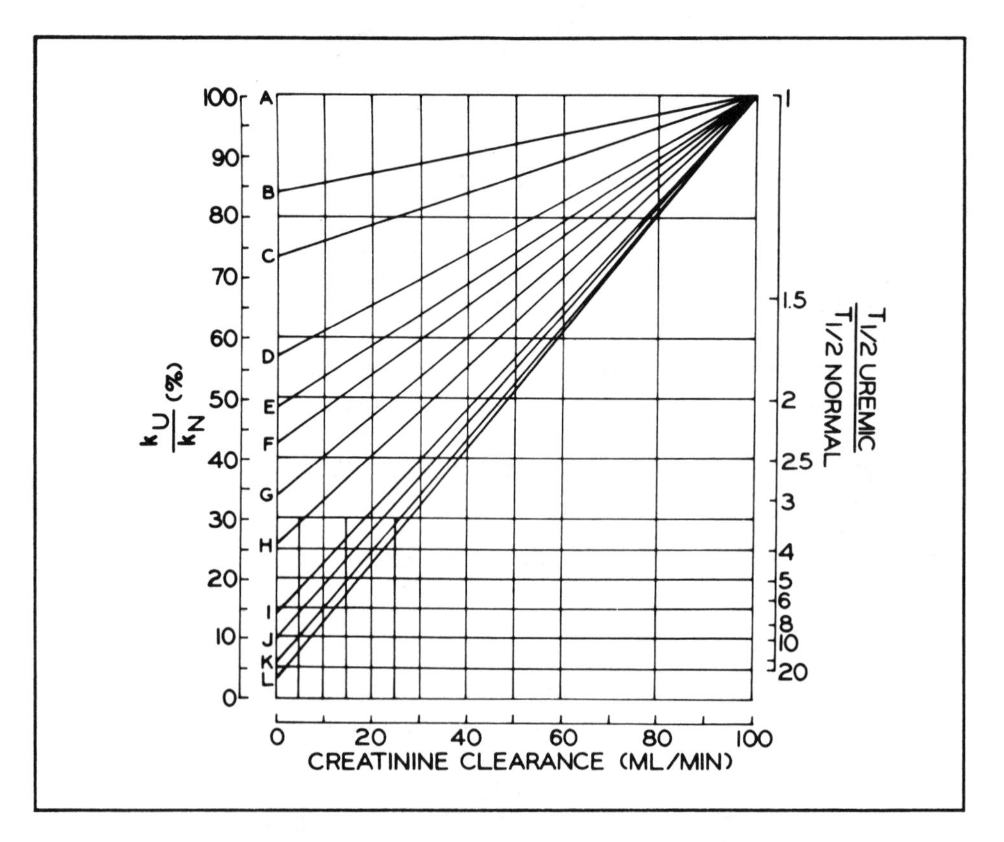

Figure 16-4. This nomograph describes the changes in the percentage of normal elimination rate constant (left ordinate) and the consequent geometric increase in elimination half-life (right ordinate) as a function of creatinine clearance. The drugs associated with the individual slopes are given in Table 16-2. (*From Welling PG, Craig WA, 1976, with permission.*[8])

TABLE 16-2. ELIMINATION RATE CONSTANTS FOR VARIOUS DRUGS*

Group	Drug	K_N (hr^{-1})	K_{nr}(hr^{-1})	K_{nr}/K_N%
A	Minocycline	0.04	0.04	100.0
	Rifampicin	0.25	0.25	100.0
	Lidocaine	0.39	0.36	92.3
	Digitoxin	0.114	0.10	87.7
B	Doxycycline	0.037	0.031	83.8
	Chlortetracycline	0.12	0.095	79.2
C	Clindamycin	0.16	0.12	75.0
	Chloramphenicol	0.26	0.19	73.1
	Propanolol	0.22	0.16	72.8
	Erythromycin	0.39	0.28	71.8
D	Trimethoprim	0.054	0.031	57.4
	Isoniazid (fast)	0.53	0.30	56.6
	Isoniazid (slow)	0.23	0.13	56.5
E	Dicloxacillin	1.20	0.60	50.0
	Sulfadiazine	0.069	0.032	46.4
	Sulfamethoxazole	0.084	0.037	44.0
F	Nafcillin	1.26	0.54	42.8
	Chlorpropamide	0.020	0.008	40.0
	Lincomycin	0.15	0.06	40.0
G	Colistimethate	0.154	0.054	35.1
	Oxacillin	1.73	0.58	33.6
	Digoxin	0.021	0.007	33.3
H	Tetracycline	0.120	0.033	27.5
	Cloxacillin	1.21	0.31	25.6
	Oxytetracycline	0.075	0.014	18.7
I	Amoxicillin	0.70	0.10	14.3
	Methicillin	1.40	0.19	13.6
J	Ticarcillin	0.58	0.066	11.4
	Penicillin G	1.24	0.13	10.5
	Ampicillin	0.53	0.05	9.4
	Carbenicillin	0.55	0.05	9.1
K	Cefazolin	0.32	0.02	6.2
	Cephaloridine	0.51	0.03	5.9
	Cephalothin	1.20	0.06	5.0
	Gentamicin	0.30	0.015	5.0
L	Flucytosine	0.18	0.007	3.9
	Kanamycin	0.28	0.01	3.6
	Vancomycin	0.12	0.004	3.3
	Tobramycin	0.32	0.010	3.1
	Cephalexin	1.54	0.032	2.1

*K_N is for patients with normal renal function; K_{nr} is for patients with severe renal impairment; and $K_{nr}/K_N\%$ = percent of normal elimination in severe renal impairment.
From Welling C, 1976, with permission.[8]

PRACTICE PROBLEMS

Lincomycin is given at 500 mg every 6 hr in a 75-kg normal patient. What doses would be used (a) in complete renal shutdown ($Cl_{Cr} = 0$) and (b) when $Cl_{Cr} = 10$ ml/min?

Solution

a. When $Cl_{Cr} = 0$,

$$K_u = K_{nr} + K_r$$

In complete renal shutdown ($K_r = 0$)

$$K_u = K_{nr} = 0.06 \text{ hr}^{-1} \text{ (Table 16-2, group F)}$$

or find K_u/K_N in Figure 16-4, group F, at $Cl_{Cr} = 0$ ml/min:

$$\frac{K_u}{K_N} = 0.425$$

$$K_u = 0.425(0.15) = 0.0638 \text{ hr}^{-1}$$

$$\text{Uremic dose} = 500 \text{ mg} \times \frac{0.0638}{0.15} = 212 \text{ mg every 6 hr}$$

b. At $Cl_{Cr} = 10$ ml,

$$\frac{K_u}{K_N} = 0.48$$

$$K_N = 0.15 \text{ hr}^{-1}$$

$$K_u = (0.48)(0.15) = 0.072 \text{ hr}^{-1}$$

$$\text{Dose} = \frac{0.072}{0.15} \times 500 \text{ mg} = 240 \text{ mg}$$

Alternatively,

$$\text{Dose} = (0.48)(500) = 240 \text{ mg}$$

The Wagner Method

This method takes advantage of the fact that the elimination constant for a patient can be obtained from the creatinine clearance, as follows.

$$K\% = a + bCl_{Cr} \tag{16.19}$$

The values of a and b are statistically determined for each drug from the pooled data on uremic patients. The method is simple to use and should provide accurate determination of elimination constants for patients when a good linear relationship exists between elimination constant and creatinine concentration. The theoretical derivation of this approach is as follows.

$$K\% = \text{total elimination rate constant}$$

$$K_{nr} = \text{nonrenal elimination rate constant } (\%)$$

$$K_r = \text{renal excretion rate constant}$$

$$R = \frac{\mathrm{Cl}_d}{\mathrm{Cl}_{Cr}} = \frac{\text{drug clearance}}{\text{creatinine clearance}} \tag{16.20}$$

$$\mathrm{Cl}_d = R\mathrm{Cl}_{cr}$$

$$K_r = \frac{R}{V_d}\mathrm{Cl}_{Cr}$$

$$K = K_{nr} + \frac{R}{V_d}\mathrm{Cl}_{Cr}$$

$$100K = 100K_{nr} + \frac{100R}{V_d}\mathrm{Cl}_{Cr}$$

$$K\% = a + b\mathrm{Cl}_{Cr} \tag{16.21}$$

Equation 16.21 can also be used with drugs that follow the two-compartment model. In such cases the terminal half-life is used and b would be substituted for $K\%$. Since the equation assumes a constant nonrenal elimination constant (K_{nr}) and volume of distribution, any changes in these two parameters will result in error in the estimated elimination constant.

PRACTICE PROBLEMS

A patient normally takes 500 mg ampicillin every 6 hr. What would the dose be for a patient with a Cl_{Cr} of 80 ml/min?

Solution

From Table 16-3, the following information on ampicillin is obtained: $a = 11$; $b = 0.59$; and normal $K\% = 70$. Using Equation 16.21, $K\%$ for the uremic patient is obtained:

$$K\% = a + b\mathrm{Cl}_{Cr} = 11 + 0.59 \times 80 = 58.2\%$$

$$\text{Uremic patient's dose} = \text{Normal dose} \times \frac{\text{patient's } K\%}{\text{normal } K\%}$$

$$\text{Dose of ampicillin} = 500 \times \frac{58.2}{70} = 416 \text{ mg (every 6 hr)}$$

TABLE 16-3. ADJUSTMENT OF DRUG DOSAGE IN PATIENTS WITH IMPAIRED RENAL FUNCTION, BASED ON ENDOGENOUS CREATININE CLEARANCE

Drug	Patient $K_{\%} = a + b \cdot Cl_{Cr}$ (%/hr)		Normal $K_{\%}$ (%/hr)	Normal $t_{1/2}$ (hr)
	a	b		
α-Acetyldigoxin	1.0	0.02	3.0	23.0
Ampicillin	11.0	0.59	70.0	1.0
Carbenicillin	6.0	0.54	60.0	1.2
Cephalexin	3.0	0.67	70.0	1.0
Cephaloridine	3.0	0.37	40.0	1.7
Cephalothin	6.0	1.34	140.0	0.5
Chloramphenicol	20.0	0.10	30.0	2.3
Chlortetracycline	8.0	0.04	12.0	5.8
Ciba 36278	3.0	0.67	70.0	1.0
Colistin	8.0	0.23	31.0	2.2
Digitoxin	0.3	0.001	0.4	173.0
Digoxin	0.8	0.009	1.7	41.0
Doxycycline	3.0	0.0	3.0	23.0
Erythromycin	13.0	0.37	50.0	1.4
5-Fluorocytosine	0.7	0.243	25.0	2.8
Gentamicin	2.0	0.28	30.0	2.3
Isoniazid—fast inactivators	34.0	0.19	53.0	1.3
Isoniazid—slow inactivators	12.0	0.11	23.0	3.0
Kanamycin	1.0	0.24	25.0	2.75
Lincomycin	6.0	0.09	15.0	4.6
Methicillin	17.0	1.23	140.0	0.5
Methyldigoxin	0.7	0.009	1.6	43.0
Oxacillin	35.0	1.05	140.0	0.5
Penicillin G	3.0	1.37	140.0	0.5
Polymyxin B	2.0	0.14	16.0	4.3
Rolitetracycline	2.0	0.04	6.0	11.6
Streptomycin	1.0	0.26	27.0	2.6
Strophanthin G	1.2	0.038	5.0	14.0
Strophanthin K	1.0	0.03	4.0	17.0
Sulfadiazine	3.0	0.05	8.0	8.7
Sulfamethoxazole	7.0	0.0	7.0	9.9
Sulfasomidine (children)	1.0	0.14	15.0	4.6
Tetracycline	0.8	0.072	8.0	8.7
Thiamphenicol	2.0	0.24	26.0	2.7
Trimethoprim	2.0	0.04	6.0	12.0
Vancomycin	0.3	0.117	12.0	5.8

From Wagner JG, 1975, with permission.[9]

The Giusti–Hayton Method

This method assumes that the effect of reduced kidney function on the renal portion of the elimination constant can be estimated from the ratio of the uremic creatinine clearance (Cl^{u}_{Cr}) to the normal creatinine clearance (Cl^{N}_{Cr}):

$$\frac{K_r^u}{K_r^N} = \frac{Cl^u_{Cr}}{Cl^N_{Cr}}$$

where K_r^u is the uremic renal excretion rate constant and K_r^N is the normal renal excretion rate constant

$$K_r^u = K_r^N \frac{\mathrm{Cl}_{\mathrm{Cr}}^u}{\mathrm{Cl}_{\mathrm{Cr}}^N} \tag{16.22}$$

since the overall uremic elimination rate constant K_u is the sum of renal and nonrenal factors:

$$K_u = K_{nr}^u + K_r^u$$

$$K_u = K_{nr}^u + K_r^N\left(\frac{\mathrm{Cl}_{\mathrm{Cr}}^u}{\mathrm{Cl}_{\mathrm{Cr}}^N}\right) \tag{16.23}$$

Dividing Equation 16.23 by K_N on both sides yields

$$\frac{K_u}{K_N} = \frac{K_{nr}^u}{K_N} + \frac{K_r^N}{K_N}\left(\frac{\mathrm{Cl}_{\mathrm{Cr}}^u}{\mathrm{Cl}_{\mathrm{Cr}}^N}\right) \tag{16.24}$$

Let $f = K_r^N/K_N$ = fraction of drug excreted unchanged in the urine and $1-f = K_{nr}^u/K_N$ = fraction of drug excreted by nonrenal routes. Substitution into Equation 16.24 yields

$$\frac{K_u}{K_N} = (1-f) + f\left(\frac{\mathrm{Cl}_{\mathrm{Cr}}^u}{\mathrm{Cl}_{\mathrm{Cr}}^N}\right)$$

or

$$\frac{K_u}{K_N} = 1 - f\left(1 - \frac{\mathrm{Cl}_{\mathrm{Cr}}^u}{\mathrm{Cl}_{\mathrm{Cr}}^N}\right) = G \tag{16.25}$$

where the G factor is a ratio that can be obtained from the fraction of drug excreted by the kidney and the creatinine clearance of the uremic patient. Equation 16.25 is known as the *Giusti—Hayton equation*.[10]

The Giusti–Hayton equation is useful for most drugs in the literature for which the fraction of drug excreted by renal or nonrenal routes has been reported.

PRACTICE PROBLEMS

The maintenance dose of gentamicin is 80 mg every 6 hr for a patient with normal renal function. What would the maintenance dose be for a uremic patient with creatinine clearance of 20 ml/min?

Solution

From the literature, gentamicin was found to be 100% excreted by the kidney—i.e., $f = 1$. Using Equation 16.25 and assuming a normal creatinine clearance of 100 ml/min,

$$G = 1 - 1\left(1 - \frac{20}{100}\right) = 0.2$$

since

$$\frac{D_u}{D_N} = \frac{K_u}{K_N} = G \qquad \text{where } D_u = \text{uremic dose, } D_N = \text{normal dose} \qquad (16.26)$$

$$D_u = D_N \times \frac{K_u}{K_N} = 80 \text{ mg} \times 0.2 = 16 \text{ mg}$$

The maintenance dose would be 16 mg every 6 hr. Alternatively, the dosing interval can be adjusted without changing the dose;

$$\frac{\tau_u}{\tau_N} = \frac{K_N}{K_u}$$

$$\tau_u = \tau_N \frac{K_N}{K_u} = 6 \text{ hr} \times \frac{1}{0.2} = 30 \text{ hr}$$

where τ_u and τ_N are dosing intervals for uremic and normal patients, respectively. Thus, the patient may be given 80 mg every 30 hr.

Comparison of the Various Methods for Dose Adjustment in Uremic Patients

All of the methods mentioned previously have the common limitations that the drug must follow dose-independent kinetics and that the volume of distribution of the drug must remain relatively constant in the uremic patient. In addition, it is usually assumed that the nonrenal routes of elimination such as hepatic clearance does not change. Since no correction for metabolites is made, any drug having an active pharmacologic metabolite must be additionally modified. Another assumption in the use of these methods is that pharmacologic response is unchanged in the uremic patient. This assumption may be unrealistic with drugs that act differently in the disease state. For example, the pharmacologic response with digoxin is dependent on the potassium level in the body, and the potassium level in the uremic patient may be rather different from that of the normal individual. In a patient undergoing dialysis, loss of potassium may increase the potential of toxic effect of the drug digoxin. With many drugs, studies have shown that the incidence of adverse effects was increased in uremic patients. It is often impossible to distinguish whether the increase in adverse effect is due to a pharmacokinetic change or to a change in the receptor sensitivity to the drug. In any event, these observations point out the fact that dose adjustment must be regarded as a preliminary estimation to be followed with further adjustments in accordance with the observed clinical response.

PRACTICE PROBLEMS

1. The normal IV dose of kanamycin is 250 mg every 6 hr. What would the dose be for a patient whose creatinine clearance has been decreased to 50 ml/min?

Solution

Since $a = 1$, $K\%$ normal $= 25$, and $b = 0.24$ (from Table 16-3),

$$\text{Uremic } K\% = 1 + 0.24 \times 50 = 13\%$$

$$\text{Uremic dose} = 250 \text{ mg} \times \frac{13}{25} = 130 \text{ mg}$$

The dose of the uremic patient would be 130 mg every 6 hr.

2. Using the Giusti–Hayton equation (Eq. 16.25), calculate the dose adjustment needed for uremic patients with (a) 75% of normal kidney function (i.e., $Cl^{u}_{Cr}/Cl^{N}_{Cr} = 75\%$); (b) 50% of normal kidney function; and (c) 25% of normal kidney function. Make calculations for (a) a drug that is 50% excreted by the kidney; (b) a drug that is 75% excreted by the kidney.

Solution

The values for percent of normal creatinine clearance in uremic patients with various renal functions are listed in Table 16-4.

The percent of dose adjustment in a given uremic state can be found using the following procedure. The important facts to remember are (a) although the elimination rate constant is usually composed of two components, only the renal components are reduced in a uremic patient and (b) the kidney function of the uremic patient may be expressed as a percent of uremic Cl_{Cr}/normal Cl_{Cr}. The reduction in the renal elimination rate constant can be estimated from the percent of kidney function remaining in the patient. The steps involved in making the calculations are as follows.

a. Determine f, or the fraction of drug excreted by the kidney.
b. Express the Cl_{Cr} of the uremic patient as a percent of the Cl_{Cr} of a normal patient—i.e., $Cl^{u}_{Cr}/100$.
c. Multiply $f(Cl^{u}_{Cr}/100)$ to obtain the uremic renal elimination constant.
d. Adding the uremic renal elimination constant to $1 - f$, the nonrenal elimination constant, will give the new overall elimination rate constant as a percent of the normal elimination constant. This also gives the fraction of normal dose required for a uremic patient.

TABLE 16-4. DOSAGE ADJUSTMENT IN UREMIC PATIENTS

Fraction of Drug Excreted Unchanged (K_r/K_N)	Percent of Normal Dose			
	50% Normal Cl_{Cr}	*25% Normal Cl_{Cr}*	*10% Normal Cl_{Cr}*	*0% Normal Cl_{Cr}*
0.25	87	81	77	75
0.50	75	62	55	50
0.75	62	44	32	25
0.90	55	32	19	10

3. What is the dose for a drug that is 75% excreted through the kidney in a uremic patient with a creatinine clearance of 10 ml/min?

Solution

$$f = 75\%$$

$$\text{Renal function of uremic patient} = \frac{10}{100} = 10\% \text{ normal}$$

$$\text{Uremic patient's renal elimination constant} = 75\% \times 10\% = 7.5\% \text{ normal}$$

$$\text{Uremic patient's overall elimination constant} = 7.5\% + (1 - 75\%)$$

$$= 7.5\% + 25\% = 32.5\%$$

Alternatively, using the Giusti–Hayton equation,

$$G = 1 - 0.75\left(1 - \frac{10}{100}\right) = 0.325$$

Therefore, the uremic patient's dose should be 32.5% of that of normal patient. It should be noted that the above method is actually the same as the Giusti–Hayton method. The intuitive approach, however, may be useful if the practitioner is unfamiliar with the Giusti–Hayton equation. Table 16-4 provides some of the calculated dosage adjustments for drugs eliminated to various degrees by renal excretion in different stages of renal failure.

DIALYSIS

Dialysis is an artificial process in which the accumulation of drugs or waste metabolites is removed by diffusion from the body into the dialysis fluid. There are two types of dialysis in common use, *peritoneal dialysis* and *hemodialysis*. Both processes work on the principle that as the uremic blood or fluid is equilibrated with the dialysis fluid, waste metabolites diffuse into the dialysis fluid and are removed.

In peritoneal dialysis the dialysis fluid is pumped into the peritoneal cavity, where waste metabolites in the body fluid are discharged rapidly since the peritoneum provides a large natural surface area for diffusion. In hemodialysis the blood is channeled through the dialysis machine, where the waste material is removed by diffusion before returning to the body. Hemodialysis is a much more effective method of drug removal and is preferred in situations where rapid removal of the drug from the body is important, as in overdose or poisoning. In practice, hemodialysis is most often applied to patients with terminal renal failure. Dialysis may be required from once every 2 days to 3 times a week, each treatment period lasting 5–6 hr.

Dosing of drugs in patients receiving hemodialysis is affected greatly by the frequency and type of dialysis involved. In general, drug removal in hemodialysis is governed by the factors listed in Table 16-5. These factors are carefully considered before dialysis is used for drug removal.

TABLE 16-5. FACTORS AFFECTING DIALYZABILITY OF DRUGS

Water solubility	Insoluble or fat-soluble drugs are not dialyzed–e.g., glutethimide, which is very water insoluble.
Protein binding	Tightly bound drugs are not dialyzed because dialysis is a passive process of diffusion—e.g., propranolol is 94% bound.
Molecular weight	Only molecules with molecular weights of less than 500 are easily dialyzed—e.g., vancomycin is poorly dialyzed and has a molecular weight of 1800.
Drugs with large volumes of distribution	Drugs widely distributed are dialyzed more slowly since the rate-limiting factor is the volume of blood entering the machine—e.g., for digoxin, $V_d = 250–300$ L. Drugs which are concentrated in the tissues are usually difficult to remove by dialysis.

In dialysis involving uremic patients receiving drugs for therapy, the rate at which a given drug is removed depends on the flowrate of blood to the dialysis machine and the performance of the dialysis machine. The term *dialysance* is used to describe the process of drug removal from the dialysis machine. Dialysance is a clearance term similar in meaning to renal clearance, and it describes the amount of blood completely cleared of drugs (in ml/min). Dialysance is defined by the equation

$$\mathrm{Cl_D} = \frac{Q(C_a - C_v)}{C_a} \tag{16.27}$$

where C_a = drug concentrations in arterial blood (blood entering kidney machine); C_v = drug concentration in venous blood (blood leaving kidney machine); Q = rate of blood flow to the kidney machine; and $\mathrm{Cl_D}$ = dialysance. Dialysance is sometimes referred to as *dialysis clearance*.

PRACTICE PROBLEMS

Assume the flow rate of blood to the dialysis machine is 40 ml/min. By chemical analysis the concentrations of drug entering and leaving the machine are 90 and 10 μg/ml, respectively. What is the dialysis clearance?

Solution

The rate of drug removal is equal to the volume of blood passed through the machine divided by the arterial difference in blood drug concentrations before and after dialysis. Thus,

$$\text{Rate of drug removal} = 40 \text{ ml/min} \times (90 - 10)\ \mu\text{g/ml} = 3200\ \mu\text{g/min}$$

Since clearance is equal to the rate of drug removal divided by the arterial concentration of drug,

$$\mathrm{Cl_D} = \frac{3200\ \mu\mathrm{g/min}}{90\ \mu\mathrm{g/ml}} = 35.6\ \mathrm{ml/min}$$

Alternatively, using Equation 16.27,

$$\mathrm{Cl_D} = 40\ \mathrm{ml/min} \times \frac{(90 - 10)}{90} = 35.6\ \mathrm{ml/min}$$

These calculations show that the two terms are the same. In practice, dialysance has to be measured experimentally by determining C_a, C_v, and Q. In dosing of drugs involving dialysis, the average plasma drug concentration of a patient is given by the equation

$$C_{av}^{\infty} = \frac{FD_0}{(\mathrm{Cl_T} + \mathrm{Cl_D})\tau} \qquad (16.28)$$

where F represents fraction of dose absorbed; $\mathrm{Cl_T}$ is total body drug clearance of the patient; C_{av}^{∞} is average steady-state plasma drug concentration; and τ is the dosing interval.

In practice, if $\mathrm{Cl_D}$ is 30% or more of $\mathrm{Cl_T}$, adjustment is usually made for the amount of drug lost in dialysis.

QUESTIONS

1. The normal dosing schedule for a patient on tetracycline is 250 mg PO (peroral) every 6 hr. Suggest a dosage regimen for this patient when laboratory analysis shows his renal function to have deteriorated from a $\mathrm{Cl_{Cr}}$ of 90 ml/mm to 20 ml/min.
2. A male patient stabilized on a digoxin maintenance dose of 0.125 mg daily has developed renal failure. The serum creatinine concentration is 5 mg%. What would you suggest for the new maintenance dose? Would you suggest changing the dosing interval and maintaining the same dose?
3. A patient receiving antibiotic treatment is on dialysis. The flowrate of serum into the kidney machine is 50 ml/min. Assays show that the concentration of drug entering the machine is 5 μg/ml and the concentration of drug in the serum leaving the machine is 2.4 μg/ml. The drug clearance for this patient is 10 ml/min. To what extent should the dose be increased if the average concentration of the antibiotic is to be maintained?
4. A uremic patient has a urine output of 1.8 L/24 hr and an average creatinine concentration of 2.2 mg%. What is the creatinine clearance? How would you adjust the dose of a drug normally given at 20 mg/kg every 6 hr in this patient (assume the urine creatinine concentration is 0.1 mg/ml and creatinine clearance is 100 ml/min)?
5. A patient on lincomycin at 600 mg every 12 hr intramuscular was found to have a creatinine clearance of 5 ml/min. Should the dose be adjusted? If so, (a) adjust the dose by keeping the dosing interval constant, (b) adjust

the dosing interval and give the same dose, and (c) adjust both dosing interval and dose. What are the significant differences in the adjustment methods?

6. Using the method of *Cockcroft and Gault*, calculate the creatinine clearance for a young adult woman (age 38 years, 62 kg) whose serum creatinine is 1.8 mg%.

7. Would you adjust the dose of cephamandole, an antibiotic which is 98% excreted unchanged in the urine, for the patient in question 6? *Why*?

8. What assumptions are usually made when adjusting a dosage regimen according to the creatinine clearance in a patient with renal failure?

9. The usual dose of gentamycin in patients with normal renal function is 1.0 mg/kg every 8 hr by multiple IV bolus injections. Using the nomogram method (Fig. 16-4), what dose of gentamycin would you recommend for a 55-year-old adult male patient weighing 72 kg with a creatinine clearance of 20 ml/min?

10. A single intravenous bolus injection (1 g) of an antibiotic was given to a male anephric patient (75 kg, age 68). During the next 48 hr, the elimination half-life of the antibiotic was 16 hr. The patient was then placed on hemodialysis for 8 hr and the elimination half-life was reduced to 4 hr.

   a. How much drug was eliminated by the end of the dialysis period?

   b. Assuming the apparent volume of distribution of this antibiotic is 0.5 L/kg, what was the plasma drug concentration just prior to and after dialysis?

11. There are several pharmacokinetic methods for the adjustment of a drug dosage regimen for patients with uremic disease based on the serum creatinine concentration in that patient. From your knowledge of clinical pharmacokinetics discuss the following:

   a. the basis of these methods for the calculation of drug dosage regimens in uremic patients and

   b. the validity of the assumptions upon which these calculations are made.

12. After assessment of the uremic condition of the patient the drug dosage regimen may be adjusted by either (a) keeping the dose constant and prolonging the dosage interval, τ, or (b) decreasing the dose and maintaining the dosage interval constant. Discuss the advantages and disadvantages for adjusting the dosage regimen using either method (a) or method (b).

REFERENCES

1. Hallynck TH, Soeph HH, Thomis VA, Boelaert J, Daneels R, Dettli L: Should clearance be normalized to body surface or lean body mass? Br J Clin Pharm 11:523–26, 1981
2. Jellife RW: Estimation of creatinine clearance when urine cannot be collected. Lancet 1:975–76 (May 8), 1971
3. Cockcroft DW, Gault MH: Prediction of creatinine clearance from serum creatinine. Nephrin 16:31–41, 1976
4. Kampmann J, Siersback-Nielsen JM: Rapid evaluation of creatinine clearance. Acta Med Scand 196:517–20, 1974

5. Bjornsson TD, Cocchetto DM, McGowan FX, Verghese CP, Sedar F: Nomogram for estimating creatinine clearance. Clin Pharmacokin 8:365–99, 1983
6. Schwartz GV, Haycock GB, Edelmann CM, Spitzer A: A simple estimate of glomerular filtration rate in children derived from body length and plasma creatinine. Pediatrics 58:259–63, 1976
7. Traub SL, Johnson CE: Comparison methods of estimating creatinine clearance in children. Am J Hosp Pharm 37:195–201, 1980
8. Welling PG, Craig WA: Pharmacokinetics in disease states modifying renal function. In Benet LZ (ed), The Effects of Disease States on Drug Pharmacokinetics. Washington, D.C., American Pharmaceutical Assoc., 1976
9. Wagner JG: Fundamentals of Clinical Pharmacokinetics. Hamilton, Ill., Drug Intelligence Publications, 1975, p. 161
10. Giusti DL, Hayton WL: Dosage regimen adjustments in renal impairment. Drug Intell Clin Pharm 7:382–87, 1973
11. Jellife RW: Creatinine clearance: Bedside estimate. Ann Int Med 79:604–05, 1973

BIBLIOGRAPHY

Anderson RJ: Drug prescribing for patients in renal failure. Hosp Prac 145–60, 1983

Benet L: The Effect of Disease States on Drug Pharmacokinetics. Washington, D.C., American Pharmaceutical Assoc., 1976

Bennett WM, Singer I: Drug prescribing in renal failure: Dosing guidelines for adults—An update. Am J Kidney Dis 3:155–93, 1983

Bjornsson TD: Use of serum creatinine concentration to determine renal function. Clin Pharmacokin 4:200–22, 1979

Brater DC: Drug Use in Renal Disease. Press Boston, ADIS Health Science, 1983

Chennavasin P, Brater DC. Nomograms for drug use in renal disease. Clin Pharmacokin 6:193–214, 1981

David K, Edwards G: Drugs affecting kidney function and metabolism. Prog Biochem Pharmacol 7, 1972

Dettli L: Elimination kinetics and dosage adjustment of drugs in patients with kidney disease. In Grobecker H et al. (eds), Progress in Pharmacology, Vol 1. New York, Gustav Fischer Verlag, 1977

Fabre J, Balant L: Renal failure, drug pharmacokinetics and drug action. Clin Pharmacokin 1:99–120, 1976

Gibaldi M: Drug distribution in renal failure. Am J Med 62:471–74, 1977

Gibson TP, Nelson HA: Drug kinetics and artificial kidneys. Clin Pharmacokin 2:403–26, 1977

Giusti DL, Hayton WL: Dosage regimen adjustments in renal impairment. Drug Intell Clin Pharm 7:382–87, 1973

Jellife RW, Jellife SM: A computer program for estimation of creatinine clearance from unstable serum creatinine concentration. Math Biosci 14:17–24, 1972

Kampmann JP, Hansen JM: Glomerular filtration rate and creatinine clearance. Brit J Clin Pharmacol 12:7–14, 1981

LeSher DA: Considerations in the use of drugs in patients with renal failure. J Clin Pharmacol 16:570, 1976

Levy G: Pharmacokinetics in renal disease. Am J Med 62:461–65, 1977

Lott RS, Hayton WL: Estimation of creatinine clearance from serum creatinine concentration —A review. Drug Intell Clin Pharm 12:140–50, 1978

Maher JF: Principle of dialysis and dialysis of drugs. Am J Med 62:475–81, 1977

Parker PR, Parker WA: Pharmacokinetic considerations in the hæmodialysis of drugs. J Clin Hosp Pharm 7:87–99, 1982

Schumacher GE: Practical pharmacokinetic techniques for drug consultation and evaluation, II: A perspective on the renal impaired patient. Am J Hosp Pharm 30:824–30, 1973

Traub SL: Creatinine and creatinine clearance. Hosp Pharm 13:715–22, 1978

Watanabe AS: Pharmacokinetic aspects of the dialysis of drugs. Drug Intell Clin Pharm 11:407–16, 1977

CHAPTER SEVENTEEN

Relationship Between Pharmacokinetic Parameters and Pharmacologic Response

PHARMACODYNAMICS AND PHARMACOKINETICS

Research on the time course of drug response have been studied independent of pharmacokinetic observations for many years. Much of the early studies were performed empirically by observing the onset, intensity, and duration of the pharmacologic response. These findings were not related quantitatively to pharmacokinetic parameters such as rate of absorption and elimination, volume of distribution, and metabolic rates of the drug. The intensity of pharmacologic responses are now related to the concentration of the active drug at the site of the drug receptor. The time course for the pharmacologic response including the onset and duration of activity is influenced by the rate of arrival and removal of the drug from the receptor site. The term *pharmacodynamics* refers to the relationship between drug concentrations at the site of action and drug effects and factors influencing this relationship.[1]

With increased knowledge of pharmacokinetics and advances in technical skills for the measurement of drug concentrations, it is now possible to relate changes in pharmacologic response to the concentration time profile of the drug and/or its active metabolites. Using the generated pharmacokinetic parameters and a pharmacodynamic model, it is possible to predict the pharmacologic response for certain drugs. Much of the mathematics and techniques used in pharmacodynamic models are highly theoretical but do supply useful information for understanding drug action.

RELATION OF DOSE TO PHARMACOLOGIC EFFECT

The intensity and duration of the pharmacologic effect are dependent on the administered dose and the distribution kinetics of the drug. For most drugs the pharmacologic effect (E) is found to be proportional to the log of the dose. Figure 17-1 shows a typical log dose–response curve. The linear region of the log–dose

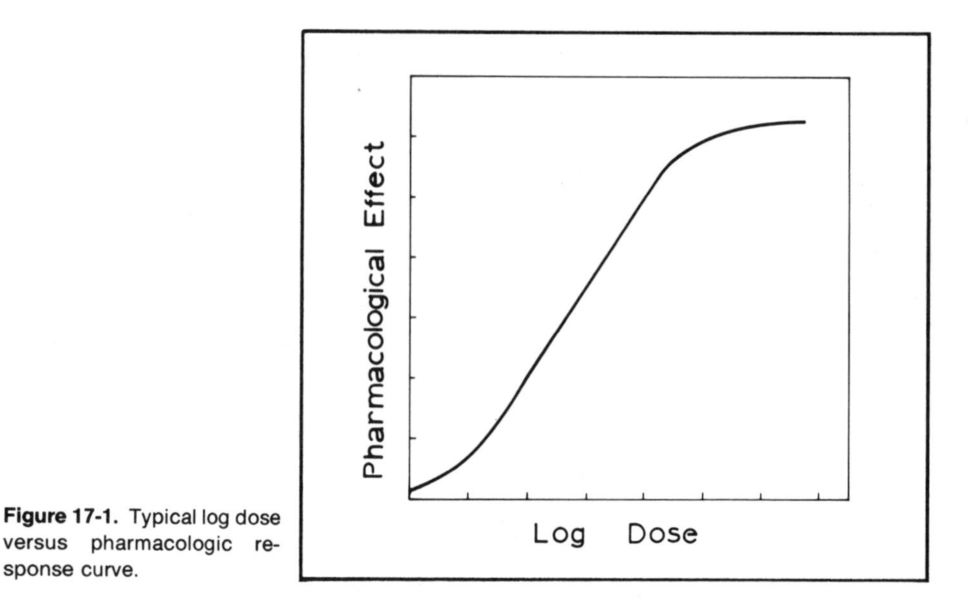

Figure 17-1. Typical log dose versus pharmacologic response curve.

response curve is usually true for a dosage range of 20–80% of the maximum pharmacologic effect. Beyond this range, this relationship is no longer linear. A relationship between pharmacologic effect (E) and the concentration of drug in the body can be obtained mathematically, since a larger dose usually produces a larger concentration of drug in the body. For a one-compartment model drug the pharmacologic response is proportional to the log concentration within a specified range, as shown in Figure 17-2.

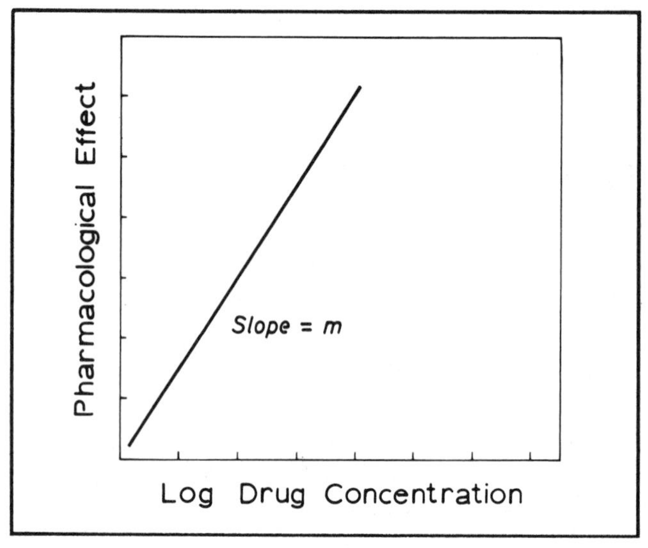

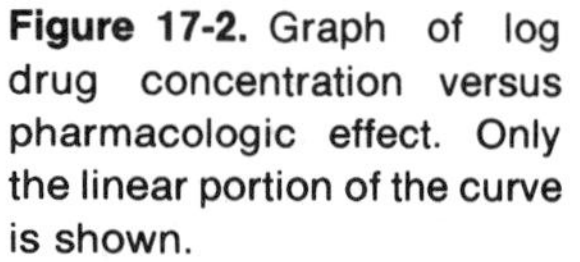

Figure 17-2. Graph of log drug concentration versus pharmacologic effect. Only the linear portion of the curve is shown.

Mathematically, the relationship in Figure 17-2 may be expressed by the following equation, where m is the slope and e is an extrapolated intercept.

$$E = m \log C + e \tag{17.1}$$

Solving for log C yields the expression

$$\log C = \frac{E - e}{m} \tag{17.2}$$

However, after an intravenous dose the concentration of a drug in the body in a one-compartment open model is described as follows.

$$\log C = \log C_0 - \frac{Kt}{2.3} \tag{17.3}$$

By substituting Equation 17.2 into Equation 17.3, we get Equation 17.4, where E_0 = effect at concentration C_0.

$$\frac{E - e}{m} = \frac{E_0 - e}{m} - \frac{Kt}{2.3}$$

$$E = E_0 - \frac{Kmt}{2.3} \tag{17.4}$$

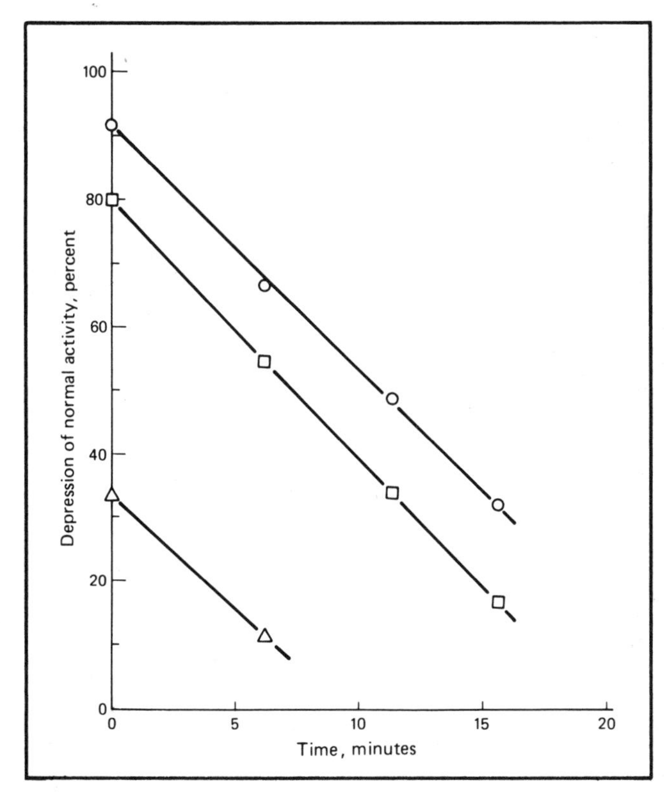

Figure 17-3. Depression of normal muscle activity as a function of time after intravenous administration of 0.1–0.2 mg (+)-tubocurarine per kilogram to unanesthetized volunteers. Circles represent head lift; squares, hand grip; and triangles inspiratory flow, presenting mean values of six experiments on five subjects. *(After Johansen SH, et al, 1964, with permission.[2])*

The pharmacologic response at any time after an intravenous dose of a drug may be calculated theoretically with Equation 17.4. From this equation, the pharmacologic effect declines with a slope of $Km/2.3$. The decrease in pharmacologic effect is affected by both the elimination constant K and the slope m. For a drug with a large m the pharmacologic response declines rapidly and requires that multiple doses be given at small intervals to maintain the pharmacologic effect. Furthermore, Equation 17.4 predicts that the pharmacologic effect will decline linearly with respect to time for a drug that follows a one-compartment model and a linear log dose–pharmacologic response.

The relationship between pharmacokinetics and pharmacologic response can be demonstrated by observing the percent depression of muscular activity after an IV dose of (+)-tubocurarine. The decline of pharmacologic effect is linear as a function of time (Fig. 17-3). For each pharmacologic response the slope of each curve is the same. Since the values for each slope, which include Km (Eq. 17.4), are the same, it is assumed that the sensitivity of the receptors for (+)-tubocurarine is the same at each site of action. Note that a plot of the log concentration of drug versus time yields a straight line.

A second example of the pharmacologic effect declining linearly with time was observed with LSD (Fig. 17-4). After an IV dose of the drug, log concentrations of drug decreased linearly with time except for a brief distribution period. Further-

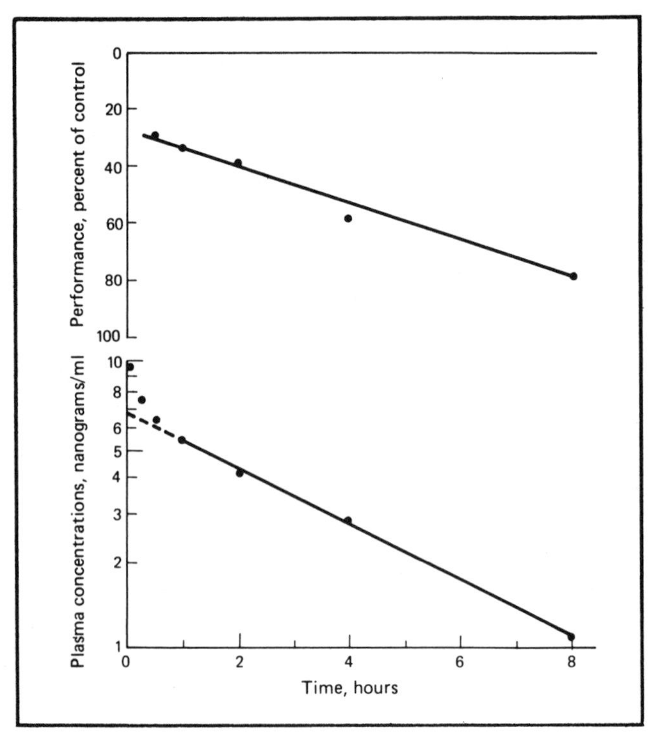

Figure 17-4. Mean plasma concentrations of lysergic acid diethylamide (LSD) and performance test scores as a function of time after intravenous administration of 2 μg LSD per kilogram to five normal human subjects. *(After Aghajanian OK, Bing OHL, 1964, with permission.*[3]*)*

more, the pharmacologic effect, as measured by the performance score of each subject, also declined linearly with time. Since the slope is governed in part by the elimination rate constant, the pharmacologic effect declines much more rapidly when the elimination rate constant is increased due to increased metabolism or renal excretion. Conversely, an increased pharmacologic response is experienced among patients with longer drug half-lives.

RELATIONSHIP BETWEEN DOSE AND DURATION OF ACTIVITY, t_{eff} SINGLE IV BOLUS INJECTION

The relationship between the duration of the pharmacologic effect and the dose can be inferred from Equation 17.3 After an intravenous dose, assuming a one-compartment model, the time needed for any drug to decline to a concentration C is given by the following equation, assuming the drug takes effect immediately.

$$t = \frac{2.3(\log C_0 - \log C)}{K} \tag{17.5}$$

Using C_{eff} to represent the minimum effective drug concentration, the duration of drug action can be obtained as follows.

$$t_{eff} = \frac{2.3\left(\log \frac{D_0}{V_d} - \log C_{eff}\right)}{K} \tag{17.6}$$

Some practical applications are suggested by this equation. For example, a doubling of the dose will not result in a doubling of the effective duration of pharmacologic action. On the other hand, a doubling of $t_{1/2}$ or a corresponding decrease in K will result in a proportional decrease in duration of action. A clinical situation is often encountered in the treatment of infections where C_{eff} is the bacteriocidal concentration of the drug, and in order to double the duration of the antibiotic, a considerably greater increase than simply doubling the dose is necessary.

PRACTICE PROBLEM

The MEC in plasma for a certain antibiotic is 0.1 μg/ml. The drug follows a one-compartment open model and has an apparent volume of distribution (V_d) of 10 L and a first-order elimination rate constant of 1.0 hr^{-1}. (a) What would be the t_{eff} for a single 100-mg IV dose of this antibiotic? (b) What would be the new t_{eff} or t'_{eff} for this drug if the dose was increased 10-fold to 1000 mg?

Solution

a. The t_{eff} for a 100-mg dose is calculated as follows:

Since $V_d = 10{,}000$ ml, then

$$C_0 = \frac{100 \text{ mg}}{10{,}000 \text{ ml}} = 10 \ \mu\text{g/ml}$$

For a one-compartment model IV dose, $C = C_0 e^{-Kt}$.
Thus

$$0.1 = 10e^{-(1.0)t_{eff}}$$

$$t_{eff} = 4.61 \text{ hr}$$

b. The t'_{eff} for a 1000-mg dose is calculated as follows: Since $V_d = 10{,}000$ ml, then

$$C'_0 = \frac{1000 \text{ mg}}{10{,}000 \text{ ml}} = 100 \ \mu\text{g/ml}$$

and

$$C'_{eff} = C'_0 e^{-Kt'_{eff}}$$

$$0.1 = 100e^{-(1.0)t'_{eff}}$$

$$t'_{eff} = 6.91 \text{ hr}$$

The percent increase in t_{eff} is therefore found by

$$\text{Percent increase in } t_{eff} = \frac{t'_{eff} - t_{eff}}{t_{eff}} \times 100$$

$$= \frac{6.91 - 4.61}{4.61} \times 100$$

$$\text{Percent increase in } t_{eff} = 50\%$$

This example shows that a 10-fold increase in the dose increases the duration of action of a drug (t_{eff}) by only 50%.

EFFECT OF BOTH DOSE AND ELIMINATION HALF-LIFE ON THE DURATION OF ACTIVITY

A single equation can be derived to describe the relationship of dose, D_0, and the elimination half-life, $t_{1/2}$, on the effective time for therapeutic activity, t_{eff}. This expression is derived below:

$$\ln C_{eff} = \ln C_0 - Kt_{eff}$$

Since $C_0 = D_0/V_d$,

$$\ln C_{eff} = \ln\left(\frac{D_0}{V_d}\right) - Kt_{eff}$$

$$Kt_{eff} = \ln\left(\frac{D_0}{V_d}\right) - \ln C_{eff}$$

$$t_{eff} = \frac{1}{K}\ln\frac{D_0/V_d}{C_{eff}} \tag{17.7}$$

Substitute $0.693/t_{1/2}$ for K:

$$t_{eff} = 1.44t_{1/2}\ln\left(\frac{D_0}{V_d C_{eff}}\right) \tag{17.8}$$

From Equation 17.8 an increase in $t_{1/2}$ will increase the t_{eff} in direct proportion. However, an increase in the dose, D_0, does not increase the t_{eff} in direct proportion. The effect of an increase in V_d or C_{eff} could be seen by using generated data. Only the positive solutions for Equation 17.8 is valid, although mathematically t_{eff} can be

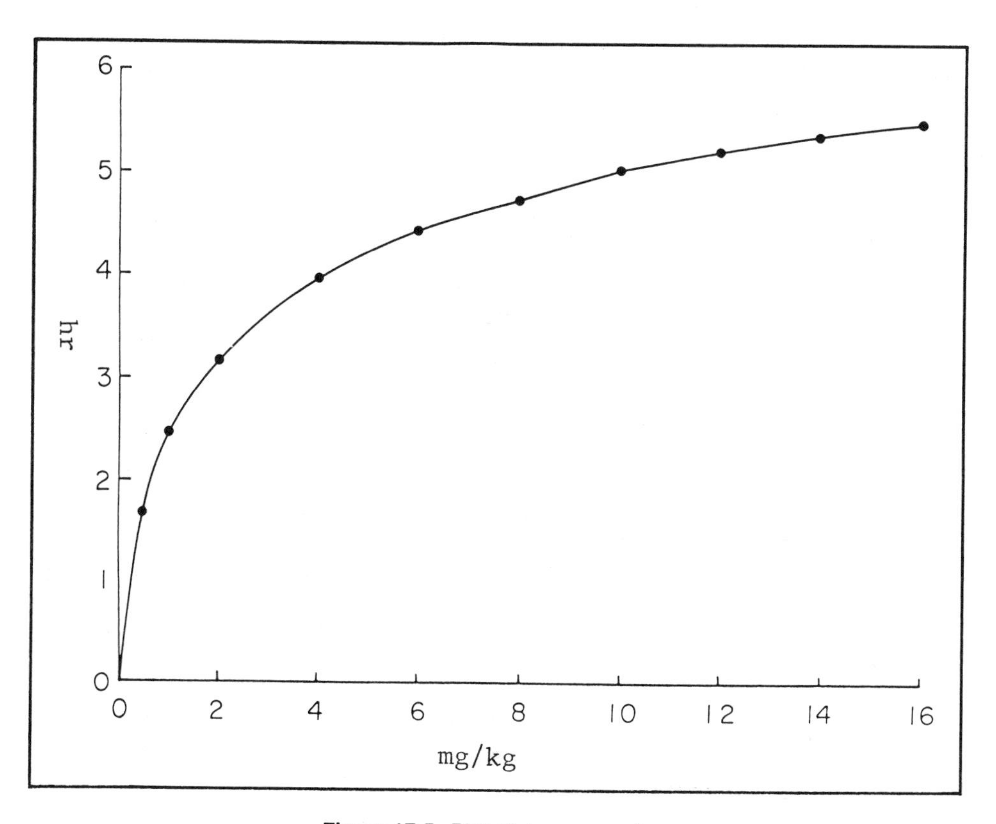

Figure 17-5. Plot of t_{eff} versus dose.

obtained by increasing C_{eff} or V_d. The effect of changing dose on t_{eff} is shown in Figure 17-5 using data generated with Equation 17.8. The nonlinear increase in t_{eff} is observed as dose increases.

EFFECT OF ELIMINATION HALF-LIFE ON DURATION OF ACTIVITY

Since elimination of drugs is due to the processes of excretion and metabolism, an alteration of any of these elimination processes will effect the $t_{1/2}$ of the drug. In certain disease states pathophysiologic changes in hepatic or renal function will decrease the elimination of a drug observed by a prolonged $t_{1/2}$. This prolonged $t_{1/2}$ will lead to retention of the drug in the body, thereby increasing the duration of activity of the drug, t_{eff}, as well as increasing the possibility of drug toxicity.

In order to improve antibiotic therapy with the penicillins and cephalosporins, clinicians have intentionally prolonged the elimination of these drugs by giving a second drug, probenecid, which competitively inhibits renal excretion of the antibiotic. This approach to prolong the duration of activity of antibiotics that are rapidly excreted through the kidney has been used successfully for a number of years. The data in Table 17-1 illustrates how a change in the elimination $t_{1/2}$ will affect the t_{eff} for a drug. For all doses a 100% increase in the $t_{1/2}$ will result in a 100% increase in the t_{eff}. For example, for a drug whose $t_{1/2}$ is 0.75 hr and is given at a dose of 2 mg/kg, the t_{eff} is 3.24 hr. If the $t_{1/2}$ is increased to 1.5 hr, the t_{eff} is increased to 6.48 hr, which is an increase of 100%. However, the effect of doubling the dose from

TABLE 17-1. THE RELATIONSHIP BETWEEN ELIMINATION HALF-LIFE AND THE DURATION OF ACTIVITY

Dose (mg/kg)	$t_{1/2}$ = 0.75 hr, t_{eff} (hr)	$t_{1/2}$ = 1.5 hr t_{eff} (hr)
2.0	3.24	6.48
3.0	3.67	7.35
4.0	3.98	7.97
5.0	4.22	8.45
6.0	4.42	8.84
7.0	4.59	9.18
8.0	4.73	9.47
9.0	4.86	9.72
10	4.97	9.95
11	5.08	10.2
12	5.17	10.3
13	5.26	10.5
14	5.34	10.7
15	5.41	10.8
16	5.48	11.0
17	5.55	11.1
18	5.61	11.2
19	5.67	11.3
20	5.72	11.4

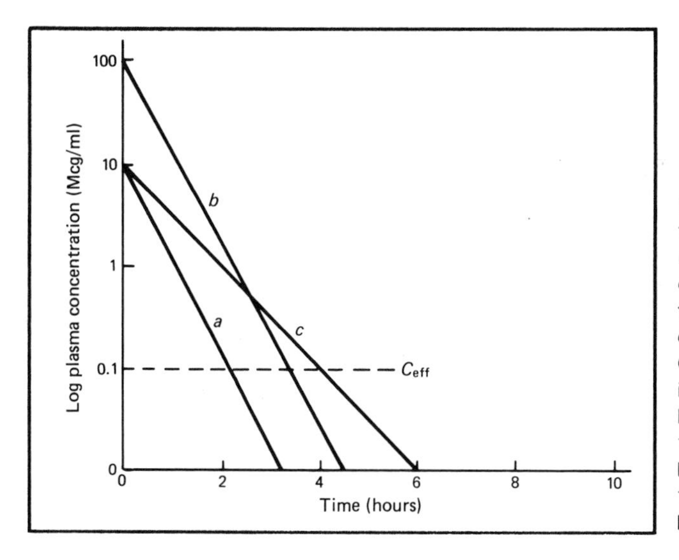

Figure 17-6. Plasma level–time curves describing the relationship of both dose and elimination half-life on duration of drug action. C_{eff} = effective concentration. Curve a = single 100 mg IV injection of drug; $K = 1.0$ hr^{-1}. Curve b = single 1000-mg IV injection; $K = 1.0$ hr^{-1}. Curve c = single 100-mg IV injection; $K = 0.5$ hr^{-1}. V_d is 10 L.

2 mg/kg to 4 mg/kg (no change in elimination processes) will only increase the t_{eff} to 3.98 hr, which is an increase of 22.8%. The effect of prolonging the elimination half-life has an extremely important effect on the treatment of infections, particularly in patients with high metabolism or clearance of the antibiotic. Therefore, antibiotics must be dosed with full consideration of the effect of alteration of the $t_{1/2}$ on the t_{eff}. Consequently, a simple proportional increase in dose will leave the patient's blood concentration below the effective antibiotic level most of the time during drug therapy.

Changes in elimination half-life will proportionately change the t_{eff}. It is interesting to note that indeed clinicians have long observed the therapeutic usefulness of combining probenecid with penicillin. The effect of a prolonged t_{eff} is shown in lines a and c in Figure 17-6. Figure 17-6 also shows the disproportionate increase in t_{eff} as the dose is increased 10-fold (a and b).

THEORETICAL TREATMENT OF PHARMACOLOGIC EFFECT AND DOSE

The relation between pharmacologic effect and dose was considered by Wagner[4] using a kinetic approach to the drug receptor theory (Fig. 17-7). The rate of change in the number of drug receptor complexes is expressed as db/dt. From Figure 17-7 a differential equation is obtained:

$$\frac{db}{dt} = K_1 c^s (a - b) - bK_2 \tag{17.9}$$

where $K_1 c^s (a - b)$ = rate of receptor complex formation and bK_2 = rate of dissociation of the receptor complex.

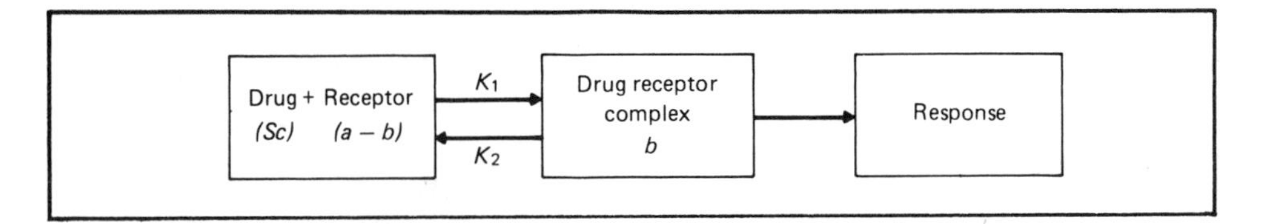

Figure 17-7. Model of the drug receptor theory: a = total number of drug receptors; c = concentration of drug; S = number of moles of drug that combine with one receptor (constant for each drug); and b = number of drug receptor complexes.

At steady state, $db/dt = 0$ and Equation 17.9 reduces to

$$K_1 c^s a - K_1 c^s b - bK_2 = 0$$

$$\frac{b}{a} = \frac{K_1 c^s}{K_1 c^s + K_2} = \frac{1}{1 + (K_2/K_1 c^s)} \qquad (17.10)$$

For many drugs the pharmacologic response (R) is proportional to the number of receptors occupied:

$$R \propto \frac{b}{a}$$

The pharmacologic response (R) is related to the maximum pharmacologic response (R_{max}), the concentration of drug, and the rate of change in the number of drug receptor complexes occupied:

$$R = \frac{R_{max}}{1 + (K_2/K_1 c^s)} \qquad (17.11)$$

A graph of Equation 17.11 constructed from the percent pharmacologic response, $(R/R_{max}) \times 100$, versus the concentration of drug gives the response–concentration curve (Fig. 17-8). This type of theoretical development explains that the pharmacologic response versus dose curve is not completely linear over the entire dosage range, as is frequently observed.

The total pharmacologic response elicited by a drug is difficult to quantitate in terms of the intensity and the duration of the drug response. The *integrated pharmacologic response* is a measure of the total pharmacologic response and is mathematically expressed as the product of these two factors (i.e., duration and intensity of drug action) summed up over a period of time. Using Equation 17.11, an integrated pharmacologic response is generated if the drug plasma concentration–time curve can be adequately described by a pharmacokinetic model.

Table 17-2 is based on a hypothetical drug that follows a one-compartment open model. The drug is given intravenously in divided doses. With this drug, the total integrated response increases considerably when the total dose is given in a greater number of divided doses. By giving the drug in a single dose, two doses, four

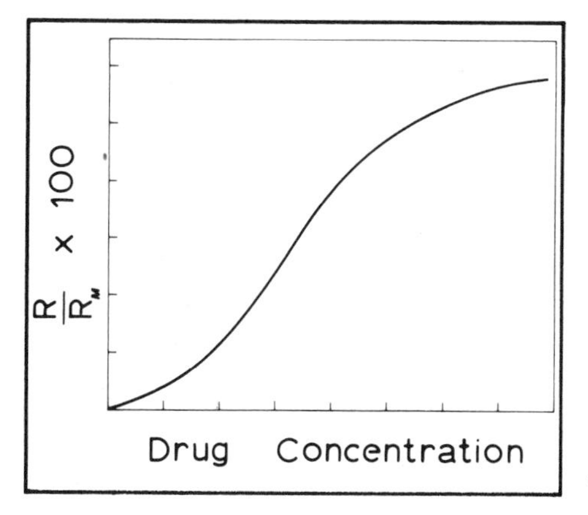

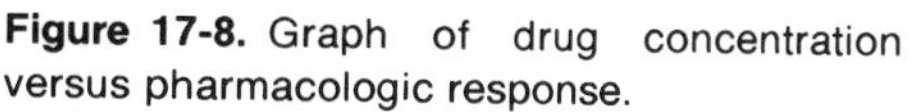
Figure 17-8. Graph of drug concentration versus pharmacologic response.

doses, and eight doses, an integrated response was obtained that ranged from 100 to 138.9%, using the single-dose response as a 100% reference. It should be pointed out that when the bolus dose is broken into a smaller number of doses, the largest percent increase in the integrated response occurs when the bolus dose is divided into two doses. Further division will cause less of an increase, proportionally. The actual percent increase in integrated response depends on the $t_{1/2}$ of the drug as well as the dosing interval.

The values in Table 17-2 were theoretically generated. However, these data illustrate that the pharmacologic response is dependent on the dosing schedule. A large total dose given in divided doses may produce a pharmacologic response quite different from that obtained by administration of the drug in a single dose.

TABLE 17-2. HYPOTHETICAL DRUG GIVEN INTRAVENOUSLY IN SINGLE AND DIVIDED DOSES*

Dose Number	Single Dose	Dose Given Initially and at 12th Hour	Dose Given at 0, 6, 12, 18 hr	Dose Given at 0, 3, 6, 9, 12, 15, 18, 21 hr
1	422	272	139.4	62.53
2		276	148.2	71.46
3			148.5	74.41
4			149.0	75.61
5				76.27
6				76.44
7				76.71
8				76.81
Total response	422	548	585.1	590.2
% Response	100	130	138.7	138.9

* The drug follows a one-compartment open model. Each value represents a unit of integrated pharmacologic response.

After Wagner J, 1968, with permission.[4]

The correlation of pharmacologic response to pharmacokinetics is not always possible with all drugs. Sometimes intermediate steps are involved in the mechanism of action of the drug that are more complex than is assumed in the model. For example, with warfarin (an anticoagulant), delayed response occurs and direct correlation of the anticoagulant activity to the plasma drug concentration is not possible. The plasma warfarin level is correlated with the inhibition of the prothrombin complex production rate. However, many of the correlations of pharmacologic effect and plasma drug concentration are performed using models proposed and discarded. The process of pharmacokinetic modeling can greatly enhance our understanding of the way drugs act in a quantitative manner.

PHARMACODYNAMIC MODELS

To predict the time course of drug response using a pharmacodynamic model, a mathematical expression is developed to describe the drug concentration time profile of the drug at the receptor site. This equation is then used to relate drug concentrations to the time course and intensity of the pharmacologic response. Most pharmacodynamic models assume that pharmacologic action is due to a drug–receptor interaction, and the magnitude of the response is quantatively related to the drug concentration in the receptor compartment. In the simplest case the drug receptor lies in the plasma compartment and pharmacologic response has been established through a one-compartment model with drug response proportional to log drug concentration (Equation 17.1). More complicated models involving a receptor compartment that lies outside the central compartment have been proposed by Sheiner et al.[5] This latter model locates the receptor in an effect compartment in which drug equilibrates from the central compartment by a first-order rate constant K_{1e}. There is no back diffusion of drug away from the effect compartment, thereby simplifying the complexity of the equations. This model was successfully applied to monitor the pharmacologic effects of the drug trimazosin.[6]

The pharmacokinetics of trimazosin is described as a two-compartment open model with conversion to a metabolite by a first-order rate constant K_{1m}. The pharmacokinetics of the metabolite is described by a one-compartment model with a first-order elimination constant K_{mo}. The drug effect may be described by two pharmacodynamic models, either model (a) or model (b). Model (a) assumes that the drug effect in the effect compartment is produced by the drug only. Model (b) assumes that both the drug and a metabolite produces drug effect (Figure 17-10).

The following equation describes the pharmacokinetics and pharmacodynamics of the drug:

$$C_p = Ae^{-at} + Be^{-bt} \tag{17.12}$$

where C_p is concentration of the drug in the central compartment.

$$C_m = \frac{V_1 K_{1m}}{V_m}\left[\frac{A}{(K_{mo} - a)}(e^{at} - e^{-K_{mo}t}) + \frac{B}{(K_{mo} - b)}(e^{-bt} - e^{-K_{mo}t})\right] \tag{17.13}$$

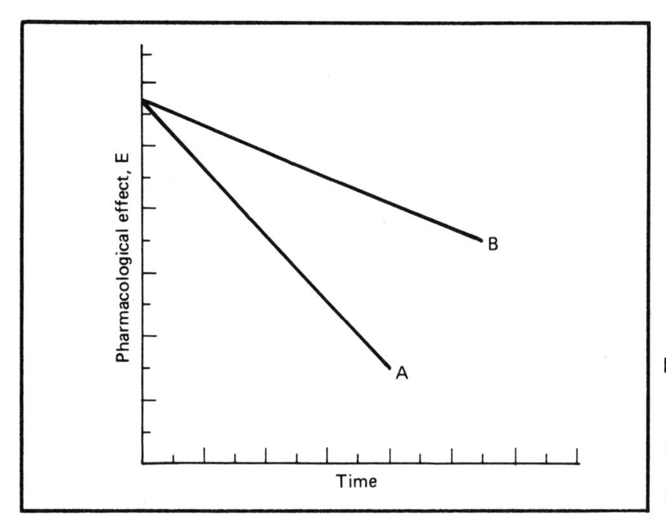

Figure 17-9. Graph of pharmacologic response *E* as a function of time for the same drug in patients with normal (*A*) and uremic (*B*) kidney function, respectively.

where C_m is concentration of the metabolite in the body; V_m is volume of distribution of the metabolite; V_1 is the volume of central compartment of the body; K_{1m} is the first-order constant for converting drug to metabolite; K_{mo} is the elimination rate constant of the metabolite; A and B are two-compartment model coefficients for the drug (see Chapter 5); and K_{1o} is elimination rate constant of the drug.

The drug concentration in the effect compartment is calculated by assuming that at equilibrium the concentration of the drug in the effect compartment and the central compartment are equal:

$$K_{1e}V_1 = K_{eq}V_e \tag{17.14}$$

Where V_e is volume of the effect compartment. Therefore, the drug concentration $C\ (e, d)$ is calculated as

$$C(e,d) = \frac{AK_{eq}}{(K_{eq} - a)}(e^{-at} - e^{-K_{eq}t}) + \frac{BK_{eq}}{(K_{eq} - b)}(e^{-bt} - e^{-K_{eq}t}) \tag{17.15}$$

The effect due to drug is assumed to be linear:

$$E = M_d C(e,d) + i \tag{17.16}$$

where M_d is the sensitivity slope to the drug, i.e., effect per unit of drug concentration in the effect compartment. The parameters M_d, i, and K_{eq} are determined by least-squares fitting of the data. For the metabolite the concentration of metabolite

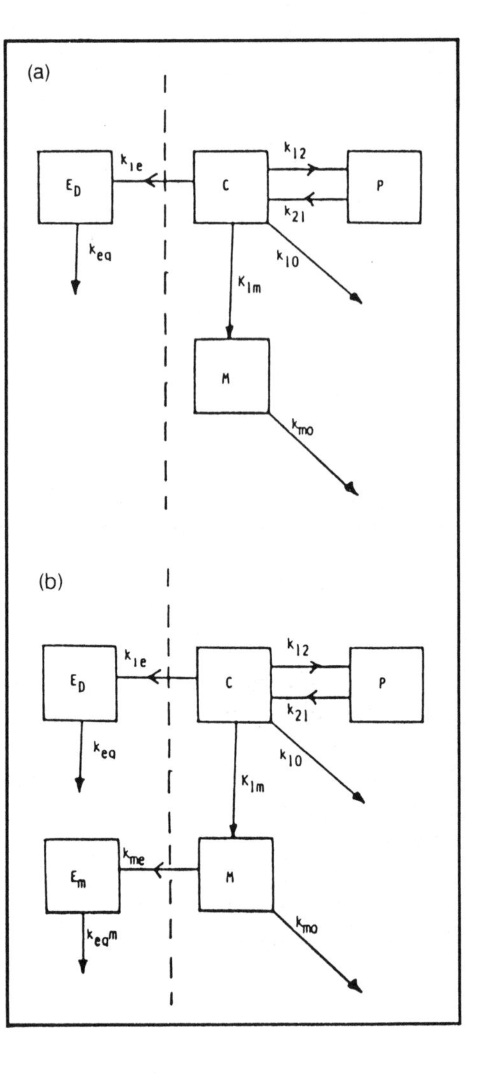

Figure 17-10. Two proposed pharmacodynamic models for describing the hypotensive effect of trimazosin. A Model (a) assumes an effect compartment (left of dotted line) for the drug. Model (b) assumes an effect compartment for the drug as well as the metabolite. (*From Meredith et al, 1983, with permission.*[6])

in the effect compartment is $C\ (e, m)$:

$$C(e,m) = \frac{AV_1K_{1m}K_{eq}m}{V_m} \times \left[\frac{e^{-at}}{(a-K_{mo})(a-K_{eq}m)} + \frac{e^{-K_{mo}t}}{(a-K_{mo})(K_{eq}m-K_{mo})} - \frac{e^{-K_{eq}mt}}{(a-K_{eq}m)(K_{eq}m-K_{mo})} + \frac{BV_1K_{im}K_{eq}m}{V_m} \frac{e^{-bt}}{(b-K_{mo})(b-K_{eq}m)} + \frac{e^{-K_{mo}t}}{(b-K_{mo})(K_{eq}m-K_{mo})} - \frac{e^{-K_{eq}mt}}{(b-K_{eq}m)(K_{eq}m-K_{mo})} \right]$$

The concentration of the metabolite in the effect compartment is in turn related to drug effect as for the parent drug. The total effect produced is

$$E_t = M_d C(e, d) + M_m C(e, m) + I \qquad (17.17)$$

From Equation 17.17 the five parameters M_d, M_m, i, K_{eq}, and $K_{eq}m$ may be estimated. Figure 17-11 shows the observed decline in systolic blood pressure compared with the theoretical decline in blood pressure predicted by the model. An excellent fit of the data was obtained by assuming that both drug and metabolite are active.

This example illustrated that for a dose of a drug, the drug concentration in the effect compartment and others may be described by a mathematical model. These equations were further developed to describe the time course of a pharmacologic event. In this case Meredith et al[6] demonstrated that both the drug and the metabolite formed in the body may affect the time course of the pharmacologic action of the drug in the body.

QUESTIONS

On the basis of the graph in Figure 17-9, answer "true" or "false" to the following statements. State the reason for your answers.

1. The pharmacologic response is directly proportional to the log plasma drug concentration.
2. The volume of distribution is not changed by uremia.
3. The drug is exclusively eliminated by hepatic biotransformation.
4. The receptor sensitivity is unchanged in the uremic patient.

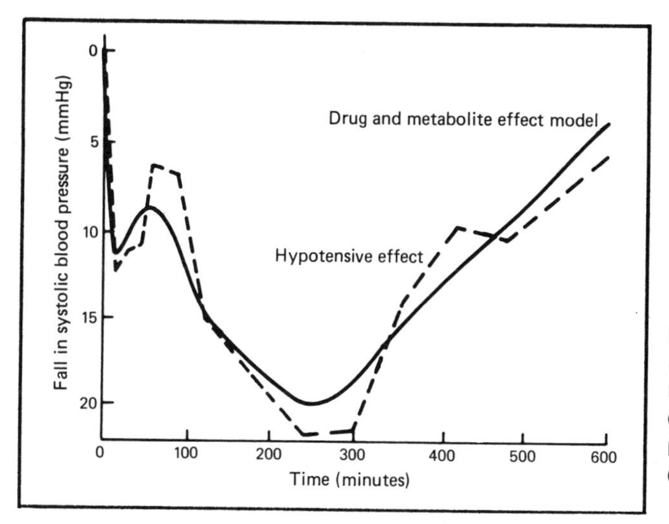

Figure 17-11. Diagram showing the agreement between hypotensive effect recorded (solid) and hypotensive effect projected by model (b). (*From Meredith et al, 1983, with permission.*[6])

REFERENCES

1. Holford NHG, Sheiner LB: Kinetics of pharmacologic response. Pharm Ther 16:143–66, 1982
2. Johansen SH, Jorgensen M, Molbech S: Effect of tubocurarine on respiratory and nonrespiratory muscle power in man. J Appl Physiol 19:990–91, 1964
3. Aghajanian OK, Bing OHL: Persistence of lysergic acid diethylamide in the plasma of human subjects. Clin Pharmacol Ther 5:611–14, 1964
4. Wagner JG: Kinetics of pharmacologic response, I: Proposed relationship between response and drug concentration in the intact animal and man. J Theor Biol 20:173–201, 1968
5. Sheiner LB, Stanski DR, Vozek S, et al: Simultaneous modeling of pharmacokinetics and pharmacodynamics: Application to *d*-tubocurarine. Clin Pharmacol Ther 25:358–370, 1979
6. Meredith PA, Kelman AW, Eliott HL, Reid JL: Pharmacokinetic and pharmacodynamic modeling of trimazosin and its major metabolite. J Pharmokinet Biopharm 11:323–34, 1983

BIBLIOGRAPHY

Gibaldi M, Levy G, Weintraub H: Drug distribution and pharmacological effects. Clin Pharmacol Ther 12:734, 1971

Jusko WJ: Pharmacodynamics of chemotherapeutic effects: Dose–time–response relationship for phase-nonspecific agents. J Pharm Sci 60:892, 1971

Levy G: Kinetics of pharmacologic effects. Clin Pharmacol Ther 1:362, 1966

CHAPTER EIGHTEEN

Controlled Release Drug Products

Most conventional drug products such as tablets and capsules are formulated to release the active drug immediately to obtain rapid and complete systemic absorption of the drug. In recent years various modified drug products have been developed to release the active drug at a controlled rate. A variety of controlled release drug products have been designed with specific therapeutic objectives based on the physiochemical, pharmacologic, and pharmacokinetic properties of the drug. Due to the variety of release characteristics for these drug products, a number of different terms are used to describe the available types of controlled release drug products.

TERMS USED IN CONTROLLED RELEASE PRODUCTS

An *enteric coated* tablet is an example of a modified dosage form, designed for release at the small intestine. For example, aspirin may irritate the gastric mucosal cells of the stomach. An enteric coating on the aspirin tablet prevents the tablet from dissolving and releasing its contents at the low pH in the stomach. The tablet will later dissolve and release the drug in the higher pH of the duodenum, where the drug is rapidly absorbed with less irritation to the mucosal cells.

Another type of controlled release drug product is the *repeat action* tablet, which is designed to release one dose of drug initially and a second dose of drug at a later time. A *prolonged action* drug product is designed to release the drug slowly and to provide a continuous supply of drug over an extended period. The prolonged action drug product prevents very rapid absorption of the drug, which could result in extremely high peak plasma drug concentration. Most prolonged release products extend the duration of action but do not release drug at a constant rate. A *sustained release* drug product is designed to deliver an initial therapeutic dose of the drug (loading dose) followed by a slower and constant release of drug. The rate of release of the maintenance dose is designed so that the amount of drug loss from the body by elimination is constantly replaced. With the sustained release product, a constant

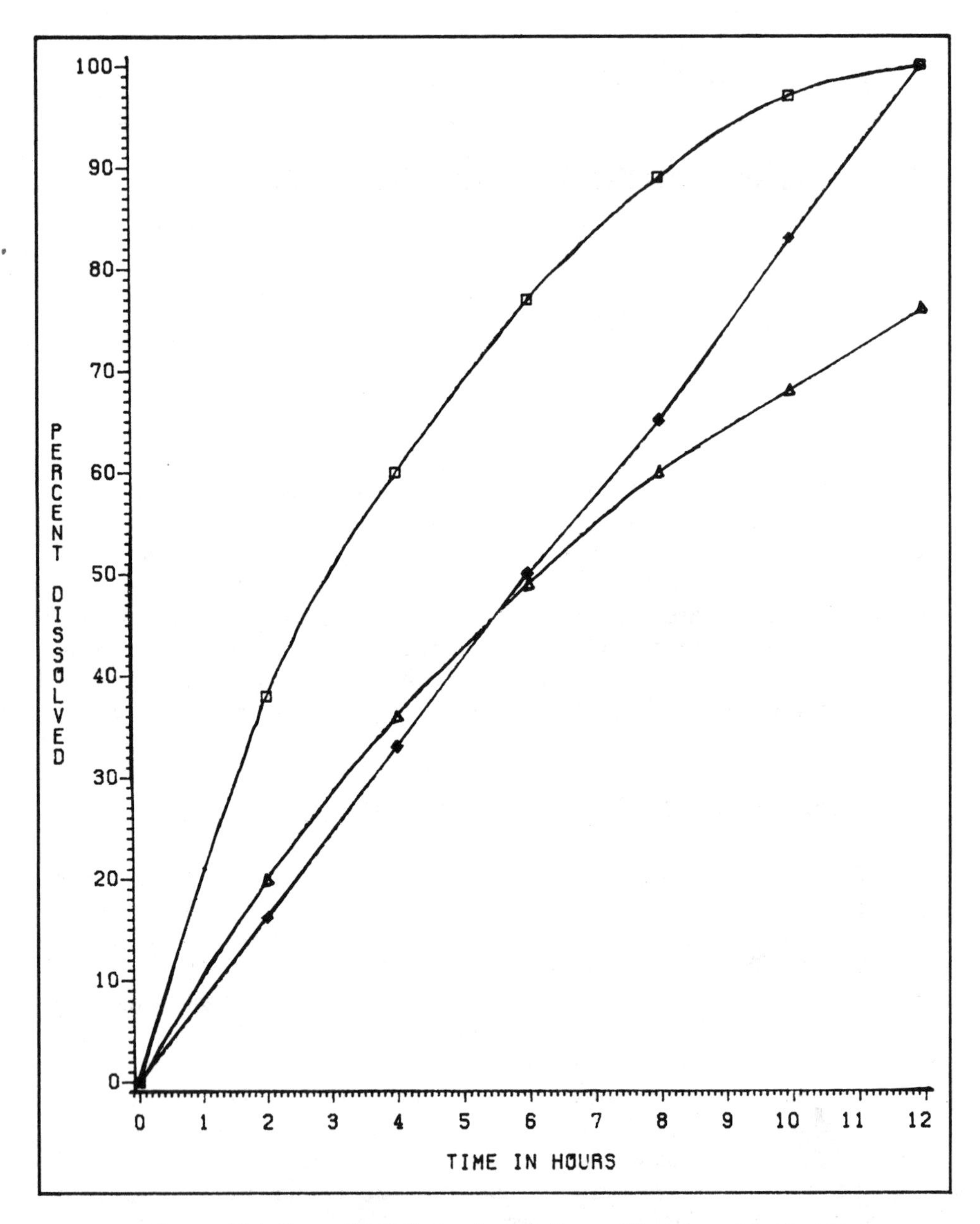

Figure 18-1. Drug dissolution rates of three different sustained release products in vitro. (□ = first-order release, ◆ = zero-order release, and △ = first-order release with incomplete dissolution after 12 hr).

plasma drug concentration may be maintained with minimal fluctuation. Figure 18-1 shows the dissolution rate of three sustained release products without loading dose. The plasma concentrations resulting from the sustained release products are shown in Figure 18-2. A prolonged action tablet with first-order release is also illustrated in the same diagram. A prolonged action tablet typically results in peak and trough drug level in the body. The product releases drug without matching the rate of drug elimination resulting in uneven plasma drug level in the body. Various other terms have been associated with controlled release drug products, including *extended action*, *timed release*, *long acting*, *drug delivery system*, and *programmed drug delivery*.

The use of these various terms does not imply zero-order drug release. Many of these drug products release drug at a first-order rate. Moreover, some drug products are formulated with materials that are more soluble at a specific pH, and the product may release drug depending on the pH of the gastrointestinal tract. Ideally, the controlled release drug product should release drug at a constant rate independent of both the pH and the ionic content within the entire segment of the gastrointestinal tract.

BIOPHARMACEUTIC FACTORS

The major objective of a controlled release drug product is to achieve a prolonged therapeutic effect while minimizing unwanted side effects due to fluctuating plasma drug levels. Ideally, the controlled release drug product should release the drug at a constant, or zero-order, rate. After release from the drug product the drug is rapidly absorbed, and the drug absorption rate should follow zero-order kinetics similar to an intravenous infusion of the drug. In all cases the drug product is designed so that the rate of systemic drug absorption is limited by the rate of drug release via the drug delivery system. Unfortunately, most controlled release drug products that release drug by zero-order kinetics in vitro do not demonstrate zero-order drug absorption when given in vivo. The lack of zero-order drug absorption from these controlled release drug products after oral administration may be due to a number of unpredictable events happening in the gastrointestinal tract during absorption.

The Stomach

The stomach is a "mixing and secreting" organ where food is mixed with digestive juice and emptied periodically into the small intestine. However, the movement of food or drug product in the stomach and small intestine are very different depending on the physiologic state. In the presence of food the stomach undergoes the digestive phase, and in the absence of food the stomach undergoes the interdigestive phase. During the digestive phase the food particles or solids larger than 2 mm are retained in the stomach, whereas smaller particles are emptied through the pyloric sphincter in a first-order rate depending on the content and size of the meals. During the interdigestive phase the stomach rests for up to a period of 30–40 min coordinated with equal resting period in the small intestine. Peristaltic contractions then occur,

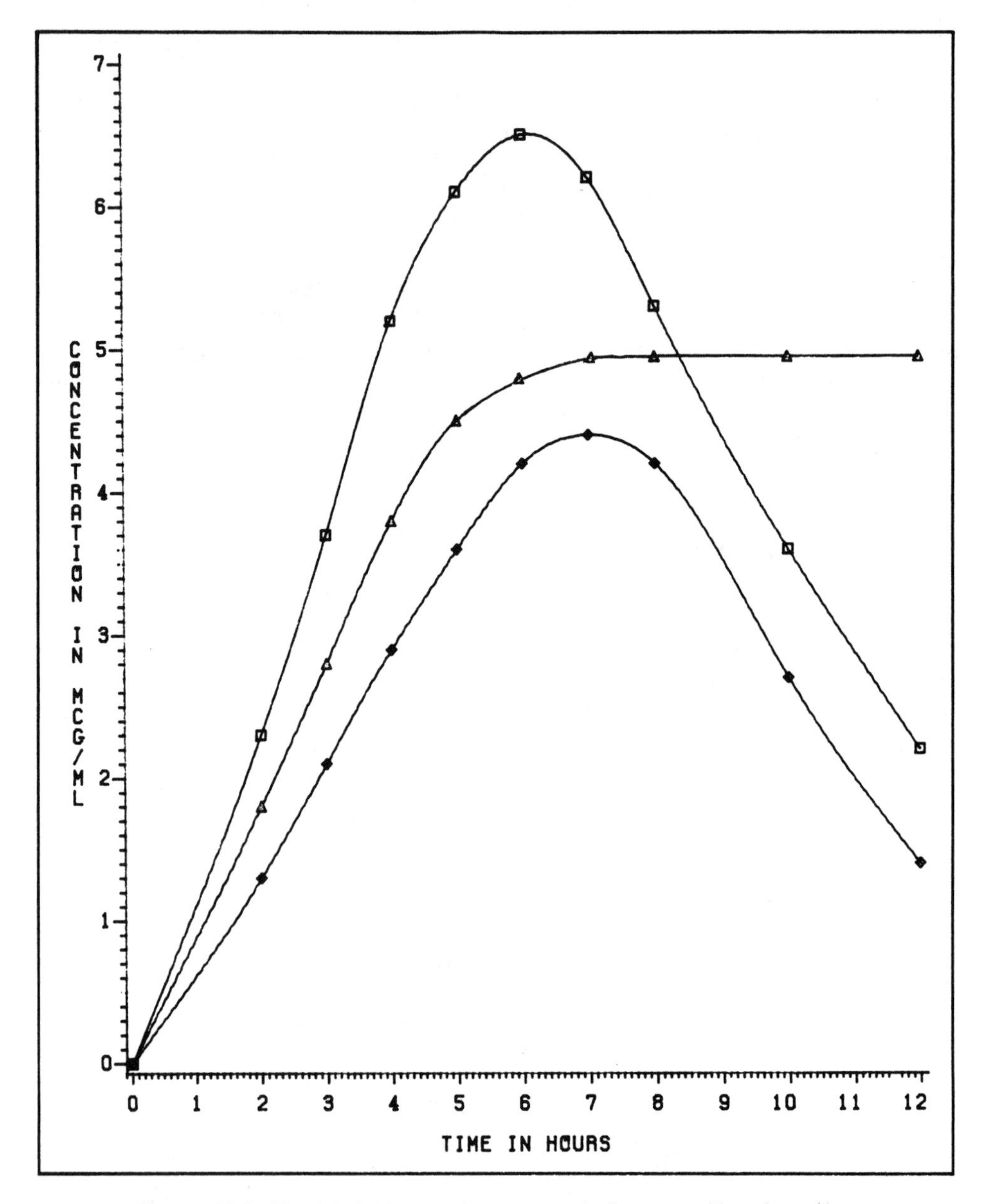

Figure 18-2. Simulated plasma drug concentrations resulting from three different sustained release products in Figure 18-1. (□ = first-order release, △ = zero-order release, and ◆ = first-order release with incomplete dissolution after 12 hr).

which ends with strong "housekeeper contractions" that move everything in the stomach through to the small intestine. Similarly, large particles in the small intestine are moved along only in the housekeeper contraction period. A drug may remain for several hours in the stomach if administered during the digestive phase. Fatty material, nutrients, and osmolality may further extend the time it stays in the stomach. On the other hand, when the drug is administered during the interdigestive phase, it may be swept along rapidly into the small intestine. Dissolution of drugs in the stomach may also be affected by the presence or absence of food. Normal resting pH of the stomach is 1; when food is present, the pH often rises to 3–5 because of buffering food substances. A drug that is tested to release at a zero-order rate in vitro with 0.1 N HCl may not release drug at the same rate at pH 3–5. The drug Theo-24 has recently been found to release drug at a higher rate in the presence of food. Whether this is related to a change in the stomach emptying rate or a food–drug interaction is not known. A longer time of retention in the stomach may expose the drug to stronger agitation in the acid environment. The stomach has been described as having "jet mixing" action that sends mixture with up to 50 mg Hg pressure toward the pyloric sphincter causing it to open and periodically release chymes to the small intestine.

The Small Intestine

The small intestine is about 10–14 ft in length. The first part is sterile, while the terminal part that connects the cecum contains some bacteria. The proximal part of the small intestine has a pH of about 6 due to neutralization of the acid by bicarbonates secreted by the duodenal mucosa and the pancreas. The small intestine provides an enormous surface area for drug absorption because of the presence of microvilli. The small intestine transit time of a solid preparation has been concluded to be about 3 hr or less in 95% of the population.[1] Transit time for meals from mouth to cecum (beginning of large intestine) has been reviewed by the same authors. Various investigators have used the "lactulose hydrogen test," which measures the appearance of hydrogen in a patient's breath (lactulose is metabolized by bacteria rapidly in the large intestine yielding hydrogen that is normally absent in a person's breath), to estimate transit time. These results confirm a relatively short GI transit time from mouth to cecum of 4–6 hr. This interval was concluded to be too short for sustained release preparations that last up to 12 hr, unless the drug is to be absorbed in the colon. The colon has little fluid and the abundance of bacteria may make drug absorption erratic and incomplete. The transit time for pellets has been studied in both disintegrating and nondisintegrating forms using both insoluble and soluble radiopaques. Most of the insoluble pellets were released from the capsule in 15 min. Scattering of pellets were seen in the stomach and along the entire length of the small intestine at 3 hr. At 12 hr most of the pellets were in the ascending colon, and at 24 hr the pellets were all in the descending colon ready to enter the rectum. With the disintegrating pellets, there was more scattering of the pellets along the GI tract. The pellets also varied widely in the rate of disintegration in vivo.[2]

The Large Intestine

The large intestine is about 4–5 ft long. This consists of the cecum and the ascending and descending colons that eventually end with the rectum. Little fluid is in the colon and drug transit is slow. Not much is known about drug absorption in this area, although unabsorbed drug that reaches this region may be metabolized by bacteria. Incompletely absorbed antibiotics may affect the normal flora of the bacteria. The rectum has a pH of about 6.8–7.0 and contains more fluid. Drugs are absorbed rapidly when administered as rectal preparation. However, the transit rate is affected by the rate of defecation. Presumably, drugs formulated for 24 hr would remain in this region to be absorbed.

There are a number of sustained release products formulated to take advantage of the physiologic conditions of the GI tract. Enteric coated beads have been found to release drug over 8 hr when taken with food due to the gradual emptying of the beads into the small intestine. Specially formulated "floating tablets" that remain in the top of the stomach have been used to extend the resident time of the product in the stomach. None of these methods, however, are consistent enough to perform reliably for potent medications. More experimental research is needed in this area.

DOSAGE FORM SELECTION

The selection of the drug and dosage is important in formulating a sustained release product. In general, a drug with low solubility should not be formulated into a nondisintegrating tablet. The risks of incomplete dissolution is high. A drug with low solubility at neutral pH should be formulated so that most of the drug is released prior to reaching the colon. The lack of fluid in the colon may make complete dissolution difficult. Erosion tablets are more reliable since the entire tablet eventually dissolves. With most single-unit dosage forms, there is a risk of erratic performance due to variable stomach emptying and GI transit time. The selection of the pellet or bead dosage form may minimize the risk of erratic stomach emptying since the pellets are usually scattered soon after ingestion. Disintegrating tablets have the same advantages since they are broken up soon after ingestion.

A drug that is highly soluble in the stomach but very insoluble at intestinal pH may be very difficult to formulate into a sustained release product. Too much protection may result in low bioavailability while too little protection may result in dose dumping in the stomach. A moderate extension of duration with enteric coated beads may be possible. However, the risk of erratic performance is higher than that of the conventional dosage form. The "osmotic type" of controlled system may be more suitable for this type of drug.

DRUG RELEASE FROM MATRIX

A matrix may be described as an inert solid vehicle in which a drug is uniformly suspended. A matrix may be formed simply by compressing or fusing the drug and the matrix material together. Generally, the drug is present in a smaller percent so that the matrix gives extended protection against water and the drug diffuses out slowly over time. Most matrix materials are water insoluble although some may swell in water slowly. Matrix type of drug release may be built into a tablet or small beads depending on the formulation composition. Figure 18-3 shows three common approaches by which the matrix mechanisms are employed. In case A the drug is coated with a soluble coating so drug release solely relies on the regulation of the matrix material. If the matrix is porous, water penetration would be rapid and the drug would diffuse out rapidly. A less porous matrix may give a longer duration of release. Unfortunately, drug release from a simple matrix tablet is not zero order.

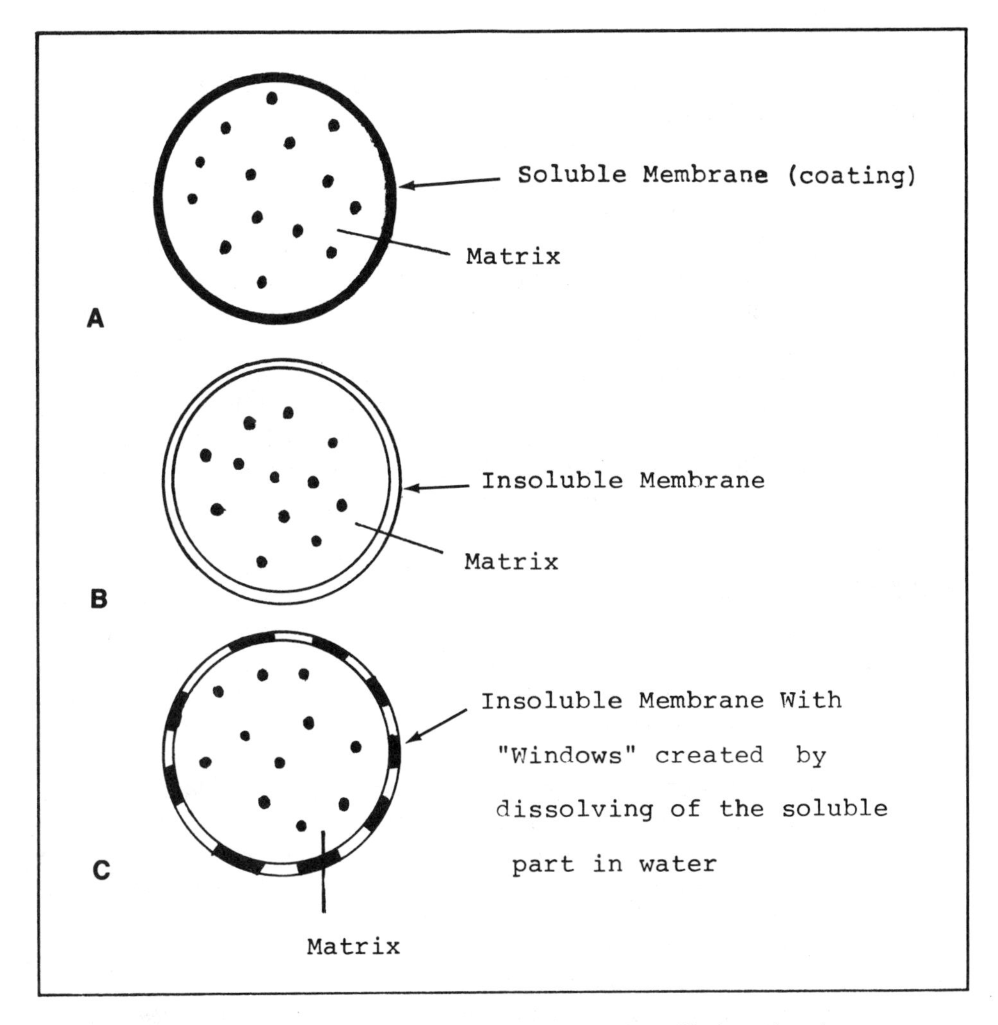

Figure 18-3. Examples of three different types of modified matrix release mechanisms.

The Higuchi equation describes the release rate of a matrix tablet:

$$Q = DS(P/\lambda)[A - 0.5SP]^{1/2}\sqrt{t} \tag{18.1}$$

where Q = amount of drug release per cm^2 of surface at time t; S = solubility of drug in g/cm^3 in dissolution media; A = content of drug in insoluble matrix; P = porosity of matrix; D = diffusion coefficient of drug; and λ = tortuosity factor.

Case B represents a matrix enclosed by an insoluble membrane so that drug release rate is regulated by the permeability of the membrane as well as the matrix. Case C represents a matrix tablet enclosed with a combined film. The film becomes porous after dissolution of the soluble part of the film. An example of this is the combined film formed by ethylcellulose and methylcellulose. Close to zero-order release has been obtained with this type of release mechanism.

ADVANTAGES AND DISADVANTAGES OF CONTROLLED RELEASE PRODUCTS

Despite the complexity of designing a controlled release drug product that behaves ideally, these dosage forms offer several important advantages over immediate release dosage forms of the same drug. Controlled release allows for sustained therapeutic blood levels of the drug, which provides for a prolonged and consistent clinical response in the patient. Moreover, if the drug input rate is constant, the blood levels should not fluctuate between a maximum and minimum as in a multiple-dose regimen with an immediate release drug product. Highly fluctuating blood concentrations of drug may produce unwanted side effects in the patient if the drug level is too high or fails to exert the proper therapeutic effect if the drug level is too low. Another advantage of controlled release is patient convenience, which leads to better patient compliance. For example, if the patient only needs to take the medication once daily, he or she will not have to remember to take additional doses at specified times during the day. Furthermore, since the dosage interval is longer, the patient needs not interrupt his sleep. The patient may also derive an economic benefit in using a controlled release drug product. A single dose of the controlled release product might cost less than an equivalent drug dose given several times a day in rapid release tablets. For patients under nursing care, the cost of nursing time required to administer medication is decreased if only one drug dosage is given to the patient each day.

For some drugs, such as chlorpheniramine, which have long elimination half-lives, the inherent duration of pharmacologic activity is long. Moreover, minimal fluctuations of blood concentrations of these drugs are observed after multiple doses are administered. Therefore, there is no rationale for controlled release formulations of these drugs. However, such drug products are marketed with the justification that controlled release products minimize toxicity, decrease adverse reactions, and provide patients with more convenience and thus better compliance.

There are also a number of disadvantages in using controlled release medication. If the patient suffers from an adverse drug reaction or becomes accidentally intoxicated, the removal of drug from the system is more difficult than with a rapid release drug product. With orally administered controlled release drug products, erratic or variable drug absorption might occur due to various interactions of the drug with the contents of the gastrointestinal tract and changes in gastrointestinal motility. The formulation of controlled release drug products for drugs usually given in large doses (> 500 mg) in conventional dosage forms may not be practical. Since the controlled release drug product may contain three or more times the dose given in more frequent intervals, the size of the controlled release drug product would have to be quite large, too large for the patient to swallow easily. For delayed or enteric drug problems, two possible problems might occur if the enteric coating is poorly formulated. First, the enteric coating might not prevent early release of the drug, which in turn could be degraded in the stomach or cause irritation to the gastric mucosal lining. Second, the enteric coating may fail to dissolve at the proper site and, therefore, the tablet might be lost prior to drug release and absorption.

KINETICS OF CONTROLLED RELEASE DOSAGE FORMS

The amount of drug required in a controlled release dosage form to provide a sustained drug level in the body is determined by the pharmacokinetics of the drug, the desired therapeutic level of the drug, and the intended duration of action. In general, the total dose required, D_{tot}, is the sum of the maintenance dose, D_m, and the initial dose, D_I, which is immediately released to provide a therapeutic blood level:

$$D_{tot} = D_I + D_m \tag{18.2}$$

In practice, D_m is released over a period of time and is equal to the product of t_d (the duration of action) and the zero-order rate K_r^0. Therefore, Equation 18.2 can be expressed as

$$D_{tot} = D_I + K_r^0 t_d \tag{18.3}$$

Ideally, the maintenance dose, D_m, is released after D_I has produced a blood level equal to the therapeutic drug level, C_p. However, due to the limits of formulations, D_m actually starts to release at $t = 0$. Therefore, D_I may be reduced from the calculated amount to avoid "topping."

$$D_{tot} = D_I - K_r^0 t_p + K_r^0 t_d \tag{18.4}$$

Equation 18.4 describes the total dose of drug needed, with t_p representing the time needed to reach peak drug concentration after the initial dose.

For a drug that follows a one-compartment open model, the rate of elimination R needed to maintain the drug at a therapeutic level C_p is

$$R = KV_d C_p \tag{18.5}$$

where K_r^0 must be equal to R in order to provide a stable blood level of the drug. Equation 18.5 provides an estimation of the release rate (K_r^0) required in the formulation. Equation 18.5 may also be rewritten as

$$R = C_p \text{Cl}_T \tag{18.6}$$

where Cl_T is the clearance of the drug. In designing a controlled release product, D_I

would be the loading dose that would raise the drug concentration in the body to C_d, and the total dose needed to maintain therapeutic concentration in the body would simply be

$$D_{tot} = D_I + C_d Cl_T \cdot \tau \tag{18.7}$$

For many sustained release drug products, there is no built-in loading dose (i.e., $D_I = 0$); the dose needed to maintain a therapeutic concentration for τ hours would be

$$D = C_p \tau Cl_T \tag{18.8}$$

EXAMPLE

What would be the dose needed to maintain a therapeutic concentration of 10 μg/ml for 12 hr in a sustained release product? 1. Assume $t_{1/2}$ of the drug is 3.46 hr and V_d is 10 L. 2. Assume $t_{1/2}$ of the drug is 1.73 hr and V_d is 5 L.

1.

$$K = 0.693/3.46 = 0.2/\text{hr}$$

$$Cl_T = 0.2 \times 10 = 2\ \text{L/hr}$$

From Equation 18.8,

$$D = 10 \times 2 \times 1000 \times 12 = 24000\ \mu\text{g or } 24\ \text{mg}$$

2.

$$K = 0.693/1.73 = 0.4\ \text{hr}$$

$$Cl_T = 0.4 \times 5 = 2\ \text{L/hr}$$

From Equation 18.8,

$$D = 10 \times 2 \times 1000 \times 12 = 24000\ \mu\text{g or } 24\ \text{mg}$$

In this example it is seen that the amount of drug needed in a sustained release product to maintain therapeutic concentration is dependent on both the V_d and the elimination half-life. In the example in part (2), although the elimination half-life is shorter, the volume of distribution is also smaller. If the volume of distribution is constant, then the amount of drug needed to maintain C_p is simply dependent on the elimination half-life.

Table 18-1 shows the influence of $t_{1/2}$ on the amount of drug needed for a controlled release drug product. Table 18-1 was constructed by assuming that the drug has a desired serum concentration of 10 μg/ml and an apparent volume of distribution of 20,000 ml. The release rate R decreases as the elimination half-life increases. Since elimination is slower for a drug with a long half-life, the input rate should be slower. The total amount of drug needed in the controlled release drug product is dependent on both the release rate R and the desired duration of activity for the drug. For a drug with an elimination half-life of 4 hr and a release rate of 17.3 mg/hr, the controlled release product must contain 207.6 mg to provide a duration of activity of 12 hr (Table 18-1). The bulk weight of the controlled release

TABLE 18-1. RELEASE RATES FOR CONTROLLED RELEASE DRUG PRODUCTS AS A FUNCTION OF ELIMINATION HALF-LIFE*

			Total mg to Achieve Duration			
$t_{1/2}$ (hr)	K (hr^{-1})	R (mg/hr)	6 hr	8 hr	12 hr	24 hr
1	0.693	69.3	415.8	554.4	831.6	1663
2	0.347	34.7	208.2	277.6	416.4	832.8
4	0.173	17.3	103.8	138.4	207.6	415.2
6	0.116	11.6	69.6	92.8	139.2	278.4
8	0.0866	8.66	52.0	69.3	103.9	207.8
10	0.0693	6.93	41.6	55.4	83.2	166.3
12	0.0577	5.77	34.6	46.2	69.2	138.5

*Assume $C_{desired}$ is 5 μg/ml and the V_d is 20,000 ml; $R = KV_dC_p$; no immediate release dose.

product will be greater than this amount due to the presence of excipients needed in the formulation. From the values in Table 18-1, in order to achieve a long duration of activity ($\geq$ 12 hr) for a drug with a very short half-life (1–2 hr), the controlled release drug product becomes quite large and impractical for most patients to swallow.

PHARMACOKINETIC SIMULATION OF SUSTAINED RELEASE PRODUCTS

The plasma drug concentration of many sustained release products has been found to fit an oral one-compartment model assuming first-order absorption and elimination. Compared to an immediate release product, the sustained release product would typically show a smaller absorption constant due to the slower absorption of the sustained release product. The time for peak concentration (t_{max}) is usually longer (Fig. 18-4) and the peak drug concentration (C_{max}) is reduced. If the drug is properly formulated, the area under the plasma drug concentration curve should be the same. These parameters conveniently show how successful the sustained release product performs in vivo. For example, a product with a t_{max} of 3 hr would not be very satisfactory if the product is intended to last 12 hr. Similarly, if the C_{max} is excessively high, it would be a sign of dose dumping due to inadequate formulation. The pharmacokinetic analysis of single- and multiple-dose plasma data have been applied to evaluate many sustained release products by the regulatory agency. The analysis is practical since many products can be fitted to this model even though the drug is not released in a first-order manner. The limitation of this type of analysis is that the absorption rate constant may not relate to the rate of drug dissolution in vivo. If the drug follows strictly zero-order release and absorption, the model may not fit the data. Various other models have been used to simulate plasma drug levels of sustained release product by P.G. Welling.[3] The plasma drug levels from a zero-order controlled release drug product may be simulated with Equation 18.9. In the absence of a loading dose, the drug level in the body rises slowly to a plateau with minimum fluctuations (Fig. 18-5).

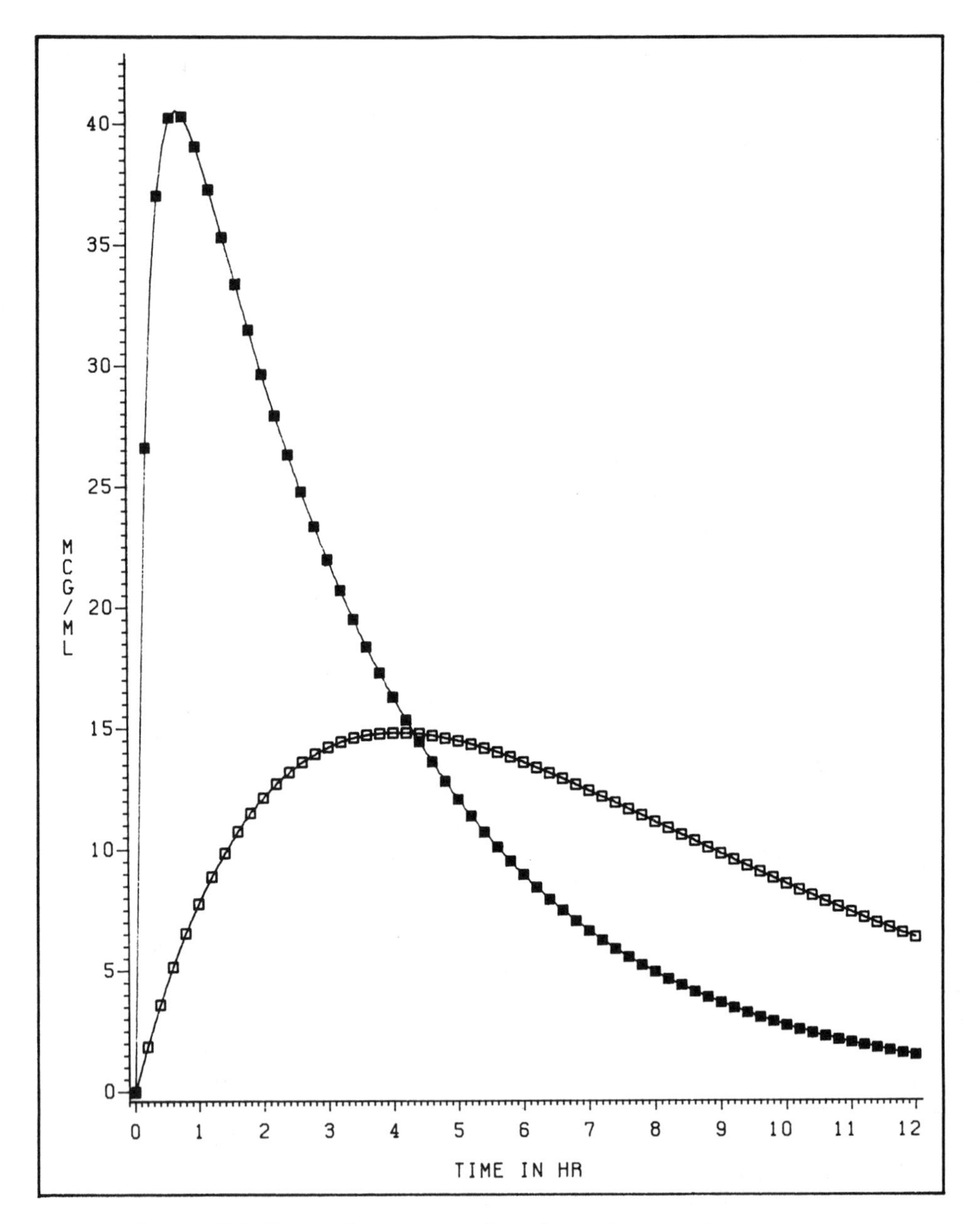

Figure 18-4. Plasma drug concentration of a sustained and regular release product. Note differences of peak time and peak concentration of the two products. (■ = rapid release; □ = sustained release.)

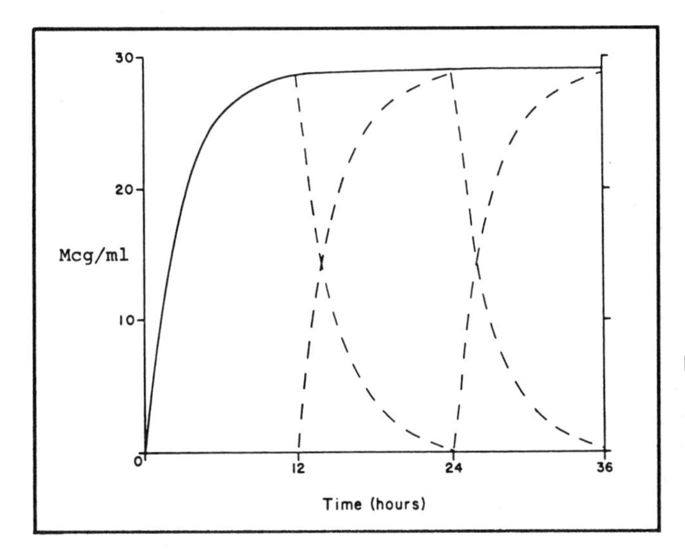

Figure 18-5. Simulated plasma drug level of a sustained release product administered every 12 hr. The plasma level shows a smooth rise to steady-state level with no fluctuations.

This simulation assumes (a) rapid drug release without delay, (b) perfect zero-order release and absorption of the drug, and (c) the drug is given exactly every 12 hr. In practice, the above assumptions are not precise and fluctuations in drug level do occur.

$$C_p = \frac{D_s}{V_d K}(1 - e^{-Kt}) \tag{18.9}$$

where D_s = maintenance dose or rate of drug release, mg/min; C_p = plasma drug concentration; K = overall elimination constant; and V_d = volume of distribution.

When a sustained release drug product with a loading dose (rapid release) and a zero-order maintenance dose is given, the resulting plasma drug concentrations are described by

$$C_p = \frac{D_i K_a}{V_d(K_a - K)}(e^{-Kt} - e^{-K_a t}) + \frac{D_s}{KV_d}(1 - e^{-Kt}) \tag{18.10}$$

where D_i = immediate release (loading dose) dose and D_s = maintenance dose (zero-order). It is obvious that this expression is the sum of the oral absorption equation (first part) and the intravenous infusion equation (second part). An example of a zero-order release product with loading dose is shown in Figure 18-6. The contribution due to the loading and the maintenance dose are shown by the dotted lines. The inclusion of a built-in loading dose in the sustained release product has only limited use.

With most sustained release products, the drug is administered for more than one dose, and there is no need for a built-in loading dose. Having a loading dose in the subsequent dosing would introduce more drug into the body than necessary due to the "topping" effect (Fig. 18-7). In situations where a loading dose is necessary, the rapid release product is used to titrate a loading dose that would bring the plasma drug level to therapeutic level.

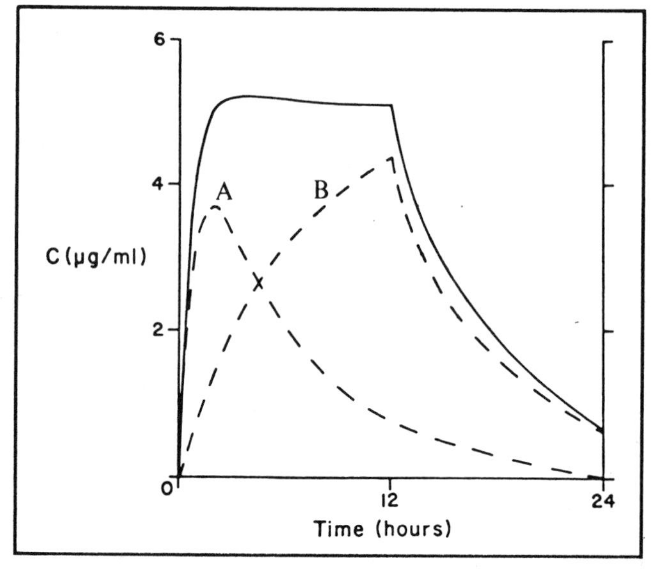

Figure 18-6. Simulated plasma drug level of a sustained release product with a fast release component (A) and a maintenance component (B). The solid line represents total plasma drug level due to the two components. (*From Welling PG, 1983, with permission.*[3])

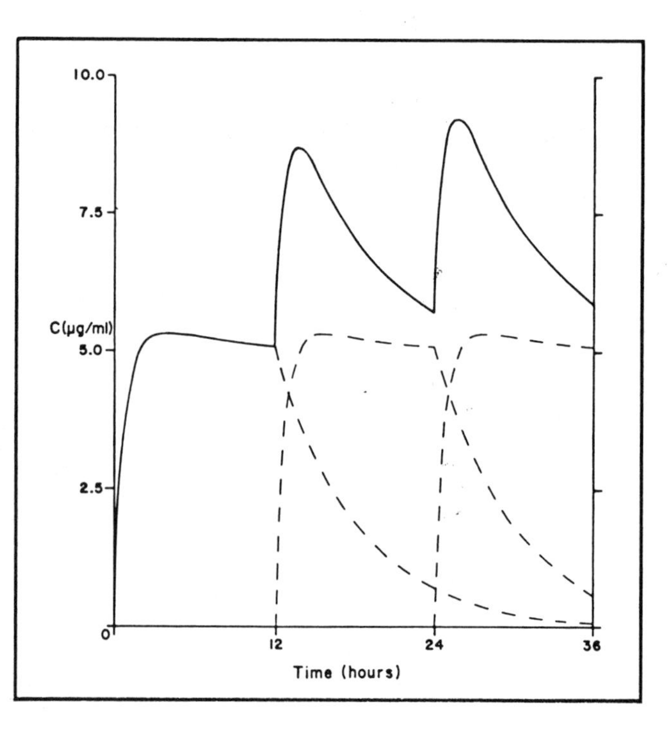

Figure 18-7. Simulated plasma level for a sustained release product given every 12 hr. The product has a built-in loading dose of 160 mg and a maintenance rate of 27.2 mg/hr. The plateau level was achieved rapidly after the first dose. Note the spiking peak following each dose due to the topping of the loading dose. (*From Welling PG, 1983, with permission.*[3])

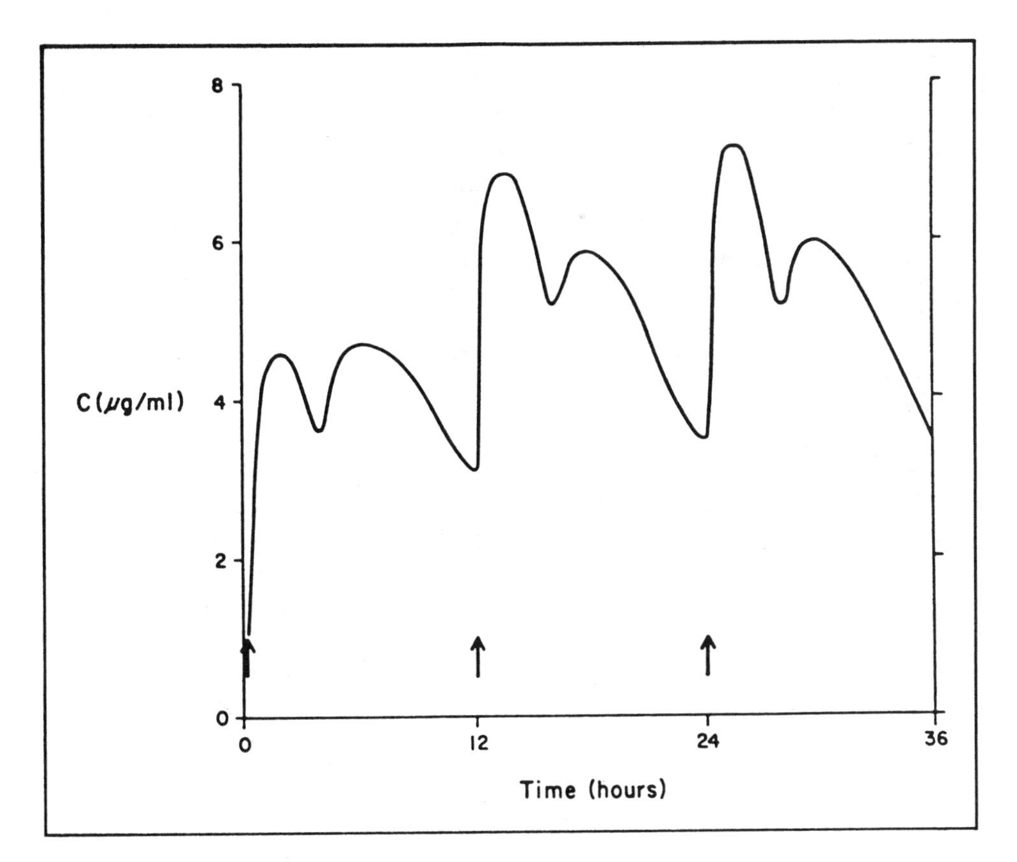

Figure 18-8. Simulated plasma drug level of the sustained release drug administered every 12 hr. The product contains a loading and a maintenance dose that are both absorbed according to first-order kinetic. Note the presence of double spikes in the plasma level. (*From Welling PG, 1983, with permission.*[3])

A pharmacokinetic model that assumes first-order absorption of the loading and maintenance dose has also been proposed. This model predicts spiking peaks due to loading dose when the drug is administered continuously (Fig. 18-8) in multiple doses.

REGULATORY CONSIDERATIONS IN CONTROLLED RELEASE PRODUCTS

There are two important requirements for preparing controlled release products: (1) demonstration of safety and efficacy and (2) demonstration of controlled drug release.

For many drugs data are available demonstrating the safety and efficacy for drugs given in a conventional dosage form. These include all those drugs in the

Federal Register that are listed as safe and effective. Bioavailability data demonstrating comparable blood level to an approved controlled release product is acceptable. The bioavailability data requirements are specified in the *Federal Register*, CFR 320.25 (f). The important points are as follows:

1. The product should demonstrate sustained release as claimed without dose dumping (abrupt release of large amount of drug in an uncontrolled manner).
2. The drug should show steady-state levels comparable to the steady-state levels reached using a conventional dosage form given as in multiple doses, which was demonstrated to be effective.
3. The drug product should show consistent pharmacokinetic performance between individual dosage units.
4. The product should allow for maximum amount of drug to be absorbed while maintaining minimum patient-to-patient variation.
5. The demonstration of steady-state drug levels after the recommended doses are given should be within the effective plasma drug levels for the drug.
6. The development of an in vitro method and data that demonstrate the reproducible controlled release nature of the product. The in vitro method usually consists of a suitable dissolution procedure that provides a meaningful in vitro–in vivo correlation.
7. In vivo pharmacokinetic data consists of single and multiple dosage comparing the controlled release product to a reference standard (usually an approved non-sustained-release or a solution product).

The pharmacokinetic data usually consists of plasma drug data and/or urinary drug excreted. Pharmacokinetic analyses are performed to determine such parameters as $t_{1/2}$, V_d, t_{max}, AUC, K, and other related parameters.

TYPES OF CONTROLLED RELEASE PRODUCTS

For the sake of discussion, all sustained release products are referred to as "controlled release products" without distinction of the precision of the release mechanisms. Table 18-2 shows some common controlled release products and the mechanisms making them sustained release.

Among the many types of commercial preparations available, there is probably hardly any one type that works only on one pure mechanism. Most of the controlled release preparations work by a combination of processes involving dissolution, permeation, and diffusion. The single most important factor is water permeation, without which none of the product release mechanisms would operate. Controlling the rate of water influx to the product generally dictates the rate at which the drug dissolves. Once the drug is dissolved, the rate of drug diffusion may be further controlled to a desirable rate.

Pellet-Type Sustained Release Preparation

The pellet type of sustained release preparation is often referred to as "bead"-type preparation. In general, the beads are prepared by coating drug powder onto

TABLE 18-2. EXAMPLES OF CONTROLLED RELEASE PRODUCTS

Type	Trade Name	Rationale
Erosion tablet	Constant-*T*	Sustained release theophylline to achieve long duration and less fluctuation in blood level
Waxy matrix tablet	Kaon Cl–10 tablet Klatrix	Controlled release potassium chloride; less GI irritation
Coated pellets in capsule	Ornade Spansule	Sustained release cold preparation
Coated pellet in tablet	Theo-Dur	Sustained release theophylline to achieve long duration and lessen fluctuation in blood level of theophylline
Flotation–diffusion	Valrelease	Long action form for diazapam
Microencapsulation	Bayer timed release	Sustained release aspirin
Leaching tablet	Ferro Gradumet	Sustained release iron preparation; reduced GI irritation
Coated ion exchange	Penkinetic	Sustained release ion exchange system
Osmotic pressure	Osmosin	Sustained release indomethacin

preformed cores called "nonpareil seeds." The nonpareil seeds are made from slurry of starch, sucrose, and lactose. Preparation of the cores are tedious. The rough core granules are rounded for hours on a coating pan and then classified according to size. The drug-coated beads generally provide a rapid release carrier for the drug depending on the coating solution used in coating the drug. Commonly, sucrose solution provides a convenient way of coating the drug without impairing the rapid release of the drug. Once the drug beads are prepared, they may be further coated with a protective coating to allow a sustained or prolonged release of the drug.

The use of various amounts of coating solution can provide beads with various coating protection. A careful blending of beads may achieve any release profile desired. Alternatively, a blend of beads coated with materials of different solubility may also provide a means of controlling dissolution of the drug.

Some products take advantage of bead blending to provide two doses of drug in one formulation. For example, a blend of rapid release beads with some pH-sensitive enteric coated material may provide a second dose of drug release when the drug reaches the intestine.

The pellet dosage form can be prepared as a capsule or tablet. When pellets are prepared as tablets, the beads must be compressed lightly so that they cannot break. Usually, a disintegrant is included in the tablet causing the beads to be released rapidly after administration. Formulation of a drug into pellet form may reduce gastric irritation since the drug is released slowly over a period of time, therefore avoiding high drug concentration in the stomach. An example of such a drug is

TABLE 18-3. INCIDENCE OF ADVERSE EFFECTS OF A SUSTAINED RELEASE THEOPHYLLINE PELLET VERSUS A THEOPHYLLINE SOLUTION*

	Volunteers Showing Side Effects	
Side Effects	***Using Solution***	***Using Sustained Release Pellets***
Nausea	10	0
Headache	4	0
Diarrhea	3	0
Gastritis	2	0
Vertigo	5	0
Nervousness	3	1

*After 5-day dosing at 600 mg theophylline/24 hr, adverse reaction points on fifth day: Solution, 135; pellets, 18.
From Breimer DD, 1980, with permission.[4]

theophylline. Table 18-3 shows the frequency of adverse reactions after theophylline is administered as solutions versus pellets.

In the case of theophylline administered as solution, high concentration of theophylline may be reached in the body due to rapid drug absorption. Some side effects may be attributed to the high concentration of theophylline reached in the body. Pellet dosage form allows drug to be absorbed gradually, therefore reducing the incidence of side effects by preventing high C_p.

A second example involves the drug bitolerol. A study in dogs has indicated that the incidence of tachycardia was reduced in a controlled release bead preparation whereas the bronchiodilation effect was not reduced. Administering the drug as pellets apparently reduced excessive high drug concentration in the body and avoided stimulated increase in heart rate. Studies have also reported reduced gastrointestinal side effects of the drug potassium chloride in pellet or in microparticulate form. Potassium chloride is irritating to the GI tract. Formulation in pellet form reduces the chance of exposing high concentrations of potassium chloride to the mucosal cells in the GI tract.

There are many examples utilizing the pellet dosage form. For example, the weight-reducing drug phenylpropanolamine is often formulated into a sustained release pellet capsule to curb appetite for 12 hr. Many long-acting cold products also employ the bead concept. A major advantage of the pellet dosage form is that the pellets are less sensitive to the effect of stomach emptying. Since there are numerous pellets within a capsule, some pellets will gradually reach the small intestine and deliver the drug; whereas a single tablet may be delayed in the stomach for a long time due to erratic stomach emptying. Stomach emptying is particularly important in the formulation of enteric coated products. Enteric coated tablets may be delayed for hours by the presence of food in the stomach; whereas the enteric coated pellets are relatively unaffected by the presence of food.

Prolonged-Action Tablet

A common way to prolong the action of a drug is to reduce the solubility of the drug so that the drug dissolves slowly over a period of several hours. The solubility of a drug is dependent on the salt form used, and an examination of the solubility of the various derivative of the drug should be the first step. In general, the base or acid form of the drug is usually much less soluble than the corresponding salt. For example, sodium phenobarbital is much more soluble than phenobarbital, the acid form of the drug. Similarly, diphenhydramine hydrochloride is more soluble than the base form diphenhydramine.

In cases where it is inconvenient to prepare a less soluble form of the drug, the drug may be granulated with an excipient to slow down dissolution of the drug. Often, fatty or waxy lipophilic materials are employed in formulations. Stearic acid, castorwax, high-molecular weight polyethylene glycol (Carbowax), glyceryl monosterate, white wax, and spermaceti oil are useful ingredients in providing an oily barrier to slow water penetration and dissolution of the tablet. Many of the lubricants used in tableting may also be used as lipophilic agents to slow dissolution. For example, magnesium stearate and hydrogenated vegetable oil (Sterotex) are actually used in high percentages to cause sustained drug release in a preparation. The major disadvantage of this type of preparation is the difficulty in maintaining a reproducible drug release from patient to patient, since oily materials may be subjected to digestion, temperature, and mechanical stress, which may affect the release rate of the drug.

Ion Exchange Preparation

Ion exchange preparations usually involve an insoluble resin capable of reacting with either an anionic or cationic drug. A cationic resin is usually negatively charged so that positively charged cationic drug may react with the resin to form an insoluble nonabsorbable resin–drug complex. Upon exposure to the gastrointestinal tract, cations in the gut such as potassium and sodium may displace the drug from the resin releasing the drug which is absorbed freely. The main disadvantage of ion exchange preparations is that the amount of cation–anion in the GI tract is not easily controllable and varies among individuals, making it difficult to be a consistent mechanism of drug release. A further disadvantage is that resins may provide a potential means of interaction with nutrients and drugs.

Ion exchange may be used in a sustained-release liquid preparation. An added advantage is that the technique provides some protection for very bitter or irritating drugs. Recently, the ion exchange approach has been combined with a coating to obtain a more effective sustained release product. For example, the drug dextromethorphan has been formulated using the ion exchange principle to mask the bitter taste and to prolong the duration of action of the drug. In the past, amphetamine has been formulated with ion exchange resins to provide prolonged release as an appetite suppressant in weight reduction.

A general mechanism for the formulation of anionic or cationic drugs is described in the following scheme:

Cationic drugs:

$$H^+ + \text{resin–}SO_3^- \text{ drug}^+ \rightleftarrows \text{resin–}SO_3^- H^+ + \text{drug}^+$$

Insoluble drug complex Soluble drug

Anionic drugs:

$$Cl^- + \text{resin–}N^+(CH_3)_3\,\text{drug}^- \rightleftarrows \text{resin–}N^+(CH_3)_3Cl^- + \text{drug}^-$$

Insoluble drug complex — Soluble drug

The insoluble drug complex containing the resin and drug dissociates in the gastrointestinal tract in the presence of the appropriate counterions. The released drug dissolves in the fluids of the gastrointestinal tract and is rapidly absorbed.

Core Tablet

A core tablet is conceptually a tablet within a tablet. The core is usually for the slow drug release; whereas the outside shell contains a rapid release dose of drug. Formulation of a core tablet requires two granulations. The core granulation is usually compressed lightly to form a loose core and then transferred to a second die cavity where a second granulation containing additional ingredients is compressed further to form the final tablet.

The core material may be surrounded by hydrophobic excipients so that the drug leaches out over a prolonged period of time. This type of preparation is sometimes called *slow erosion core* tablet since the core generally contains either no disintegrant or insufficient disintegrant to fragment the tablet. The composition of the core may range from waxy to gummy or polymeric material. Numerous slow erosion tablets have been patented and are commercially sold under various trade names.

The success of core tablets depends very much on the nature of the drug and the excipients used. As a general rule, this preparation is very much hardness dependent in release rate. Critical control of hardness and processing variables are important in producing a tablet with a consistent release rate.

Core tablets are occasionally used to avoid incompatibility in preparations containing two physically incompatible ingredients. For example, buffered aspirin has been formulated into a core and shell to avoid a yellowing discoloration of the two ingredients upon aging.

Gum-type Matrix Tablet

Some excipients have a remarkable ability to swell in the presence of water and form gel-like consistency. When this happens, the gel provides a natural barrier for drug diffusion from the tablet to occur. Since the gellike material is quite viscous and may not disperse for hours, this provides a means of sustaining the drug for hours until all the drug has been dissolved and diffused out into the intestinal fluid. A common gelling material is gelatin. However, gelatin will dissolve rapidly after the gel is formed. Drug excipients such as methylcellulose, gum tragacanth, Veegum, and alginic acid will form a viscous mass and provide a useful matrix for controlling drug dissolution. Drug formulation with these excipients provides sustained drug release for hours. The drug diazepam, for example, has been formulated using methylcellulose to provide sustained release. In the case of sustained release diazepam, claims were made that the hydrocolloid (gel) floated in the stomach to give sustained release. In other studies material of various densities were emptied from the stomach without any difference as to whether the drug product was floating on top or sitting at the bottom of the stomach.

The most important consideration in this type of formulation appears to be the gelling strength of the gum material and the concentration of gummy material used. Modification of the release rates of the product may further be achieved with various amounts of talc or other lipophilic lubricant.

Microencapsulation

Microencapsulation is a process of encapsulating microscopic drug particles with a special coating material, therefore making the drug particles more desirable in terms of physical and chemical characteristics. A common drug that has been encapsulated is aspirin. Aspirin has been microencapsulated with ethylcellulose, making the drug superior in flow characteristics; when compressed into a tablet, the drug releases more gradually.

Many techniques are used in microencapsulating a drug. One process used in microencapsulating acetaminophen involves suspending the drug in aqueous solution while stirring. The coating material, ethylcellulose, is dissolved in cyclohexane, and the two liquids are added together with stirring and heating. As the cyclohexane is evaporated by heat, the ethylcellulose coats the microparticles of the acetaminophen. The microencapsulated particles have a slower dissolution rate because the ethylcellulose is not water soluble and provides a barrier for diffusion of drug. The amount of coating material deposited on the acetaminophen will determine the rate of drug dissolution. The coating also serves as a means of reducing the bitter taste of the drug. In practice, microencapsulation is not consistent enough to produce a reproducible batch of product, and it may be necessary to blend the microencapsulated material in order to obtain a desired release rate.

Polymeric Matrix Tablet

The use of polymeric material in prolonging the release rate of drug has received increased attention. The most important characteristic of this type of preparation is that the prolonged release may last days and weeks rather than for a shorter duration (as with other techniques). The first example of an oral polymeric matrix tablet is the Gradumet (Abbott Labs.) which is marketed as an iron preparation. The plastic matrix provides a rigid geometric surface for drug diffusion so that a relatively constant rate of drug release is obtained. In the case of the iron preparation the matrix reduces the exposure of the irritating drug to the gastrointestinal mucosal tissues. The matrix is usually expelled unchanged in the feces after all the drug has been leached out.

The matrix tablets for oral use are generally quite safe. However, for certain patients with reduced gastrointestinal motility caused by disease, the polymeric matrix tablet should be avoided since accumulation or obstruction of the gastrointestinal tract by the matrix tablet has been reported. As an oral sustained release product, the matrix tablet has not been popular. In contrast, the use of the matrix tablet in implantation has been much more popular.

The use of biodegradable polymeric material for controlled release have been the focus of intensive research. One such example is the use of polylactic acid copolymer, which degrades to natural lactic acid and eliminates the problem of retrieval after implantation.

Osmotic Controlled Release

The osmotic pump represents a new concept in controlled release preparations. Drug delivery is precisely controlled by the use of an osmotically controlled device that pumps a constant amount of water through the system dissolving and releasing a constant amount of drug per unit time.

This device consists of an outside layer of semipermeable membrane filled with a mixture of drug and osmotic agent. When the device is placed in water, osmotic pressure generated by the osmotic agent within the core causes water to move into the device, which forces the dissolved drug to move out of the delivery orifice. The process continues until all the drug is released. The rate of drug delivery is relatively unaffected by the pH of the environment. The osmotic preparation available for implantation is known as the osmotic minipumps, whereas the system designed for oral use is called the gastrointestinal therapeutic system (Fig. 18-9). It was developed by the Alza Corp.

One example of the gastrointestinal therapeutic system uses acetazolamide for the treatment of ocular hypertension in glaucoma. The drug was delivered from the system at zero-order rate for 12 hr at 15 mg/hr, as shown in Figure 18-10.

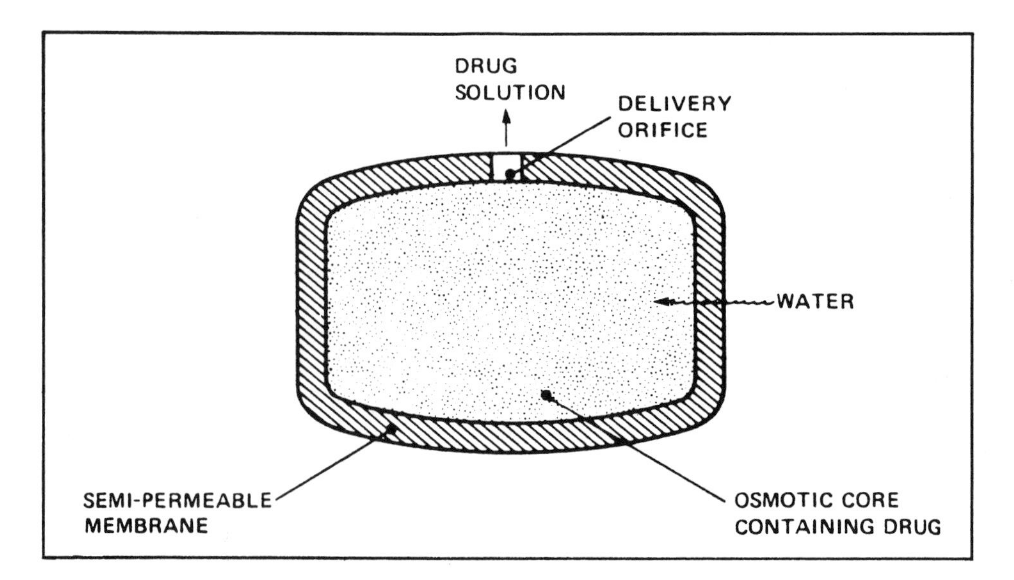

Figure 18-9. Cross-sectional diagram of gastrointestinal therapeutic system. (*From Shaw JE, Chandrasekaran SK, 1978, with permission.*[5])

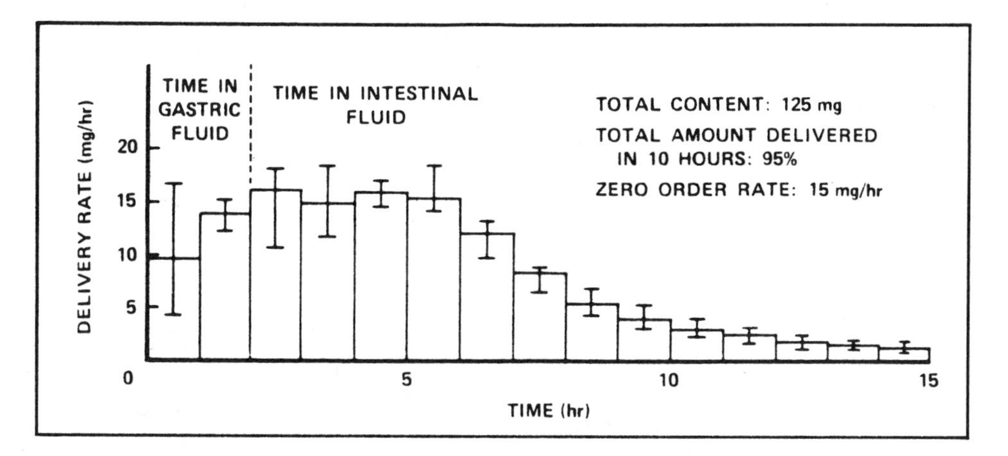

Figure 18-10. Pattern of delivery of acetazolamide from elementary osmotic pump therapeutic system delivering 70% of the total content (125 mg) at specified rate of 15 mg/hr in 6 hr and 80% in 8 hr. (*From Shaw JE, Chandrasekaran SK, 1978, with permission.*[5])

The frequency of side effect experienced by the patients using the gastrointestinal therapeutic system was considerably less than that of the conventional tablet (Fig. 18-11). When the therapeutic system was compared to the regular 250-mg tablet given twice daily, ocular pressure was effectively controlled by the osmotic system. The blood level of acetazolanine using the gastrointestinal therapeutic system, however, was considerably below that from the tablet. In fact, the therapeutic index of the drug was considerably increased by using the therapeutic system. The use of controlled release drug products, which release drug consistently, may provide promise for administering many drugs that previously had frequent adverse side effects because of the drug's narrow therapeutic index.

Transdermal Delivery Systems

Transdermal preparation refers to drugs administered topically for systemic absorption through the skin in a controlled rate over an extended period of time. In general, the preparation consists of drugs impregnated on a reservoir layer supported by a backing. Drug diffusion is controlled by a semipermeable membrane above the reservoir layer. Nitroglycerin is commonly administered by transdermal delivery. Transdermal delivery systems of nitroglycerin may provide hours of protection against angina, whereas the duration of nitroglycerin given in a sublingual tablet may only last a few minutes. Presently, three commercial transdermal preparations are available. These are Nitro-Disc (Searle), Transderm-nitro (Ciba Geigy), and Nitro-Dur (Key Lab). These preparations are placed over the chest area and provide up to 12 hr of duration. In a recent study comparing these three dosage forms in patients, no substantial difference was observed among the three preparations. In all case the skin was found to be the rate-limiting step of nitroglycerin absorption. Variations among products were found to be less than variations of the same product among different patients.

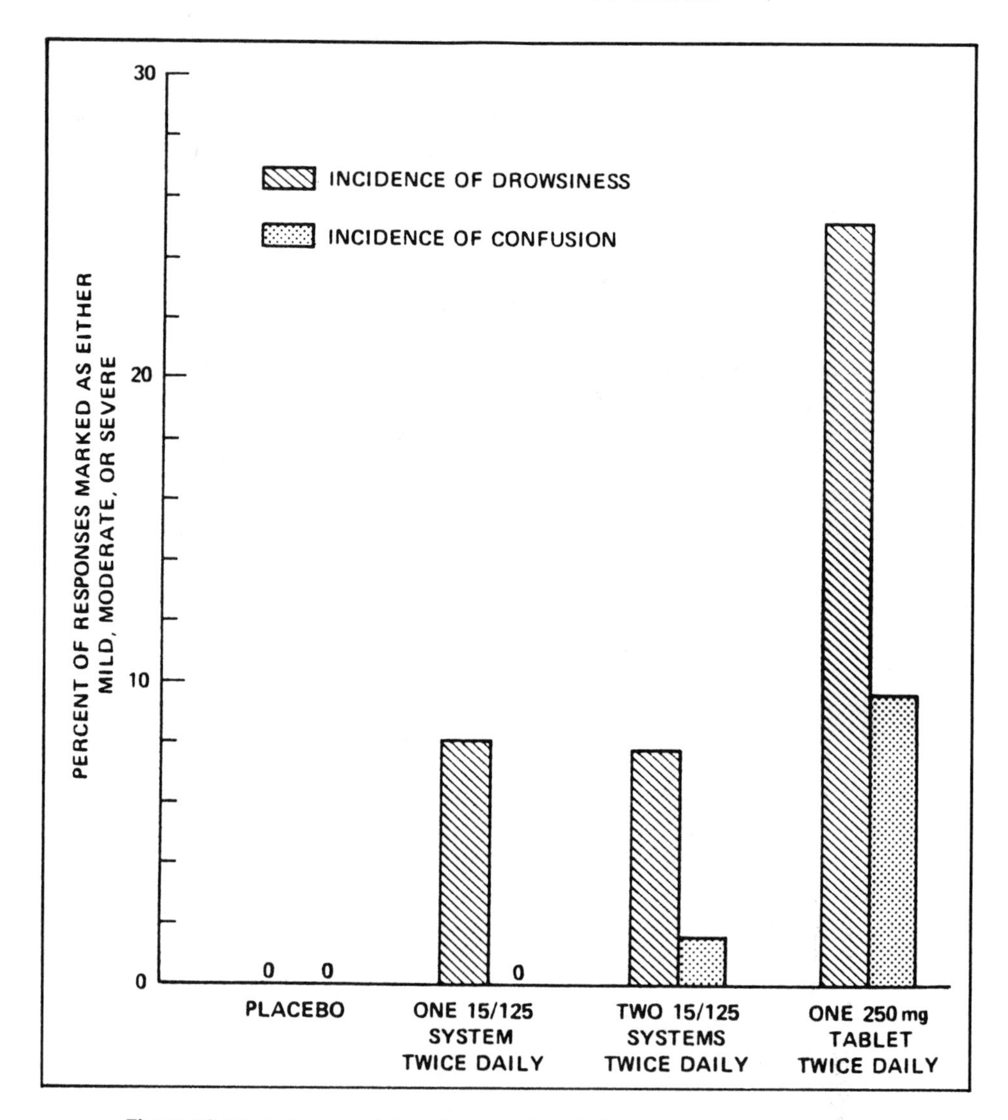

Figure 18-11. Incidence of drowsiness and confusion on acetazolamide given in three regimens. More frequent incidence of side effects were seen with the tablet over the osmotic system. (*From Shaw JE, Chandrasekaran SK, 1978, with permission.*[5])

An important limitation of transdermal preparation is quantitation of the dose. In general, drugs given at a dose of over 100 mg will require too large a patch to be used practically. However, new advances in pharmaceutic solvents may provide a mechanism for an increased amount of drug to be absorbed transdermally. Azone is a solvent that increases the absorption of many drugs through the skin. This solvent is relatively nontoxic. More applications of absorption enhancers may be available in the future.

QUESTIONS

1. The dissolution profile of a three-drug product is illustrated in Figure 18-12.
   a. Which of the drug products in Figure 18-12 release drug at a zero-order rate of about 8.3% every hour?
   b. Which of the drug products does not release drug at a zero-order rate?
   c. Which of the drug products has an almost zero rate of drug release during certain hours of the dissolution process?
   d. Suggest a common cause of slowing drug dissolution rate of many rapid release drug products toward the end of dissolution.
   e. Suggest a common cause of slowing drug dissolution of a sustained release product toward the end of dissolution test.
2. A drug is normally given 10 mg four times a day. Suggest an approach for designing a 12-hr zero-order release product.
   a. Calculate the desired zero-order release rate.
   b. Calculate the concentration of the drug in an osmotic pump type of oral dosage form that delivers 0.5 ml/hr of fluid.
3. An industrial pharmacist would like to design a sustained release drug product to be given every 12 hr. The active drug ingredient has an apparent

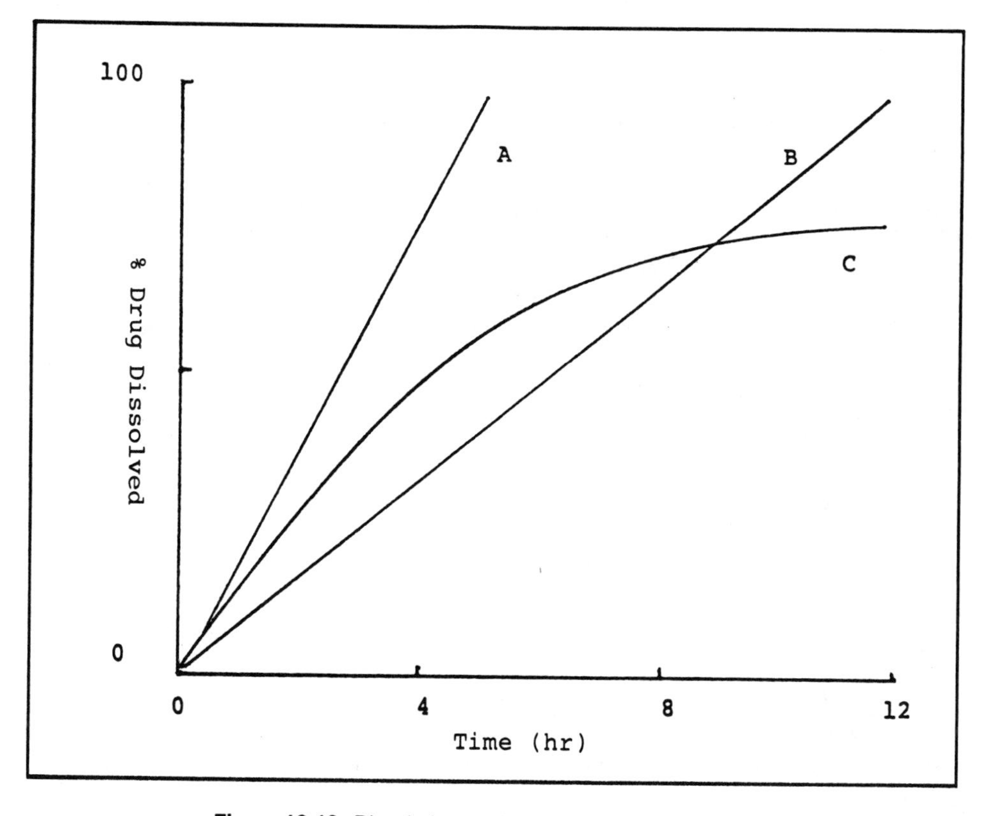

Figure 18-12. Dissolution profile of a three-drug product.

volume of distribution of 10 L, an elimination half-life of 3.5 hr, and a desired therapeutic plasma drug concentration of 20 mg/ml. Calculate the zero-order release rate of the sustained release drug product and the total amount of drug needed assuming no loading dose is required.

REFERENCES

1. Hofmann FF, Pressman JH, Code CF, Witztum KF: Controlled entry of orally administered drugs: Physiological considerations. Drug Devel Indust Pharm 9:1077–199, 1983
2. Galeone M, Nizzola L, Cacioli D, Moise G: In vivo demonstration of delivery mechanisms from sustained-release pellets. Cur Therapeut Res 29:217–34, 1981
3. Welling PG: Pharmacokinetic considerations of controlled release drug products. Drug Devel Indus Pharm 9:1185–225, 1983
4. Breimer DD, Dauhof M: Towards Better Safety of Drugs and Pharmaceutical Products. Amsterdam, Elsevier/North-Holland Biomedical Press, 1980, pp. 117–42
5. Shaw JE, Chandrasekaran SK: Controlled topical delivery systems for systemic action. Drug Met Rev 8:223–33, 1978

BIBLIOGRAPHY

Boxenbaum HG: Physiological and pharmacokinetic factors affecting performance of sustained release dosage forms, Drug Devel Ind Pharm 8:1–25, 1982

Bruck S (ed): CRC Controlled Drug Delivery. CRC Press, Boca Raton, FL, 1983

Chien YW: Oral controlled drug administration. Drug Devel Ind Pharm 9, 1983

Chien YW: Novel Drug Delivery Systems. Marcel Dekker, New York, 1982

Cabana BE: Bioavailability regulations and biopharmaceutic standard for controlled release drug delivery. Proceedings of 1982 Research and Scientific Development Conference, The Proprietary Association, Washington, DC, 1983, pp 56–69.

Hunter E, Fell JT, Sharma H: The gastric emptying of pellets contained in hard gelatin capsules. Drug Devel Ind Pharm 8:151–57, 1982

Malinowski HJ: Biopharmaceutic aspects of the regulatory review of oral controlled-release drug products. Drug Devel Ind Pharm 9:1255–79, 1983

Mueller Lissner SA, Blum AL: The effect of specific gravity and eating on gastric emptying of slow-release capsules. N Engl J Med 304:1365–66, 1981

Robinson JR: Oral drug delivery systems. Proceedings of 1982 Research and Scientific Development Conference, The Proprietary Association, Washington, DC, 1983, pp 54–69

Robinson JR: Sustained and Controlled Release Drug Delivery Systems. Marcel Dekker, New York, 1978

Robinson, JR, Eriksen SP: Theoretical formulation of sustained release dosage forms. J Pharm Sci 53:1254–63, 1966

Rosement TJ, Mansdorf SZ: Controlled Release Delivery Systems. Marcel Dekker, New York, 1983

Urquhart J: Controlled-Release Pharmaceuticals. American Pharmaceutical Association, Washington, DC, 1981

APPENDIX A

SOLUTIONS TO PROBLEMS

CHAPTER 2

1. a. Zero-order process (Fig. A-1).

b. Rate constant, K_0:

Method 1

Values obtained from the graph (Fig. A-1):

t(min)	*A(mg)*
40	71
80	41

$$K_0 = \text{slope} = \frac{\Delta Y}{\Delta X}$$

$$K_0 = \frac{71 - 41}{40 - 80} = 0.75 \text{ mg/min}$$

Method 2

By extrapolation: $A_0 = 103.5$ at $t = 0$; $A = 71$ at $t = 40$ min.

$$A = -K_0 t + A^0$$

$$71 = -40K_0 + 103.5$$

$$K_0 = 0.81 \text{ mg/min}$$

Notice that the answer differs in accordance with the method used.

c. $t_{1/2}$

For zero-order kinetics, the larger the initial amount of drug A^0, the longer the $t_{1/2}$.

Method 1

$$t_{1/2} = \frac{0.5A^0}{K_0}$$

$$= \frac{0.5(103.5)}{0.78} = 66 \text{ min}$$

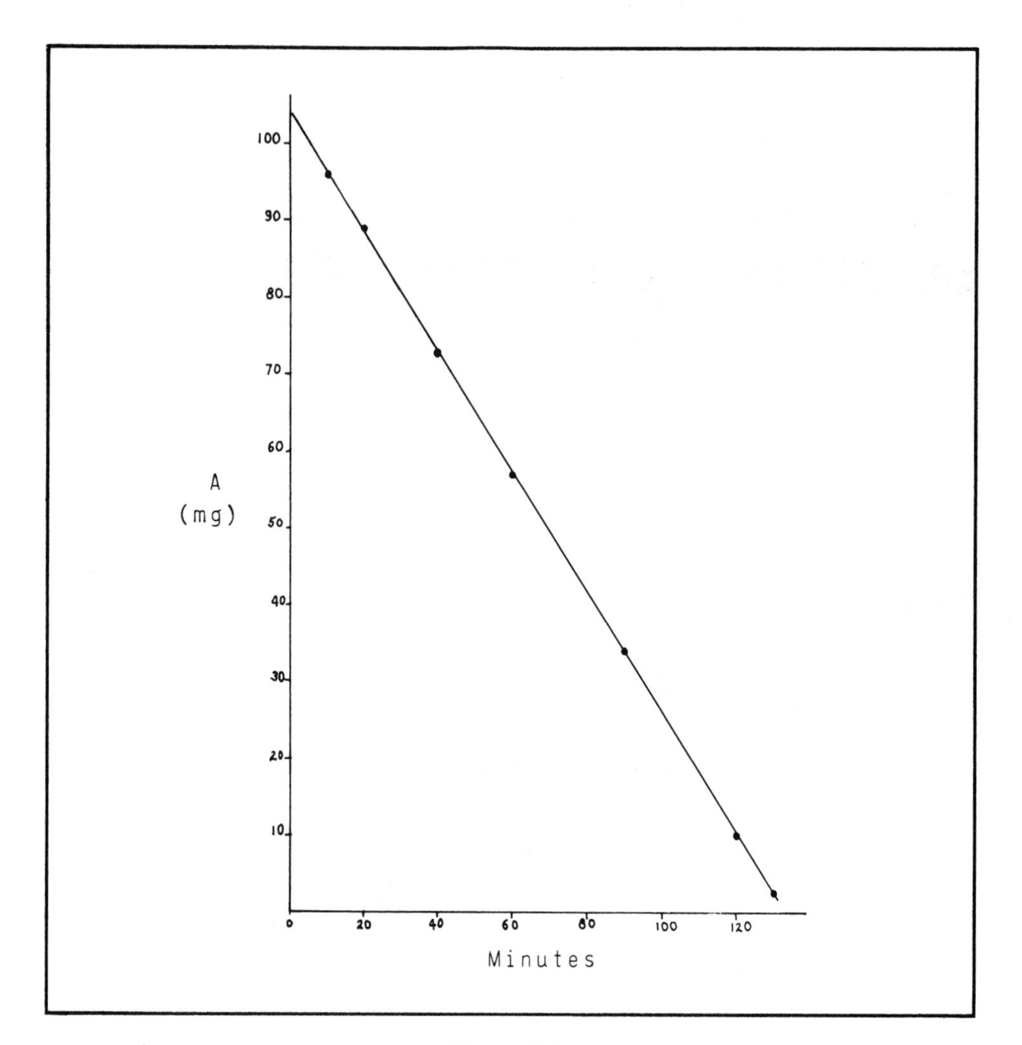

Figure A-1.

Method 2

The zero-order $t_{1/2}$ may be read directly from the graph:

At $t = 0$, $A^0 = 103.5$ mg

At $t_{1/2}$, $A = 51.8$ mg

Therefore, $t_{1/2} = 66$ min

d. The amount of drug A does extrapolate to zero on the x axis.

e. The equation of the line is:

$$A = -Kt + A^0$$
$$= -0.78t + 103.5$$

2. a. First-order process (Fig. A-2).

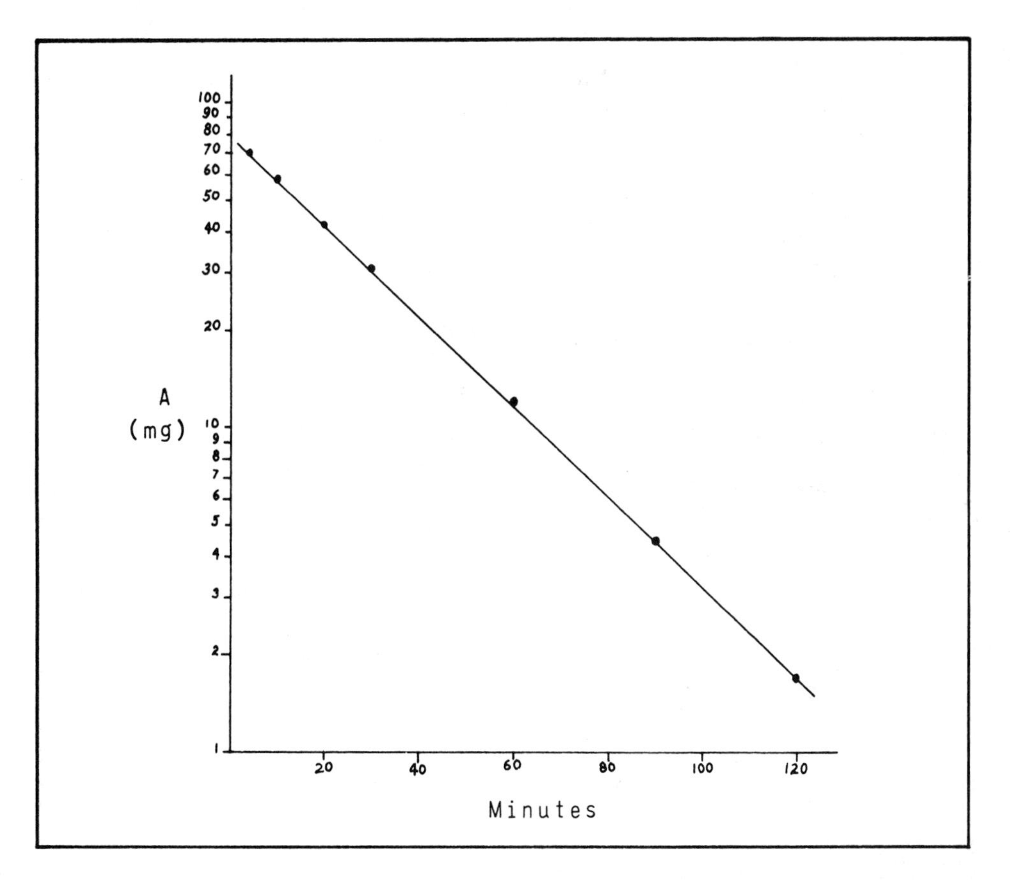

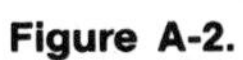
Figure A-2.

b. Rate constant, K:

Method 1

Obtain the first-order $t_{1/2}$ from the graph (Fig. A-2):

t(min)	*A(mg)*
30	30
53	15

$$t_{1/2} = 23 \text{ min}$$

$$K = \frac{0.693}{t_{1/2}} = \frac{0.693}{23} = 0.03 \text{ min}^{-1}$$

Method 2

$$\text{Slope} = \frac{-K}{2.3} = \frac{\log Y_2 - \log Y_1}{X_2 - X_1}$$

$$K = \frac{-2.3(\log 15 - \log 30)}{53 - 30} = 0.03 \text{ min}^{-1}$$

c. $t_{1/2} = 23$ min (see 2b above).
d. The amount of drug A does *not* extrapolate to zero on the x axis.
e. The equation of the line is

$$\log A = -\frac{Kt}{2.3} + \log A^0$$

$$= -\frac{0.03t}{2.3} + \log 78$$

$$A = 78e^{-0.03t}$$

$A = A_0 e^{-Kt}$

3. a. Zero-order process (Fig. A-3).
b.

$A = A_0 - Kt$ 0 ORDER

$$K_0 = \text{Slope} = \frac{\Delta Y}{\Delta X}$$

Values obtained from the graph (Fig. A-3),

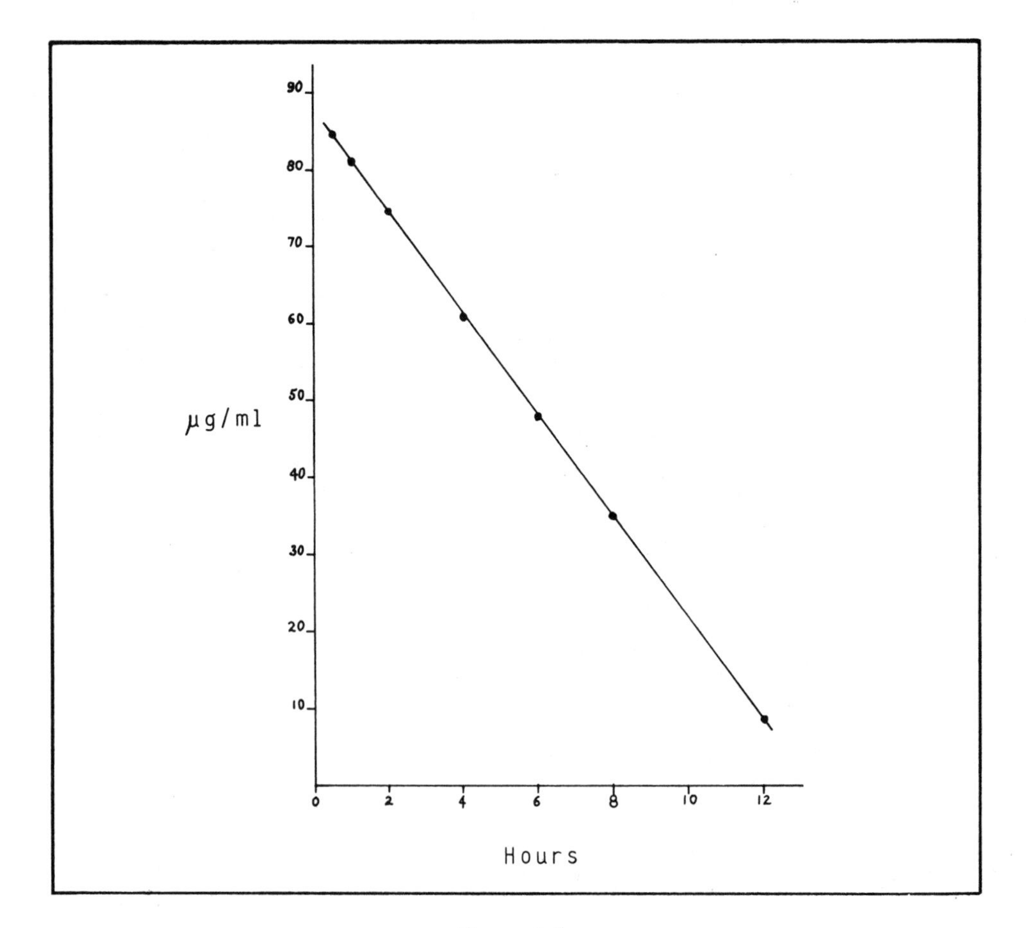

Figure A-3.

t(hr)	*C(μg/ml)*
1.2	80
4.2	60

It is always best to plot the data. Obtain a regression line (i.e., the line of best fit), then use points C and t from that line.

$$-K_0 = \frac{80 - 60}{1.2 - 4.2}$$

$$K_0 = 6.67\ \mu\text{g/ml hr}$$

c. By extrapolation:

At t_0, $C_0 = 87.5\ \mu\text{g/ml}$

d. The equation (using ruler only) is:

$$A = -Kt + A^0$$
$$= -6.67t + 87.5$$

4. Given:

C(mg/ml)	*t(days)*
300	0
75	30

a.

$$\log C = \frac{-Kt}{2.3} + \log C_0$$

$$\log 75 = \frac{-30K}{2.3} + \log 300$$

$$K = 0.046\ \text{days}^{-1}$$

$$t_{1/2} = \frac{0.693}{K} = \frac{0.693}{0.046} = 15\ \text{days}$$

b. *Method 1*

$300\ \text{mg/ml} = C_0$ at $t = 0$

$75\ \text{mg/ml} = C$ at $t = 30$ days

$225\ \text{mg/ml}$ = difference between initial and final drug concentration

$$K_0 = \frac{225\ \text{mg/ml}}{30\ \text{days}} = 7.5\ \text{mg/ml day}$$

The time, $t_{1/2}$, for the drug to decompose to $\frac{1}{2}C_0$ (from 300 to 150 mg/ml) is calculated by

$$t_{1/2} = \frac{150\ \text{mg/ml}}{7.5\ \text{mg/ml day}} = 20\ \text{days}$$

Method 2

$$C = -K_0 t + C_0$$

$$75 = -30K_0 + 300$$

$$K_0 = 7.5 \text{ mg/ml day}$$

At $t_{1/2}$, $C = 150$ mg/ml

$$150 = -7.5t_{1/2} + 300$$

$$t_{1/2} = 20 \text{ days}$$

Method 3

A $t_{1/2}$ value of 20 days may be obtained directly from the graph by plotting C against t on rectangular coordinates.

5. Assume an original concentration of drug to be 1000 mg/ml.

Method 1

mg/ml	*No. of Half-lives*	*mg/ml*	*No. of Half-lives*
1000	0	15.6	6
500	1	7.81	7
250	2	3.91	8
125	3	1.95	9
62.5	4	0.98	10
31.3	5		

99.9% of 1000 = 999

Concentration of drug remaining = 0.1% of 1000

1000 − 999 = 1 mg/ml

It takes approximately 10 half-lives to eliminate all but 0.1% of the original concentration of drug.

Method 2

Assume any $t_{1/2}$ value:

Let

$$t_{1/2} = 1.0 \text{ hr}$$

Then

$$K = \frac{0.693}{1} = 0.693 \text{ hr}^{-1}$$

$$\log C = \frac{-Kt}{2.3} + \log C_0$$

$$\log 1.0 = \frac{-0.693t}{2.3} + \log 1000$$

$$t = 9.96 \text{ hr}$$

$$t_{1/2} = 1.0 \text{ hr}$$

$$\frac{9.96}{1} = 9.96t_{1/2}, \text{ or } 10t_{1/2}$$

6.

$$t_{1/2} = 12 \text{ hr}$$

$$K = \frac{0.693}{t_{1/2}} = \frac{0.693}{12} = 0.058 \text{ hr}^{-1}$$

If 30% of the drug decomposes, 70% is left.

$$70\% \text{ of } 125 \text{ mg} = (0.70)(125) = 87.5 \text{ mg}$$

$$A_0 = 125 \text{ mg}$$

$$A = 87.5 \text{ mg}$$

$$K = 0.058 \text{ hr}^{-1}$$

$$\log A = -\frac{Kt}{2.3} + \log A_0$$

$$\log 87.5 = -\frac{0.058t}{2.3} + \log 125$$

$$t = 6.1 \text{ hr}$$

7. Immediately after the drug dissolves, the drug degrades at a constant, or zero-order, rate. Since concentration is equal to mass divided by volume, it is necessary to calculate the initial drug concentration (at $t = 0$) to determine the original volume in which the drug was dissolved. From the data calculate the zero-order rate constant, K_0:

$$K_0 = \text{slope} = \frac{\Delta Y}{\Delta X} = \frac{0.45 - 0.3}{0.5 - 2.0} = 0.1 \text{ mg/ml hr}$$

Then calculate the initial drug concentration, C_0, using the following equation:

$$C = -K_0 t - C_0$$

at $t = 2$ hr

$$0.3 = -0.1(2) - C_0$$

$$C_0 = 0.5 \text{ mg/ml}$$

Alternatively, at $t = 0.5$ hr

$$0.45 = -0.1(0.5) - C_0$$

$$C_0 = 0.5 \text{ mg/ml}$$

Since the initial mass of drug D_0 dissolved is 300 mg and the initial drug concentration C_0 is 0.5 mg/ml, the original volume may be calculated from the following relationship:

$$C_0 = \frac{D_0}{V}$$

$$0.5 \text{ mg/ml} = \frac{300 \text{ mg}}{V \text{ (ml)}}$$

$$V = 600 \text{ ml}$$

8. First order.

CHAPTER 3

3.

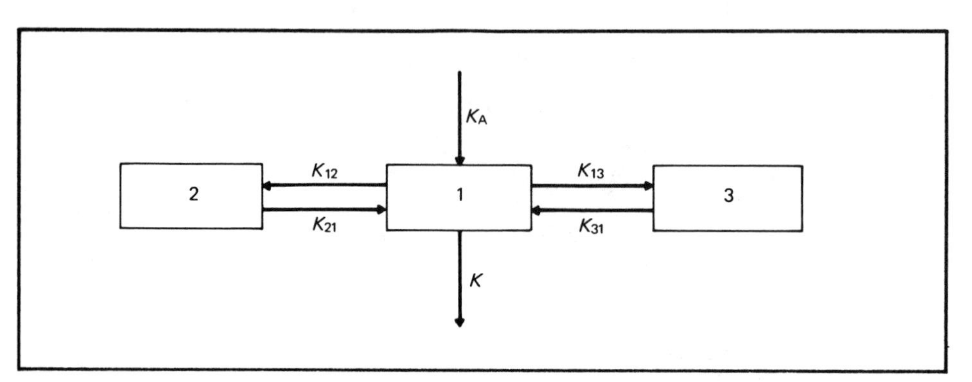

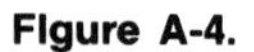

Figure A-4.

4. **a.** Nine parameters: $V_1, V_2, V_3, K_{12}, K_{21}, K_e, K_b, K_m, K_u$

b. Compartment 1 and compartment 3 may be sampled.

c.

$$K = K_b + K_m + K_e$$

d.

$$\frac{dC_1}{dt} = K_{21}C_2 - (K_{12} + K_m + K_e + K_b)C_1$$

CHAPTER 4

1. The C_p decreased from 1.2 to 0.3 μg/ml in 3 hr.

t(hr)	*C_p(μg/ml)*
2	1.2
5	0.3

$$\log C_p = -\frac{Kt}{2.3} + \log C_p^0$$

$$\log 0.3 = -\frac{K(3)}{2.3} + \log 1.2$$

$$K = 0.462 \text{ hr}^{-1}$$

$$t_{1/2} = \frac{0.693}{K} = \frac{0.693}{0.462}$$

$$t_{1/2} = 1.5 \text{ hr}$$

2. Dose (IV bolus) = 6 mg/kg × 50 kg = 300 mg

a. $V_d = \dfrac{\text{dose}}{C_p^0} = \dfrac{300 \text{ mg}}{8.4\ \mu\text{g/ml}} = \dfrac{300 \text{ mg}}{8.4 \text{ mg/L}}$

t(hr)	C_p *(µg/ml)*
2	6
6	3

$V_d = 35.7$ L

$t_{1/2}$(from graph) = 4 hr

$K = \dfrac{0.693}{4} = 0.173 \text{ hr}^{-1}$

b. $C_p^0 = 8.4\ \mu\text{g/ml} \qquad C_p = 2\ \mu\text{g/ml} \qquad K = 0.173 \text{ hr}^{-1}$

$$\log C_p = -\frac{Kt}{2.3} + \log C_p^0$$

$$\log 2 = -\frac{0.173t}{2.3} + \log 8.4$$

$$t = 8.29 \text{ hr}$$

Alternately, time t may be found from a graph of C_p versus t.

c. Time required for 99.9% of the drug to be eliminated:

(1) Approximately $10t_{1/2}$

$$t = 10(4) = 40 \text{ hr}$$

(2)

$$C_p^0 = 8.4\ \mu\text{g/ml}$$

With 0.1% of drug remaining,

$$C_p = 0.001(8.4\ \mu\text{g/ml}) = 0.0084\ \mu\text{g/ml}$$

$$K = 0.173 \text{ hr}^{-1}$$

$$\log 0.0084 = \frac{0.173t}{2.3} + \log 8.4$$

$$t = 39.9 \text{ hr}$$

d. If the dose doubled, then C_p^0 will also double. However, the elimination half-life or first-order rate constant will remain the same. Therefore:

$C_p^0 = 16.8\ \mu\text{g/ml} \qquad C_p = 2\ \mu\text{g/ml} \qquad K = 0.173 \text{ hr}^{-1}$

$$\log 2 = -\frac{0.173t}{2.3} + \log 16.8$$

$$t = 12.3 \text{ hr}$$

Notice that doubling the dose does not double the duration of activity.

3. $D_0 = 200$ mg

$$V_d = 10\% \text{ of body weight}$$
$$= 0.1(80 \text{ kg}) = 8000 \text{ ml}$$

At 6 hr

$$C_p = 1.5 \text{ mg}/100 \text{ ml}$$
$$V_d = \frac{\text{drug in body } (D_B)}{C_p}$$
$$D_B = C_p V_d = \frac{1.5 \text{ mg}}{100 \text{ ml}}(8000 \text{ ml})$$
$$= 120 \text{ mg}$$
$$\log D_B = -\frac{Kt}{2.3} + \log D_B^0$$
$$\log 120 = -\frac{K(6)}{2.3} + \log 200$$
$$K = 0.085 \text{ hr}^{-1}$$
$$t_{1/2} = \frac{0.693}{K} = \frac{0.693}{0.085}$$
$$= 8.1 \text{ hr}$$

4. $C_p = 78e^{-0.46t}$ [equation is in the form of $C_p = C_p^0 e^{-Kt}$]

$$\ln C_p = \ln 78 - 0.46t$$
$$\log C_p = -\frac{0.46t}{2.3} + \log 78$$

Thus $K = 0.46 \text{ hr}^{-1}$, $C_p^0 = 78\ \mu\text{g/ml}$.

a.

$$t_{1/2} = \frac{0.693}{K} = \frac{0.693}{0.46} = 1.5 \text{ hr}$$

b.

$$V_d = \frac{\text{dose}}{C_p^0} = \frac{300{,}000\ \mu\text{g}}{78\ \mu\text{g/ml}} = 3846 \text{ ml}$$

$$\text{Dose} = 4 \text{ mg/kg} \times 75 \text{ kg} = 300 \text{ mg}$$

c.

(1) $$\log C_p = -\frac{0.46(4)}{2.3} + \log 78$$
$$= 1.092$$
$$C_p = 12.4\ \mu\text{g/ml}$$

(2) $$C_p = 78e^{-0.46(4)}$$
$$= 78e^{-1.84}$$
$$= 78(0.165) \quad \text{[From Appendix Table 3]}$$
$$C_p = 12.9\ \mu\text{g/ml}$$

d. At 4 hr

$$D_B = C_p V_d$$
$$= 12.4\ \mu g/ml \times 3846\ ml$$
$$= 47.69\ mg$$

e.

$$V_d = 3846\ ml$$

Average weight = 75 kg

Percent body wt. = 3.846 kg/75 kg × 100 = 5.1%

The apparent V_d is the same as the plasma volume.

f.

$$C_p = 2\ \mu g/ml$$

Find t.

$$\log 2 = -\frac{0.46t}{2.3} + \log 78$$
$$t = -\frac{2.3(\log 2 - \log 78)}{0.46}$$
$$= 7.96\ hr \approx 8\ hr$$

Alternate method

$$2 = 78e^{-0.46t}$$
$$\frac{2}{78} = 0.0256 = e^{-0.46t}$$
$$-3.7 = -0.46t \qquad \text{[From Appendix Table 3]}$$
$$t = \frac{3.7}{0.46} = 8\ hr$$

6. For first-order elimination kinetics, one-half of the initial quantity is lost each $t_{1/2}$. The following table may be developed:

Time (hr)	Number of $t_{1/2}$	Amount of Drug in Body (mg)	Percent of Drug in Body	Percent of Drug Lost
0	0	200	100	0
6	1	100	50	50
12	2	50	25	75
18	3	25	12.5	87.5
24	4	12.5	6.25	93.75

Method 1

From the above table the percent of drug remaining in the body after each $t_{1/2}$ is equal to 100% times $(\frac{1}{2})^n$ as shown below:

Number of $t_{1/2}$	Percent of Drug in Body	Percent of Drug Remaining in Body after $n\ t_{1/2}$
0	100	
1	50	$100 \times \frac{1}{2}$
2	25	$100 \times \frac{1}{2} \times \frac{1}{2}$
3	12.5	$100 \times \frac{1}{2} \times \frac{1}{2} \times \frac{1}{2}$
n		$100 \times (\frac{1}{2})^n$

$$\text{Percent of drug remnining} = \frac{100}{2^n} \quad \text{where } n = \text{number of } t_{1/2}$$

$$\text{Percent of drug excreted} = 100 - \frac{100}{2^n}$$

At 24 hr $n = 4$ since $t_{1/2} = 6$ hr.

$$\text{Percent of drug lost} = 100 - \frac{100}{16} = 93.75\%$$

Method 2

The equation for a first-order elimination after IV bolus injection is

$$\log D_B = \frac{-Kt}{2.3} + \log D_0$$

where

$$D_B = \text{amount of drug remaining in the body}$$

$$D_0 = \text{dose} = 200 \text{ mg}$$

$$K = \text{elimination rate constant} = 0.693/t_{1/2}$$

$$= 0.1155 \text{ hr}^{-1}$$

$$t = 24 \text{ hr}$$

$$\log D_B = \frac{-0.1155(24)}{2.3} + \log 200$$

$$D_B = 12.47 \text{ mg} \sim 12.5 \text{ mg}$$

$$\% \text{ of drug lost} = \frac{200 - 12.5}{200} \times 100 = 93.75\%$$

7. The zero-order rate constant for alcohol is 10 ml/hr. Since the specific gravity for alcohol is 0.8, then

$$0.8 \text{ g/ml} = X\text{(g)}/10 \text{ ml} \qquad X = 8 \text{ g/ml}$$

Therefore, the zero-order rate constant, K_0, is 8 g/hr.

Drug in body at $t = 0$:

$$D_B^0 = C_p V_d = 210 \text{ mg}/0.100 \text{ L} \times (0.60)(75) = 94.5 \text{ g}$$

Drug in body at time t:

$$D_B = C_p V_d = 100\ \text{mg}/0.100\ \text{L} \times (0.60)(75) = 45.0\ \text{g}$$

For a zero-order reaction:

$$D_B = -K_0 t + D_B^0$$
$$45 = -8t + 94.5$$
$$t = 6.19\ \text{hr}$$

8. a. $$C_p^0 = \text{dose} = \frac{500\ \text{mg}}{(0.1\ \text{L/kg})(55\ \text{kg})} = 90.9\ \text{mg/L}$$

b. $$\log D_B = \frac{-Kt}{2.3} + \log D_B^0$$
$$= \frac{(0.693/0.75)(4)}{2.3} + \log 500$$
$$D_B = 12.3\ \text{mg}$$

c. $$\log 0.5 = \frac{-(0.693/0.75)t}{2.3} + \log 90.9$$
$$t = 5.62\ \text{hr}$$

9.

$$\log D_B = \frac{-Kt}{2.3} + \log D_0$$
$$\log 25 = \frac{-K(8)}{2.3} + \log 100$$
$$K = 0.173\ \text{hr}^{-1}$$
$$t_{1/2} = \frac{0.693}{0.173} = 4\ \text{hr}$$

10. $$\log D_B = \frac{-Kt}{2.3} + \log D_0$$
$$= \frac{(0.693/8)(24)}{2.3} + \log 600$$
$$D_B = 74.9\ \text{mg}$$
$$\text{Percent drug lost} = \frac{600 - 74.9}{600} \times 100 = 87.5\%$$

C_p at $t = 24$ hr:

$$C_p = \frac{74.9\ \text{mg}}{(0.4\ \text{L/kg})(62\ \text{kg})} = 3.02\ \text{mg/L}$$

12. Set up the following table:

Time(hr)	D_u*(mg)*	D_u/t	mg/hr	t^*
0	0			
4	100	100/4	25	2
8	26	26/4	6.5	6

The elimination half-life may be obtained graphically after plotting mg/hr versus t^*. The $t_{1/2}$ obtained graphically is approximately 2 hr.

$$\log \frac{dD_u}{dt} = \frac{-Kt}{2.3} + \log K_e D_B^0$$

$$\text{Slope} = \frac{-K}{2.3} + \frac{\log Y_2 - \log Y_1}{X_2 - X_1} = \frac{\log 25 - \log 6.5}{2 - 6}$$

$$K = 0.336 \text{ hr}^{-1}$$

$$= \frac{0.693}{K} = \frac{0.693}{0.336} = 2.06 \text{ hr}$$

CHAPTER 5

1. Equation for the curve:

$$C_p = 52e^{-1.39t} + 18e^{-0.135t}$$

$$K = 0.41 \text{ hr}^{-1}$$

$$K_{12} = 0.657$$

$$K_{21} = 0.458 \text{ hr}^{-1}$$

2. Equation for the curve:

$$C_p = 28e^{-0.63t} + 10.5e^{-0.46t} + 14e^{-0.077t}$$

Note: When feathering curves by hand, a minimum of three points should be used to determine the line. Moreover, the rate constants and y intercepts may vary according to the individual's skill. Therefore, values for C_p should be checked by substitution of various times for t, using the derived equation. The theoretical curve should fit the observed data.

3.

$$C_p = 11.14\ \mu\text{g/ml}$$

7.

$$C_p = Ae^{-at} + Be^{-bt}$$

After substitution:

$$C_p = 4.62e^{8.94t} + 0.64e^{-0.19t}$$

a. $$V_p = \frac{D_0}{A + B} = \frac{75000}{4.62 + 0.64} = 14259 \text{ ml}$$

b. $$V_t = \frac{V_p K_{12}}{K_{21}} = \frac{(14259)(6.52)}{(1.25)} = 74375 \text{ ml}$$

c. $$K_{12} = \frac{AB(b-a)^2}{(A+B)(Ab+Ba)} = \frac{(4.62)(0.64)(0.19-8.94)^2}{(4.62+0.64)[(4.62)(0.19)+(0.64)(8.94)]}$$

$$= 6.52\ \text{hr}^{-1}$$

$$K_{21} = \frac{Ab+Ba}{A+B} = \frac{(4.62)(0.19)+(0.64)(8.94)}{4.62+0.64}$$

$$= 1.25\ \text{hr}^{-1}$$

d. $$K = \frac{ab(A+B)}{Ab+Ba} = \frac{(8.94)(0.19)[(4.62+0.64)]}{(4.62)(0.19)+(0.64)(8.94)}$$

$$= 1.35\ \text{hr}^{-1}$$

8. The tissue compartments may not be sampled directly to obtain the drug concentration. Theoretical concentration C_t represents the average concentration in all the tissues outside of the central compartment. The amount of drug in the tissue, D_t, represents the total amount of drug outside of the central or plasma compartment. Occasionally C_t may be equal to a particular tissue drug concentration in an organ. However, this C_t may be equivalent by chance only.

CHAPTER 7

1. The following equations were obtained:

$$C_p = Be^{-kt} - Ae^{-K_a t}$$

$$C_p = 2.15e^{-0.126t} - 3.5e^{-0.924t} \quad \text{[Authors]}$$

$$C_p = 2.4e^{-0.13t} - 3.0e^{-0.81t} \quad \text{[Wagner]}$$

$$C_p = 2.8e^{-0.15t} - 3.6e^{-0.72t} \quad \text{[Computer]}$$

6. Plot C_p versus t on a semilog plot and use the technique of feathering to find K_a and K.

a. Find the slope of the terminal portion of the curve.

$$K = 0.092\ \text{hr}^{-1}$$

Find intercept I.

$$I = 150$$

b. Find K_a from the feathered line.

$$K_a = 0.2\ \text{hr}^{-1}$$

c. Find the volume of distribution using the following equation.

$$\text{Intercept } I = \frac{D_0 F K_a}{V_d(K_a - K)}$$

Substitute.

$$D = 10{,}000\ \mu\text{g}$$
$$F = 0.8$$
$$K_a = 0.2$$
$$K = 0.092$$
$$I = 150$$
$$V_d = \frac{DFK_a}{I(K_a - K)}$$
$$= \frac{10{,}000 \times 0.8 \times 0.2}{150(0.2 - 0.092)}$$
$$= 99\ \text{ml/kg}$$

d.

$$t_{max} = \frac{\ln(K_a/K)}{K_a - K}$$
$$= \frac{\ln(0.2/0.092)}{(0.2 - 0.092)}$$
$$= 7.1\ \text{hr}$$

7. The general equation for a one-compartment open model with oral absorption is:

$$C_p = \frac{FD_0}{V_d(K_a - K)}(e^{Kt} - e^{-K_a t})$$

From

$$C_p = 45(e^{-0.17t} - e^{-1.5t})$$
$$\frac{FD_0K_a}{V_d(K_a - K)} = 45$$
$$K = 0.17\ \text{hr}^{-1}$$
$$K_a = 1.5\ \text{hr}^{-1}$$

a.

$$t_{max} = \frac{\ln(K_a/K)}{K_a - K} = \frac{\ln(1.5/0.17)}{1.5 - 0.17}$$
$$= 1.64\ \text{hr}$$

b.

$$C_{p,\,max} = 45(e^{-(0.17)(1.64)} - e^{-(1.5)(1.64)})$$
$$= 30.2\ \mu\text{g/ml}$$

c.

$$t_{1/2} = \frac{0.693}{K} = \frac{0.693}{0.17} = 4.08\ \text{hr}$$

8. a.

Drug A $t_{\max} = \dfrac{\ln(1.0/0.2)}{1.0 - 0.2} = 2.01 \text{ hr}$

Drug B $t_{\max} = \dfrac{\ln(0.2/1.0)}{0.2 - 1.0} = 2.01 \text{ hr}$

b.

$$C_{p,\max} = \frac{FD_0 K_a}{V_d(K_a - K)}\left(e^{-Kt_{\max}} - e^{-K_a t_{\max}}\right)$$

Drug A $C_{p,\max} = \dfrac{(1)(500)(1)}{(10)(1 - 0.2)}\left(e^{-(0.2)(2)} - e^{-(1)(2)}\right)$

$C_{p,\max} = 33.4\ \mu\text{g/ml}$

Drug B $C_{p,\max} = \dfrac{(1)(500)(0.2)}{(20)(0.2 - 1.0)}\left(e^{-1(2)} - e^{-(0.2)(2)}\right)$

$C_{p,\max} = 3.34\ \mu\text{g/ml}$

CHAPTER 8

3. a. Oral solution. The drug is in the most bioavailable form.

b. Oral solution. Same reason as above.

c.

$$\text{Absolute bioavailability} = \frac{[\text{AUC}]\text{oral solution/dose}}{[\text{AUC}]_{\text{IV}}/\text{dose}} = \frac{145/10}{29/2} = 1.0$$

d.

$$\text{Relative bioavailability} = \frac{[\text{AUC}]\text{tablet/dose}}{[\text{AUC}]\text{solution/dose}} = \frac{116/10}{145/10} = 0.80$$

e. (1)

$C_p^0 = 6.67\ \mu\text{g/ml}$ [by extrapolation of IV curve]

$$V_d = \frac{2000\ \mu\text{g/kg}}{6.67\ \mu\text{g/ml}} = 300 \text{ ml/kg}$$

(2) $t_{1/2} = 3.01$ hr

(3) $K = 0.23 \text{ hr}^{-1}$

(4) $\text{Cl}_T = KV_d = 69$ ml/kg hr

4. Plot the data on both rectangular and semilog graph paper. The following answers were obtained from estimates from the plotted plasma level–time curves. More exact answers may be obtained mathematically by substitution into the proper formulae.

a. 1.37 hr
b. 13.6 hr
c. 8.75 hr
d. 5 hr
e. 4.21 μg/ml
f. 77.98 μg hr/ml

5.

Patient	Drug Product		
	Week I	*Week II*	*Week III*
1	A	B	C
2	B	C	A
3	C	A	B
4	A	C	B
5	C	B	A
6	B	A	C

6.

a.

$$\text{Absolute bioavailability} = \frac{D^{\infty}_{\text{u,PO}}/\text{dose PO}}{D^{\infty}_{\text{u,IV}}/\text{dose IV}}$$

$$= \frac{340/4}{20/0.2} = 0.85 \quad \text{or } 85\%$$

b.

$$\text{Relative bioavailability} = \frac{D^{\infty}_{\text{u}}\ \text{cap}/\text{dose cap}}{D^{\infty}_{\text{u}}\ \text{sol}/\text{dose sol}}$$

$$= \frac{360/4}{380/4} = 0.947 \quad \text{or } 94.7\%$$

7. The fraction of drug absorbed systemically is the absolute bioavailability.

$$\text{Fraction of drug absorbed} = \frac{\%\text{ of dose excreted after PO}}{\%\text{ of dose excreted after IV}}$$

$$= \frac{48\%}{75\%} = 0.64$$

CHAPTER 9

1. a.

$$\text{Cl}_{\text{T}} = V_{\text{d}}K = V_{\text{d}}\frac{0.693}{t_{1/2}}$$

$$\text{Average Cl}_{\text{T}} = \frac{30 \times 0.693}{3.4} = 6.11 \text{ L/hr}$$

$$\text{Upper Cl}_{\text{T}} \text{ limit} = \frac{30 \times 0.693}{1.8} = 11.55 \text{ L/hr}$$

$$\text{Lower Cl}_{\text{T}} \text{ limit} = \frac{30 \times 0.693}{6.8} = 3.06 \text{ L/hr}$$

b.

$$\text{Cl}_r = K_e V_d = 0.36 \text{ L/hr}$$

$$K_e = \frac{0.36}{30} = 0.012 \text{ hr}^{-1}$$

$$\text{Cl}_{nr} = \text{Cl}_T - \text{Cl}_r$$

$$\text{Cl}_{nr} = 6.11 - 0.36 = 5.75 \text{ L/hr}$$

$$\text{Cl}_{nr} = K_m V_d$$

$$K_m = \frac{5.75}{30} = 0.192 \text{ hr}^{-1}$$

2. a.

$$\begin{aligned}\text{Apparent } V_d &= (0.21)(78{,}000 \text{ ml}) \\ &= 16{,}380 \text{ ml} \\ \text{Cl}_T &= KV_d \\ &= \left(\frac{0.693}{2}\right)(16{,}380) \\ &= 5676 \text{ ml/hr} = 94.6 \text{ ml/min}\end{aligned}$$

b.

$$K_e = 70\% \text{ of the elimination constant}$$

$$K_e = (0.7)\left(\frac{0.693}{2}\right) = 0.243 \text{ hr}^{-1}$$

$$\text{Cl}_r = K_e V_d$$

$$\text{Cl}_r = (0.243)(16{,}380) = 3980 \text{ ml/hr} = 66.3 \text{ ml/min}$$

c.

$$\text{Normal GFR} = \text{creatinine clearance} = 122 \text{ ml/min}$$

$$\text{Cl}_r \text{ of drug} = 66.3 \text{ ml}$$

Since the Cl_r of the drug is less than the creatinine clearance, the drug is filtered at the glomerulus and is partially reabsorbed.

3. a. During intravenous infusion, the drug levels will reach more than 99% of the plasma steady-state concentration after seven half-lives of the drug.

$$\begin{aligned}\text{Cl}_T &= \frac{R}{C_p^{\infty}} \\ &= \frac{300{,}000 \ \mu\text{g/hr}}{11 \ \mu\text{g/ml}} = 27{,}272 \text{ ml/hr}\end{aligned}$$

b.

$$\text{Cl}_T = KV_d$$

$$V_d = \frac{27{,}272}{0.693} = 39{,}354 \text{ ml}$$

c.

$$\text{Since } K_m = 0, \qquad K_e \cong K$$
$$Cl_T = Cl_r = 27{,}272 \text{ ml/hr}$$

d.

$$Cl_r = 27{,}272 \text{ ml/hr} = 454 \text{ ml/min}$$

Normal GFR is 100–130 ml/min. The drug is probably filtered and actively secreted in the kidney.

4.

$$Cl_r = \frac{\text{excretion rate}}{C_p} = \frac{200 \text{ mg/2 hr}}{2.5 \text{ mg/100 ml}}$$
$$= 4000 \text{ ml/hr}$$

5.

$$Cl_T = \frac{R}{C_{ss}} \quad \text{(see Chapter 12)}$$
$$= \frac{5.3 \text{ mg/kg hr}}{17 \text{ mg/L}} = 0.312 \text{ L/kg hr}$$

For 71.7-kg adults

$$Cl_T = (0.312 \text{ L/kg hr})(71.7 \text{ kg}) = 22.4 \text{ L/hr}$$

CHAPTER 10

1. a.

$$K = K_m + K_e + K_b$$
$$= 0.20 + 0.25 + 0.15 = 0.60 \text{ hr}^{-1}$$
$$t_{1/2} = \frac{0.693}{K} = \frac{0.693}{0.60} = 1.16 \text{ hr}$$

b.

$$K = K_m + K_e = 0.45 \text{ hr}^{-1}$$
$$t_{1/2} = 1.54 \text{ hr}$$

c.

$$K = 0.35 \text{ hr}^{-1}$$
$$t_{1/2} = 1.98 \text{ hr}$$

d.

$$K = 0.80 \text{ hr}^{-1}$$
$$t_{1/2} = 0.87 \text{ hr}$$

2. a.

$$K = 0.347 \text{ hr}^{-1}$$
$$K_e = (0.9)(0.347) = 0.312 \text{ hr}^{-1}$$

b. Renal excretion

5. Normal hepatic clearance, Cl_H:

$$\text{Cl}_H = Q\left(\frac{\text{Cl}_{\text{int}}}{Q + \text{Cl}_{\text{int}}}\right) \qquad Q = 1.5 \text{ L/min}, \qquad \text{Cl}_{\text{int}} = 0.040 \text{ L/min}$$
$$= 1.5\left(\frac{0.040}{1.5 + 0.040}\right) = 0.039 \text{ L/min}$$

a. Congestive heart failure:

$$\text{Cl}_H = 1.0\left(\frac{0.040}{1.0 + 0.040}\right) = 0.038 \text{ L/min}$$

b. Enzyme induction:

$$\text{Cl}_H = 1.5\left(\frac{0.090}{1.5 + 0.090}\right) = 0.085 \text{ L/min}$$

Note: A change in blood flow Q did not markedly affect Cl_H for a drug with low Cl_{int}.

6. Normal hepatic clearance:

$$\text{Cl}_H = 1.5\left(\frac{12}{1.5 + 12}\right) = 1.33 \text{ L/min}$$

Congestive heart failure:

$$\text{Cl}_H = 1.0\left(\frac{12}{1.0 + 12}\right) = 0.923 \text{ L/min}$$

a.

$$\text{Cl}_H = Q(\text{ER}) = Q\left(\frac{\text{Cl}_{\text{int}}}{Q + \text{Cl}_{\text{int}}}\right)$$

$$\text{ER} = \frac{\text{Cl}_{\text{int}}}{Q + \text{Cl}_{\text{int}}}$$

$$\text{Normal ER} = \frac{12}{1.5 + 12} = 0.89 \text{ L/min}$$

$$\text{CHF ER} = \frac{12}{1.0 + 12} = 0.92 \text{ L/min}$$

b.

$$F = 1 - \text{ER}$$
$$= 1 - 0.89$$
$$F = 0.11 \quad \textit{or} \quad 11\%$$

CHAPTER 11

1. The zone of inhibition for the antibiotic in serum is smaller due to drug–protein binding.
2. Calculate r/D versus r and graph the results on rectangular coordinates.

r	$r/D(\times 10^4)$
0.4	1.21
0.8	0.90
1.2	0.60
1.6	0.30

The y intercept $= nK_a = 1.5 \times 10^4$
The x intercept $= n = 2$
Therefore,

$$K_a = 1.5 \times 10^4/2 = 0.75 \times 10^4$$

K_a may also be found from the slope.

CHAPTER 12

1. a. To reach 95% of C_p^∞:

$$4.32t_{1/2} = (4.32)(7) = 30.2 \text{ hr}$$

b.

$$D_L = C_p^\infty V_d = (10)(0.231)(65000) = 150 \text{ mg}$$

c.

$$R = C_p^\infty V_d K$$
$$= (10)(15000)(0.099) = 14.85 \text{ mg/hr}$$

d.

$$\text{Cl}_T = V_d K = (15000)(0.099) = 1485 \text{ ml/hr}$$

e. To establish a new C_p^∞ would still take $4.32t_{1/2}$, or 30.2 hr.

f. If Cl_T is decreased by 50%, then the infusion rate R should be decreased proportionately:

$$R = 10(0.50)(1485) = 7.425 \text{ mg/hr}$$

2. a. The steady-state level can be found by plotting the IV infusion data. The plasma–drug time curves plateau at 10 μg/ml. Alternatively, V_d and K can be found from the single IV dose data:

$$V_d = 100 \text{ ml/kg}$$

$$K = 0.2 \text{ hr}^{-1}$$

b. Using equations developed in Example 2, Chapter 12,

$$0.95 \frac{R}{V_d K} = \frac{R}{V_d K}(1 - e^{-Kt})$$

$$0.95 = 1 - e^{-0.2t}$$

$$0.05 = e^{-0.2t}$$

$$t_{95\%\,ss} = \frac{\ln 0.05}{-0.2} = 15 \text{ hr}$$

c.

$$\begin{aligned} Cl_T &= V_d K \\ &= 100 \times 0.2 \\ &= 20 \text{ ml/kg hr} \end{aligned}$$

d. The drug level 4 hr after infusion can be found by considering the drug concentration at the termination of infusion as C_p^0. At the termination of the infusion the drug level will decline by a first-order process.

$$\begin{aligned} C_p &= C_p^0 e^{-Kt} \\ &= 9.9e^{-(0.2)(4)} \\ &= 4.5\ \mu\text{g/ml} \end{aligned}$$

e. The infusion rate producing a C_{ss} of 10 μg/ml is 0.2 mg/kg hr. Therefore, the infusion rate needed for this patient is

$$0.2 \text{ mg/kg hr} \times 75 \text{ kg} = 15 \text{ mg/hr}$$

f. From the data shown, 4 hr after IV infusion the drug concentration is 5.5 μg/ml, and the drug concentration after an IV bolus of 1 mg/kg is 4.5 μg/ml. Therefore, if a 1-mg dose was given and the drug is then infused at 0.2 mg/kg hr, the plasma drug concentration would be 4.5 + 5.5 = 10 μg/ml.

3. Infusion rate R for a 75-kg patient:

$$R = 1 \text{ mg/kg hr} \times 75 \text{ kg} = 75 \text{ mg/hr}$$

Sterile drug solution contains 25 mg/ml. Therefore, 3 ml contains 3 ml × 25 mg/ml, or 75 mg. The patient should receive 3 ml (75 mg)/hr by IV infusion.

4.

$$C_{ss} = \frac{R}{V_d K} \qquad R = C_{ss} V_d K$$

$$R = 20 \text{ mg/L} \times 0.5 \text{ L/kg} \times 75 \text{ kg} \times \frac{0.693}{3 \text{ hr}}$$

$$= 173.25 \text{ mg/hr}$$

Drug is supplied as 125 mg/ml. Therefore,

$$125 \text{ mg/ml} = \frac{173.25 \text{ mg}}{X} \qquad X = 1.386 \text{ ml}$$

$$R = 1.386 \text{ ml/hr}$$

$$D_L = C_{SS} V_d = 20 \text{ mg/L} \times 0.5 \text{ L/kg} \times 75 \text{ kg} = 750 \text{ mg}$$

5.

$$C_{ss} = \frac{R}{KV_d} = \frac{R}{Cl_T} \qquad Cl_T = C_{ss}R$$

a.

$$Cl_T = 17 \text{ mg/L} \times 5.3 \text{ mg/kg hr} \times 71.7 \text{ kg} = 22.4 \text{ L/hr}$$

b. At end of IV infusion, $C_p = 17\ \mu g/ml$. Assuming first-order elimination kinetics:

$$\begin{aligned} C_p &= C_p^0 e^{-Kt} \\ 1.5 &= 17e^{-K(2.5)} \\ 0.0882 &= e^{-2.5K} \\ \ln 0.0882 &= -2.5K \\ -2.43 &= -2.5K \\ K &= 0.971 \text{ hr}^{-1} \\ t_{1/2} &= \frac{0.693}{0.971} = 0.714 \text{ hr} \end{aligned}$$

c.

$$Cl_T = KV_d \qquad V_d = Cl_T/K$$

$$V_d = \frac{22.4}{0.971} = 23.1 \text{ L}$$

d. Probenecid blocks active tubular secretion of cephradine.

6. At steady state the rate of elimination should equal the rate of absorption. Therefore, the rate of elimination would be 30 mg/hr. The C_{ss} is directly proportional to the rate of infusion R, as shown by

$$C_{ss} = \frac{R}{KV_d} \qquad KV_d = \frac{R}{C_{ss}}$$

$$\frac{R_{old}}{C_{ss,old}} = \frac{R_{new}}{C_{ss,new}}$$

$$\frac{30 \text{ mg/hr}}{20\ \mu g/ml} = \frac{40 \text{ mg/hr}}{C_{ss,new}}$$

$$C_{ss,new} = 26.7\ \mu g/ml$$

The new elimination rate would be 40 mg/hr.

CHAPTER 13

1.

$$V_d = 0.20(50 \text{ kg}) = 10{,}000 \text{ ml}$$

a.

$$D_{\max} = \frac{D_0}{1-f} = \frac{50 \text{ mg}}{1 - e^{-(0.693/2)(8)}} = 53.3 \text{ mg}$$

$$C_{\text{p, max}} = \frac{D_{\max}}{V_{\text{d}}} = \frac{53.3 \text{ mg}}{10{,}000 \text{ ml}} = 5.33 \ \mu\text{g/ml}$$

b.

$$D_{\min} = 53.3 - 50 = 3.3 \text{ mg}$$

$$C_{\text{p, min}} = \frac{3.3 \text{ mg}}{10{,}000 \text{ ml}} = 0.33 \ \mu\text{g/ml}$$

c.

$$C_{\text{av}}^{\infty} = \frac{FD_0 1.44 t_{1/2}}{V_{\text{d}}\tau} = \frac{(50)(1.44)(2)}{(10{,}000)(8)} = 1.8 \ \mu\text{g/ml}$$

2. a.

$$D_0 = \frac{C_{\text{av}}^{\infty} V_{\text{d}} \tau}{1.44 t_{1/2}}$$

$$= \frac{(10)(40{,}000)(6)}{(1.44)(5)} = 333 \text{ mg every 6 hr}$$

b.

$$\tau = \frac{FD_0 1.44 t_{1/2}}{V_{\text{d}} C_{\text{av}}^{\infty}}$$

$$= \frac{(225{,}000)(1.44)(5)}{(40{,}000)(10)} = 4.05 \text{ hr}$$

6. Dose the patient with 225 mg every 4 hr.

$$D_{\text{L}} = \frac{D_0}{1 - e^{-K\tau}} = \frac{200}{1 - e^{-(0.23)(3)}} = 400 \text{ mg}$$

Notice that D_{L} is twice the maintenance dose, since the drug is given at a dosage interval equal approximately to the $t_{1/2}$ of 3 hr.

CHAPTER 14

1. Capacity-limited processes for drugs include:

Absorption

- Active transport
- Intestinal metabolism by microflora

Distribution

- Protein binding

Elimination
  Hepatic elimination
  Biotransformation
  Active biliary secretion
Renal excretion
  Active tubular secretion
  Active tubular reabsorption

3.

$$C_p^0 = \frac{\text{dose}}{V_d} = \frac{10{,}000\ \mu g}{20{,}000\ \text{ml}} = 0.5\ \mu g/\text{ml}$$

From Equation 14.1

$$\text{Elimination rate} = -\frac{dC_p}{dt} = \frac{V_m C_p}{K_m + C_p}$$

Since $K_m = 50\ \mu g/\text{ml}$, $C_p \ll K_m$ and the reaction rate is first order. Thus, the above equation reduces to Equation 14.3:

$$-\frac{dC_p}{dt} = \frac{V_m C_p}{K_m} = K^1 C_p$$

$$K^1 = \frac{V_m}{K_m} = \frac{20\ \mu g/\text{hr}}{50\ \mu g} = 0.4\ \text{hr}^{-1}$$

For first-order reactions:

$$t_{1/2} = \frac{0.693}{K^1} = \frac{0.693}{0.4} = 1.73\ \text{hr}$$

The drug will be 50% metabolized in 1.73 hr.

6. When INH is coadministered, plasma phenytoin concentration is increased due to a reduction in metabolic rate V. Equation 14.1 shows that V and K_m are inversely related (K_m in denominator). An increase in K_m would be accompanied by an increase in plasma drug concentration. Figure 14.4 shows that an increase in K_m is accompanied by an increase in amount of drug in the body at any time t. Equation 14.4 relates drug concentration to K_m, and it can be seen that the two are proportionally related although they are not linearly proportional to each other due to the complexity of the equation. An actual study in the literature shows that K is increased several-fold in the presence of INH in the body.
7. The K_m has the unit of concentration. In laboratory studies K_m is expressed in moles per liter or micromolar per milliliter since reactions occur in moles and not milligrams. In dosing, drugs are given in milligram and plasma drug concentrations are expressed as milligrams per liter or micrograms per milliliter. The units of K_m for pharmacokinetic models are estimated from in vivo data. They are therefore commonly expressed accordingly as milligrams per liter, which is preferred over micrograms per milliliter because dose is usually expressed in milligrams. The two terms may be shown to be equivalent. Occasionally, when simulating amount of drug metabolized in the

body as a function of time, the amount of drug in the body has been assumed to follow Machaelis–Menten kinetics and K_m would assume the unit of D (i.e., mg). In this case K_m, would take on a very different meaning.

CHAPTER 15

1.

$$C_{max}^{\infty} = \frac{D_0}{V_d}\left(\frac{1}{1-e^{-K\tau}}\right)$$

$$= \frac{250{,}000}{42{,}000}\left(\frac{1}{1-e^{-(6)(1.034)}}\right)$$

$$= \frac{250{,}000}{42{,}000}\left(\frac{1}{0.998}\right) = 5.96\ \mu g/ml$$

At steady state the peak concentration of penicillin G would be 5.96 μg/ml.

2.

$$C_{av}^{\infty} = \frac{D}{KV_d\tau}$$

$$= \frac{250{,}000}{0.99 \times 20{,}000 \times 6} = 2.10\ \mu g/ml$$

Free drug concentration at steady state = 2.10(1 − 0.97) = 0.063 μg/ml

3.

$$C_{av}^{\infty} = \frac{1.44DFt_{1/2}}{V_d\tau}$$

For the normal patient

$$V_d = 0.392 \times 1 \times 1000 = 392\ ml/kg$$

$$C_{av}^{\infty} = \frac{1.44 \times D \times 1 \times 1.49}{392 \times 6} = 2\ \mu g/ml$$

$$D = \frac{392 \times 6 \times 2}{1.44 \times 1.49} = 2192\ \mu g/kg$$

$$= 2.2\ mg/kg$$

For the uremic patient

$$V_d = 23.75 \times 1 \times 1000 = 237.5\ ml/kg$$

$$C_{av}^{\infty} = \frac{1.44 \times D \times 1 \times 6.03}{237.5 \times 6} = 2\ \mu g/ml$$

$$D = \frac{2 \times 237.5 \times 6}{1.44 \times 6.03} = 328.2\ \mu g/kg$$

$$= 0.3\ mg/kg$$

4. a.

$$V_d = 306{,}000 \text{ ml}$$

$$\text{Dose} = 0.5 \times 10^6 \text{ ng}$$

$$C_{av}^{\infty} = \frac{1.44 \times DFt_{1/2}}{V_d \tau} = \frac{1.44 \times 0.5 \times 10^6 \times 0.56 \times 0.95}{306{,}000 \times 1}$$

$$= 1.25 \text{ ng/ml}$$

b. The patient is adequately dosed.

c. $F = 1$; using the above equation, the C_{av}^{∞} would be 2.2 ng/ml, although still effective, but the C_{av}^{∞} will be closer to the toxic serum concentration of 3 ng/ml.

9. Assume desired $C_{av}^{\infty} = 0.0015\ \mu\text{g/ml}$ and $\tau = 24$ hr.

$$C_{av}^{\infty} = \frac{FD_0 \times 1.44 t_{1/2}}{V_d \tau}$$

$$D_0 = \frac{C_{av}^{\infty} V_d \tau}{F \times 1.44 t_{1/2}}$$

$$= \frac{(0.0015)(4)(68)(24)}{(0.80)(1.44)(30)} = 0.283 \text{ mg}$$

Give 0.283 mg every 24 hr.

a. For a dosage regimen of one 0.30-mg tablet daily

$$C_{av}^{\infty} = \frac{(0.80)(0.3)(1.44)(30)}{(4)(68)(24)} = 0.0016\ \mu\text{g/ml}$$

which is within the therapeutic window.

b. A dosage regimen of 0.15 mg/12 hr would provide smaller fluctuations between the C_{max}^{∞} and C_{min}^{∞} compared to a dosage regimen of 0.30 mg/24 hr.

c. Since the elimination half-life is long (30 hr), a loading dose is advisable.

$$D_L = D_m \left(\frac{1}{1 - e^{-K\tau}} \right)$$

$$= 0.30 \left(\frac{1}{1 - e^{-(0.693/30)(24)}} \right)$$

$$= 0.70 \text{ mg}$$

For cardiotonic drugs related to the digitalis glycosides, it is recommended that the loading dose be administered in several portions with approximately half the total as the first dose. Additional fractions may be given at 6–8 hr intervals with careful assessment of the clinical response before each additional dose.

d. There is no rationale for a controlled release drug product due to the long elimination half-life of 30 hr inherent in the drug.

10. a.

$$C_{av}^{\infty} = \frac{FD_0 \times 1.44t_{1/2}}{V_d\tau}$$

$$= \frac{(1500)(1.44)(6)}{(1.3)(63)(4)} = 39.6\ \mu g/ml$$

b.

$$D_L = D_m\left(\frac{1}{1 - e^{-K\tau}}\right)$$

$$= 1.5\left(\frac{1}{1 - e^{-(0.693/6)(4)}}\right)$$

$$= 4.05\ g$$

c. A D_L of 4.05 g is needed that is equivalent to eight tablets containing 0.5 g each.

d. The time to achieve between 95 and 99% of steady state is approximately $5t_{1/2}$ without a loading dose. Therefore,

$$5 \times 6 = 30\ hr$$

11. a.

$$C_{ss} = \frac{R}{KV_d} \qquad R = C_{ss}KV_d$$

$$R = (5)\left(\frac{0.693}{2}\right)(0.173)(75) = 22.479\ mg/hr$$

$$D_L = C_{ss}V_d = (5)(0.173)(75) = 64.875\ mg$$

b.

$$\frac{R_{old}}{C_{ss,old}} = \frac{R_{new}}{C_{ss,new}}$$

$$\frac{22.479}{2} = \frac{R_{new}}{5} \qquad R_{new} = 56.2\ mg/hr$$

c. $4.32t_{1/2} = 4.32(2) = 8.64$ hr

CHAPTER 16

1. The normal dose of tetracycline is 250 mg PO every 6 hr. The dose of tetracycline for the uremic patient is determined by the K_u/K_N ratio, which is determined by the kidney function, as in Figure 16-4. From line H in Figure 16-4, at Cl_{Cr} of 20 ml, $K_u/K_N = 40\%$. In order to maintain the average concentration of tetracycline at the same level as in normal patients, the dose of tetracycline must be reduced.

$$\frac{D_u}{D_N} = \frac{K_u}{K_N} = 40\%$$

$$D_u = 250 \times 40\% = 100 \text{ mg}$$

Therefore, 100 mg of tetracycline should be given PO every 6 hr.

2. Since the age of the patient is not available, we can determine the $\mathrm{Cl}_{\mathrm{Cr}}$ only approximately, and the dose of digoxin determined must also be an approximation.

$$C_{\mathrm{Cr}} = 5 \text{ mg}\%$$

Using Equation 16.14,

$$\mathrm{Cl}_{\mathrm{Cr}} = \frac{100}{C_{\mathrm{Cr}}} - 12 = \frac{100}{5} - 12$$

$$= 8 \text{ ml/min } 1.73 \text{ M}^2$$

In Table 16-2 digoxin is classified under group *G*. In Figure 16-4 line *G* shows that $K_u/K_N = 38\%$. Therefore.

$$\frac{K_u}{K_N} = \frac{D_u}{D_N} = 38\%$$

$$D_u = 0.125 \times 38\%$$

$$= 0.048 \text{ mg}$$

3. The drug in this patient is eliminated by the kidneys and the dialysis machine. Therefore,

$$\text{Total drug clearance} = \mathrm{Cl_T} + \mathrm{Cl_D}$$

Using Equation 16.27,

$$\mathrm{Cl_D} = \frac{Q(C_a - C_v)}{C_a}$$

$$= \frac{50(5 - 2.4)}{5} = 26 \text{ ml/min}$$

$$\text{Total drug clearance} = 10 + 26$$

$$= 36 \text{ ml/min}$$

Since the drug clearance is increased from 10 to 36 ml/min, the dose should be increased if dialysis is going to continue. Since dose is directly proportional to clearance,

$$\frac{D_u}{D_N} = \frac{36}{10} = 3.6$$

The new dose should be 3.6 times the dose given before dialysis if the same level of antibiotics is to be maintained.

4. The creatinine clearance of a patient is determined experimentally by using Equation 16.11:

$$\mathrm{Cl}_{\mathrm{Cr}} = \frac{C_u V 100}{C_{\mathrm{Cr}} 1440}$$

$$= \frac{0.1 \times 1800 \times 100}{2.2 \times 1440}$$

$$= 5.68 \text{ ml/min}$$

Assuming the normal $\mathrm{Cl}_{\mathrm{Cr}}$ in this patient is 100 ml/min, the uremic dose should be 5.7% of the normal dose, since kidney function is drastically reduced:

$$5.7\% \times 20 \text{ mg/kg} = 1.14 \text{ mg/kg every 6 hr}$$

5. From Figure 16-4, line *F*, at a $\mathrm{Cl}_{\mathrm{Cr}}$ of 5 ml/min,

$$\frac{K_u}{K_N} = 45\%$$

a. The dose given should be

$$45\% \times 600 \text{ mg} = 270 \text{ mg every 12 hr}$$

b. Alternatively, the dose of 600 mg should be given every

$$12 \times \frac{100}{45} = 26.7 \text{ hr}$$

c. Since it may be desirable to give the drug once every 24 hr, both dose and dosing interval may be adjusted so that the patient will still maintain an average therapeutic blood level of the drug, which can then be given at a convenient time. Using the equation for C_{av}^{∞},

$$C_{av}^{\infty} = \frac{D}{KV_d\tau}$$

$$D = 600 \text{ mg}$$

$$\tau = 26.7 \text{ hr}$$

$$C_{av}^{\infty} = \frac{600}{KV_d \times 26.7}$$

To maintain C_{av}^{∞} the same, calculate a new dose, D_N, with a new dosing interval, τ_N, of 24 hr.

$$C_{av}^{\infty} = \frac{D_N}{KV_D \times 24}$$

Thus,

$$\frac{600}{26.7} = \frac{D_N}{24}$$

Therefore,

$$D_N = \frac{24}{26.7} \times 600 = 539 \text{ mg}$$

The drug can also be given at 540 mg daily.

6. For females use 85% of the Cl_{Cr} value obtained in males.

$$Cl_{Cr} = \frac{0.85[140 - \text{age (yrs)}]\ \text{body weight (kg)}}{72\ (Cl_{Cr})}$$

$$= \frac{0.85[140 - 38]62}{(72)(1.8)} = 41.5\ \text{ml/min}$$

9. Gentamycin is listed in group K (Table 16-2). From Nomogram (Fig. 16-4)

$$Cl_{Cr} = 20\ \text{ml/min} \quad \frac{K_u}{K_n} = 25\%$$

Uremic dose = 25% of normal dose

$$= (0.25)(1\ \text{mg/kg}) = 0.25\ \text{mg/kg}$$

For 72-kg patient

$$\text{Uremic dose} = (0.25)(75) = 18.8\ \text{mg}$$

Patient should receive 18.8 mg every 8 hr by multiple IV bolus injections.

10. a. During the first 48 hr postdose, $t_{1/2} = 16$ hr. For IV bolus injection, assuming first-order elimination:

$$D_B = D_0 e^{-Kt}$$

$$= 1000 e^{-(0.693/16)(48)}$$

$= 125$ mg remaining in body just prior to dialysis

During dialysis, $t_{1/2} = 4$ hr:

$$D_B = 125 e^{-(0.693/4)(8)}$$

$= 31.3$ mg after dialysis

b.

$$V_d = 0.5\ \text{L/kg} \times 75\ \text{kg} = 37.5\ \text{L}$$

Drug concentration just prior to dialysis:

$$C_p = 125\ \text{mg}/37.5\ \text{L} = 3.33\ \text{mg/L}$$

Drug concentration just after dialysis:

$$C_p = 31.3\ \text{mg}/3.75\ \text{L} = 0.83\ \text{mg/L}$$

CHAPTER 18

1. a. Both A and B release drug at a zero-order rate (straight line). Curve B shows 100% of drug is released in 12 hr, or about 8.3% per hour.

b. Product C.

c. Product C initially releases drug at a zero-order rate (first 3 hr).

d. Drug release usually slows down toward the end because most tablets gets smaller as dissolution proceeds, resulting in a smaller surface for water penetration inward and drug diffusion outward. Also, as drug dissolution occurs, the concentration gradient (Fick's law) gets progressively smaller due to the build-up of drug in the bulk solution.

e. For a sustained release product, as the surface drug are dissolved, the interior drug would have to traverse a longer or more tortuous path to reach the outside, resulting in the slowing in rate of dissolution.

2. a. A drug given 10 mg four times daily would be equivalent to 40 mg/day or 20 mg/12 hr at the rate of 1.67 mg/hr.

b. 0.5 ml/hr should deliver 1.67 mg of drug. Therefore, the concentration should be

$$1.67/0.5 = 3.34 \text{ mg/ml}$$

3. Using the infusion equation:

$$K = \frac{0.693}{3.5} = 0.198 \text{ hr}^{-1}$$

$$V_d = 10 \text{ L}$$

$$C_p = 20 \text{ mg/L}$$

$$\begin{aligned} R &= C_p V_d K \\ &= 20 \times 10 \times 0.198 \\ &= 39.6 \text{ mg/hr} \end{aligned}$$

$$\begin{aligned} \text{Total drug needed} &= R \times 12 \text{ hr} \\ &= 39.6 \times 12 \\ &= 475.2 \text{ mg} \end{aligned}$$

APPENDIX B

GLOSSARY OF TERMS

A, B, C	Intercepts for compartments 1, 2, and 3, respectively
a, b, c	Rate constants for compartments 1, 2, and 3, respectively
AUC	Area under the plasma level–time curve
C_{av}^{∞}	Average steady-state plasma drug concentration
C_C	Concentration of drug in the central compartment
C_{Cr}	Serum creatinine concentration, usually expressed as mg%
C_d	Concentration of drug
C_{eff}	Minimum effective drug concentration (MTC)
C_{max}	Maximum concentration of drug
C_{max}^{∞}	Maximum steady-state drug concentration
C_{min}	Minimum concentration of drug
C_{min}^{∞}	Minimum steady-state drug concentration
C_p	Concentration of drug in plasma
C_p^0	Concentration of drug in plasma at zero time ($t = 0$)
C_p^{∞}	Steady-state plasma drug concentration (equivalent to C_{ss})
C_{ss}	Concentration of drug at steady-state
C_t	Concentration of drug in tissue
Cl_{Cr}	Creatinine clearance
Cl_d	Dialysis clearance
Cl_h	Hepatic clearance
Cl_{int}	Intrinsic clearance
Cl_{nr}	Nonrenal clearance
Cl_r	Renal clearance
Cl_T	Total body clearance
D	Amount of drug
D_A	Amount of drug absorbed
D_B	Amount of drug in body
D_e	Drug eliminated
D_{GI}	Amount of drug in gastrointestinal track
D_L	Loading (initial) dose
D_m	Maintenance dose
D_0	Dose of drug
D^0	Amount of drug at zero time ($t = 0$)
D_u	Amount of drug in urine
D_t	Amount of drug in tissue
E	Pharmacologic effect
e	Intercept on y-axis of graph

relating pharmacologic response against log drug concentration

F Fraction of dose absorbed (bioavailability factor)

f Fraction of dose remaining in body

K Overall drug elimination rate constant (first-order)

K_a Association constant, first-order absorption rate constant

K_e Excretion rate constant (first-order)

K_m Metabolism rate constant (first-order)

K_M Michaelis–Menten constant

K_N Normal elimination rate constant (first-order)

K_0 Zero-order availability rate constant

K_u Uremic elimination rate constant (first-order)

K_{12} Transfer rate constant (from the central to the tissue compartment)

K_{21} Transfer rate constant (from the tissue to the central compartment)

m Slope

MEC Minimum effective concentration

MTC Minimum toxic concentration

P Amount of protein

Q Blood flow

R Pharmacologic response, infusion rate

r Ratio of moles of drug bound to total moles of protein

R_{max} Maximum pharmacologic response

τ Time interval between doses

t Time

t_{eff} Duration of pharmacologic response to drug

t_{max} Time of occurrence for maximum (peak) drug concentration

t^0 Initial or zero time

$t_{1/2}$ Half-life

V_C Volume of central compartment

V_d Volume of distribution

$(V_d)_{ss}$ Steady-state volume of distribution

$(V_d)_{exp}$ Extrapolated volume of distribution

V_m Maximum metabolic rate

V_p Volume of plasma (central) compartment

V_t Volume of tissue compartment

APPENDIX C

Reference Material

APPENDIX TABLE 1. TABLE OF LOGARITHMS

Natural No.											Proportional Parts								
	0	1	2	3	4	5	6	7	8	9	*1*	*2*	*3*	*4*	*5*	*6*	*7*	*8*	*9*
10	0000	0043	0086	0128	0170	0212	0253	0294	0334	0374	4	8	12	17	21	25	29	33	37
11	0414	0453	0492	0531	0569	0607	0645	0682	0719	0755	4	8	11	15	19	23	26	30	34
12	0792	0828	0864	0899	0934	0969	1004	1038	1072	1106	3	7	10	14	17	21	24	28	31
13	1139	1173	1206	1239	1271	1303	1335	1367	1399	1430	3	6	10	13	16	19	23	26	29
14	1461	1492	1523	1553	1584	1614	1644	1673	1703	1732	3	6	9	12	15	18	21	24	27
15	1761	1790	1818	1847	1875	1903	1931	1959	1987	2014	3	6	8	11	14	17	20	22	25
16	2041	2068	2095	2122	2148	2175	2201	2227	2253	2279	3	5	8	11	13	16	18	21	24
17	2304	2330	2355	2380	2405	2430	2455	2480	2504	2529	2	5	7	10	12	15	17	20	22
18	2553	2577	2601	2625	2648	2672	2695	2718	2742	2765	2	5	7	9	12	14	16	19	21
19	2788	2810	2833	2856	2878	2900	2923	2945	2967	2989	2	4	7	9	11	13	16	18	20
20	3010	3032	3054	3075	3096	3118	3139	3160	3181	3201	2	4	6	8	11	13	15	17	19
21	3222	3243	3263	3284	3304	3324	3345	3365	3385	3404	2	4	6	8	10	12	14	16	18
22	3424	3444	3464	3483	3502	3522	3541	3560	3579	3598	2	4	6	8	10	12	14	15	17
23	3617	3636	3655	3674	3692	3711	3729	3747	3766	3784	2	4	6	7	9	11	13	15	17
24	3802	3820	3838	3856	3874	3892	3909	3927	3945	3962	2	4	5	7	9	11	12	14	16
25	3979	3997	4014	4031	4048	4065	4082	4099	4116	4133	2	3	5	7	9	10	12	14	15
26	4150	4166	4183	4200	4216	4232	4249	4265	4281	4298	2	3	5	7	8	10	11	13	15
27	4314	4330	4346	4362	4378	4393	4409	4425	4440	4456	2	3	5	6	8	9	11	13	14
28	4472	4487	4502	4518	4533	4548	4564	4579	4594	4609	2	3	5	6	8	9	11	12	14
29	4624	4639	4654	4669	4683	4698	4713	4728	4742	4757	1	3	4	6	7	9	10	12	13
30	4771	4786	4800	4814	4829	4843	4857	4871	4886	4900	1	3	4	6	7	9	10	11	13
31	4914	4928	4942	4955	4969	4983	4997	5011	5024	5038	1	3	4	6	7	8	10	11	12
32	5051	5065	5079	5092	5105	5119	5132	5145	5159	5172	1	3	4	5	7	8	9	11	12
33	5185	5198	5211	5224	5237	5250	5263	5276	5289	5302	1	3	4	5	6	8	9	10	12
34	5315	5328	5340	5353	5366	5378	5391	5403	5416	5428	1	3	4	5	6	8	9	10	11

(*Continued*)

APPENDIX TABLE 1. TABLE OF LOGARITHMS (*Continued*)

Natural No.	0	1	2	3	4	5	6	7	8	9	Proportional Parts 1	2	3	4	5	6	7	8	9
35	5441	5453	5465	5478	5490	5502	5514	5527	5539	5551	1	2	4	5	6	7	9	10	11
36	5563	5575	5587	5599	5611	5623	5635	5647	5658	5670	1	2	4	5	6	7	8	10	11
37	5682	5694	5705	5717	5729	5740	5752	5763	5775	5786	1	2	3	5	6	7	8	9	10
38	5798	5809	5821	5832	5843	5855	5866	5877	5888	5899	1	2	3	5	6	7	8	9	10
39	5911	5922	5933	5944	5955	5966	5977	5988	5999	6010	1	2	3	4	5	7	8	9	10
40	6021	6031	6042	6053	6064	6075	6085	6096	6107	6117	1	2	3	4	5	6	8	9	10
41	6128	6138	6149	6160	6170	6180	6191	6201	6212	6222	1	2	3	4	5	6	7	8	9
42	6232	6243	6253	6263	6274	6284	6294	6304	6314	6325	1	2	3	4	5	6	7	8	9
43	6335	6345	6355	6365	6375	6385	6395	6405	6415	6425	1	2	3	4	5	6	7	8	9
44	6435	6444	6454	6464	6474	6484	6493	6503	6513	6522	1	2	3	4	5	6	7	8	9
45	6532	6542	6551	6561	6571	6580	6590	6599	6609	6618	1	2	3	4	5	6	7	8	9
46	6628	6637	6646	6656	6665	6675	6684	6693	6702	6712	1	2	3	4	5	6	7	7	8
47	6721	6730	6739	6749	6758	6767	6776	6785	6794	6803	1	2	3	4	5	5	6	7	8
48	6812	6821	6830	6839	6848	6857	6866	6875	6884	6893	1	2	3	4	4	5	6	7	8
49	6902	6911	6920	6928	6937	6946	6955	6964	6972	6981	1	2	3	4	4	5	6	7	8
50	6990	6998	7007	7016	7024	7033	7042	7050	7059	7067	1	2	3	3	4	5	6	7	8
51	7076	7084	7093	7101	7110	7118	7126	7135	7143	7152	1	2	3	3	4	5	6	7	8
52	7160	7168	7177	7185	7193	7202	7210	7218	7226	7235	1	2	2	3	4	5	6	7	7
53	7243	7251	7259	7267	7275	7284	7292	7300	7308	7316	1	2	2	3	4	5	6	6	7
54	7324	7332	7340	7348	7356	7364	7372	7380	7388	7396	1	2	2	3	4	5	6	6	7
55	7404	7412	7419	7427	7435	7443	7451	7459	7466	7474	1	2	2	3	4	5	5	6	7
56	7482	7490	7497	7505	7513	7520	7528	7536	7543	7551	1	2	2	3	4	5	5	6	7
57	7559	7566	7574	7582	7589	7597	7604	7612	7619	7627	1	2	2	3	4	5	5	6	7
58	7634	7642	7649	7657	7664	7672	7679	7686	7694	7701	1	1	2	3	4	4	5	6	7
59	7709	7716	7723	7731	7738	7745	7752	7760	7767	7774	1	1	2	3	4	4	5	6	7
60	7782	7789	7796	7803	7810	7818	7825	7832	7839	7846	1	1	2	3	4	4	5	6	6
61	7853	7860	7868	7875	7882	7889	7896	7903	7910	7917	1	1	2	3	4	4	5	6	6
62	7924	7931	7938	7945	7952	7959	7966	7973	7980	7987	1	1	2	3	3	4	5	6	6
63	7993	8000	8007	8014	8021	8028	8035	8041	8048	8055	1	1	2	3	3	4	5	5	6
64	8062	8069	8075	8082	8089	8096	8102	8109	8116	8122	1	1	2	3	3	4	5	5	6
65	8129	8136	8142	8149	8156	8162	8169	8176	8182	8189	1	1	2	3	3	4	5	5	6
66	8195	8202	8209	8215	8222	8228	8235	8241	8248	8254	1	1	2	3	3	4	5	5	6
67	8261	8267	8274	8280	8287	8293	8299	8306	8312	8319	1	1	2	3	3	4	5	5	6
68	8325	8331	8338	8344	8351	8357	8363	8370	8376	8382	1	1	2	3	3	4	4	5	6
69	8388	8395	8401	8407	8414	8420	8426	8432	8439	8445	1	1	2	2	3	4	4	5	6
70	8451	8457	8463	8470	8476	8482	8488	8494	8500	8506	1	1	2	2	3	4	4	5	6
71	8513	8519	8525	8531	8537	8543	8549	8555	8561	8567	1	1	2	2	3	4	4	5	5
72	8573	8579	8585	8591	8597	8603	8609	8615	8621	8627	1	1	2	2	3	4	4	5	5
73	8633	8639	8645	8651	8657	8663	8669	8675	8681	8686	1	1	2	2	3	4	4	5	5
74	8692	8698	8704	8710	8716	8722	8727	8733	8739	8745	1	1	2	2	3	4	4	5	5
75	8751	8756	8762	8768	8774	8779	8785	8791	8797	8802	1	1	2	2	3	3	4	5	5
76	8808	8814	8820	8825	8831	8837	8842	8848	8854	8859	1	1	2	2	3	3	4	5	5
77	8865	8871	8876	8882	8887	8893	8899	8904	8910	8915	1	1	2	2	3	3	4	4	5
78	8921	8927	8932	8938	8943	8949	8954	8960	8965	8971	1	1	2	2	3	3	4	4	5
79	8976	8982	8987	8993	8998	9004	9009	9015	9020	9026	1	1	2	2	3	3	4	4	5

(*Continued*)

APPENDIX TABLE 1. TABLE OF LOGARITHMS (*Continued*)

Natural No.	0	1	2	3	4	5	6	7	8	9	Proportional Parts *1*	*2*	*3*	*4*	*5*	*6*	*7*	*8*	*9*
80	9031	9036	9042	9047	9053	9058	9063	9069	9074	9079	1	1	2	2	3	3	4	4	5
81	9085	9090	9096	9101	9106	9112	9117	9122	9128	9133	1	1	2	2	3	3	4	4	5
82	9138	9143	9149	9154	9159	9165	9170	9175	9180	9186	1	1	2	2	3	3	4	4	5
83	9191	9196	9201	9206	9212	9217	9222	9227	9232	9238	1	1	2	2	3	3	4	4	5
84	9243	9248	9253	9258	9263	9269	9274	9279	9284	9289	1	1	2	2	3	3	4	4	5
85	9294	9299	9304	9309	9315	9320	9325	9330	9335	9340	1	1	2	2	3	3	4	4	5
86	9345	9350	9355	9360	9365	9370	9375	9380	9385	9390	1	1	2	2	3	3	4	4	5
87	9395	9400	9405	9410	9415	9420	9425	9430	9435	9440	0	1	1	2	2	3	3	4	4
88	9445	9450	9455	9460	9465	9469	9474	9479	9484	9489	0	1	1	2	2	3	3	4	4
89	9494	9499	9504	9509	9513	9518	9523	9528	9533	9538	0	1	1	2	2	3	3	4	4
90	9542	9547	9552	9557	9562	9566	9571	9576	9581	9586	0	1	1	2	2	3	3	4	4
91	9590	9595	9600	9605	9609	9614	9619	9624	9628	9633	0	1	1	2	2	3	3	4	4
92	9638	9643	9647	9652	9657	9661	9666	9671	9675	9680	0	1	1	2	2	3	3	4	4
93	9685	9689	9694	9699	9703	9708	9713	9717	9722	9727	0	1	1	2	2	3	3	4	4
94	9731	9736	9741	9745	9750	9754	9759	9763	9768	9773	0	1	1	2	2	3	3	4	4
95	9777	9782	9786	9791	9795	9800	9805	9809	9814	9818	0	1	1	2	2	3	3	4	4
96	9823	9827	9832	9836	9841	9845	9850	9854	9859	9863	0	1	1	2	2	3	3	4	4
97	9868	9872	9877	9881	9886	9890	9894	9899	9903	9908	0	1	1	2	2	3	3	4	4
98	9912	9917	9921	9926	9930	9934	9939	9943	9948	9952	0	1	1	2	2	3	3	4	4
99	9956	9961	9965	9969	9974	9978	9983	9987	9991	9996	0	1	1	2	2	3	3	3	4

APPENDIX TABLE 2. NATURAL LOGARITHMS OF NUMBERS

n	$\log_e n$	n	$\log_e n$	n	$\log_e n$
0.0	*	4.5	1.5041	9.0	2.1972
0.1	7.6974	4.6	1.5261	9.1	2.2083
0.2	8.3906	4.7	1.5476	9.2	2.2192
0.3	8.7960	4.8	1.5686	9.3	2.2300
0.4	9.0837	4.9	1.5892	9.4	2.2407
0.5	9.3069	5.0	1.6094	9.5	2.2513
0.6	9.4892	5.1	1.6292	9.6	2.2618
0.7	9.6433	5.2	1.6487	9.7	2.2721
0.8	9.7769	5.3	1.6677	9.8	2.2824
0.9	9.8946	5.4	4.6864	9.9	2.2925
1.0	0.0000	5.5	1.7047	10	2.3026
1.1	0.0953	5.6	1.7228	11	2.3979
1.2	0.1823	5.7	1.7405	12	2.4849
1.3	0.2624	5.8	1.7579	13	2.5649
1.4	0.3365	5.9	1.7750	14	2.6391
1.5	0.4055	6.0	1.7918	15	2.7081
1.6	0.4700	6.1	1.8083	16	2.7726
1.7	0.5306	6.2	1.8245	17	2.8332
1.8	0.5878	6.3	1.8405	18	2.8904
1.9	0.6419	6.4	1.8563	19	2.9444
2.0	0.6931	6.5	1.8718	20	2.9957
2.1	0.7419	6.6	1.8871	25	3.2189
2.2	0.7885	6.7	1.9021	30	3.4012
2.3	0.8329	6.8	1.9169	35	3.5553
2.4	0.8755	6.9	1.9315	40	3.6889
2.5	0.9163	7.0	1.9459	45	3.8067
2.6	0.9555	7.1	1.9601	50	3.9120
2.7	0.9933	7.2	1.9741	55	4.0073
2.8	1.0296	7.3	1.9879	60	4.0943
2.9	1.0647	7.4	2.0015	65	4.1744
3.0	1.0986	7.5	2.0149	70	4.2485
3.1	1.1314	7.6	2.0281	75	4.3175
3.2	1.1632	7.7	2.0412	80	4.3820
3.3	1.1939	7.8	2.0541	85	4.4427
3.4	1.2238	7.9	2.0669	90	4.4998
3.5	1.2528	8.0	2.0794	95	4.5539
3.6	1.2809	8.1	2.0919	100	4.6052
3.7	1.3083	8.2	2.1041		
3.8	1.3350	8.3	2.1163		
3.9	1.3610	8.4	2.1282		
4.0	1.3863	8.5	2.1401		
4.1	1.4110	8.6	2.1518		
4.2	1.4351	8.7	2.1633		
4.3	1.4586	8.8	2.1748		
4.4	1.4816	8.9	2.1861		

*Subtract 10 from $\log_e n$ entries for $n < 1.0$

APPENDIX TABLE 3. EXPONENTIAL FUNCTIONS

X	e^x	e^{-x}	X	e^x	e^{-x}
0.00	1.0000	1.0000	2.5	12.182	0.0821
0.05	1.0513	0.9512	2.6	13.464	0.0743
0.10	1.1052	0.9048	2.7	14.880	0.0672
0.15	1.1618	0.8607	2.8	16.445	0.0608
0.20	1.2214	0.8187	2.9	18.174	0.0550
0.25	1.2840	0.7788	3.0	20.086	0.0498
0.30	1.3499	0.7408	3.1	22.198	0.0450
0.35	1.4191	0.7047	3.2	24.533	0.0408
0.40	1.4918	0.6703	3.3	27.113	0.0369
0.45	1.5683	0.6376	3.4	29.964	0.0334
0.50	1.6487	0.6065	3.5	33.115	0.0302
0.55	1.7333	0.5769	3.6	36.598	0.0273
0.60	1.8221	0.5488	3.7	40.447	0.0247
0.65	1.9155	0.5220	3.8	44.701	0.0224
0.70	2.0138	0.4966	3.9	49.402	0.0202
0.75	2.1170	0.4724	4.0	54.598	0.0183
0.80	2.2255	0.4493	4.1	60.340	0.0166
0.85	2.3396	0.4274	4.2	66.686	0.0150
0.90	2.4596	0.4066	4.3	73.700	0.0136
0.95	2.5857	0.3867	4.4	81.451	0.0123
1.0	2.7183	0.3679	4.5	90.017	0.0111
1.1	3.0042	0.3329	4.6	99.484	0.0101
1.2	3.3201	0.3012	4.7	109.95	0.0091
1.3	3.6693	0.2725	4.8	121.51	0.0082
1.4	4.0552	0.2466	4.9	134.29	0.0074
1.5	4.4817	0.2231	5	148.41	0.0067
1.6	4.9530	0.2019	6	403.43	0.0025
1.7	5.4739	0.1827	7	1096.6	0.0009
1.8	6.0496	0.1653	8	2981.0	0.0003
1.9	6.6859	0.1496	9	8103.1	0.0001
2.0	7.3891	0.1353	10	22026	0.00005
2.1	8.1662	0.1225			
2.2	9.0250	0.1108			
2.3	9.9742	0.1003			
2.4	11.023	0.0907			

APPENDIX TABLE 4. RECOMMENDATIONS FROM THE DECLARATION OF HELSINKI.

I. Basic Principles

1. Clinical research must conform to the moral and scientific principles that justify medical research and should be based on laboratory and animal experiments or other scientifically established facts.
2. Clinical research should be conducted only by scientifically qualified persons and under the supervision of a qualified medical person.
3. Clinical research cannot legitimately be carried out unless the importance of the objective is in proportion to the inherent risk to the subject.
4. Every clinical research project should be preceded by careful assessment of inherent risks in comparison to foreseeable benefits to the subject or to others.
5. Special caution should be exercised by the doctor in performing clinical research in which the personality of the subject is liable to be altered by drugs or experimental procedure.

II. Clinical Research Combined with Professional Care

1. In the treatment of the sick person, the doctor must be free to use a new therapeutic measure, if in his judgment it offers hope of saving life, reestablishing health, or alleviating suffering.

   If at all possible, consistent with patient psychology, the doctor should obtain the patient's freely given consent after the patient has been given a full explanation. In case of legal incapacity consent should also be procured from the legal guardian; in case of physical incapacity the permission of the legal guardian replaces that of the patient.
2. The doctor can combine clinical research with professional care, the objective being the acquisition of new medical knowledge, only to the extent that clinical research is justified by its therapeutic value for the patient.

III. Nontherapeutic Clinical Research

1. In the purely scientific application of clinical research carried out on a human being, it is the duty of the doctor to remain the protector of the life and health of that person on whom clinical research is being carried out.

2. The nature, the purpose, and the risk of clinical research must be explained to the subject by the doctor.

3a. Clinical research on a human being cannot be undertaken without his free consent after he has been informed; if he is legally incompetent, the consent of the legal guardian should be procured.

3b. The subject of clinical research should be in such a mental, physical, and legal state as to be able to exercise fully his power of choice.

3c. Consent should, as a rule, be obtained in writing. However, the responsibility for clinical research always remains with the research worker; it never falls on the subject even after consent is obtained.

4a. The investigator must respect the right of each individual to safeguard his personal integrity, especially if the subject is in a dependent relationship to the investigator.

4b. At any time during the course of clinical research the subject or his guardian should be free to withdraw permission for research to be continued.

The investigator or the investigating team should discontinue the research if in his or their judgment, it may, if continued, be harmful to the individual.

Source: Guiding principles approved by the Federation of Societies for Experimental Biology. Printed with permission.

APPENDIX TABLE 5. GUIDING PRINCIPLES IN THE CARE AND USE OF ANIMALS

Animal experiments are to be undertaken only with the purpose of advancing knowledge. Consideration should be given to the appropriateness of experimental procedures, species of animals used, and number of animals required.

Only animals that are lawfully acquired shall be used in the laboratory, and their retention and use shall be in every case in compliance with federal, state, and local laws and regulations and in accordance with the NIH Guide.

Animals in the laboratory must receive every consideration for their comfort; they must be properly housed, fed, and their surroundings kept in a sanitary condition.

Appropriate anesthetics must be used to eliminate sensibility to pain during all surgical procedures. Where recovery from anesthesia is necessary during the study, acceptable technique to minimize pain must be followed. Muscle relaxants or paralytics are not anesthetics and they should not be used alone for surgical restraint. They may be used for surgery in conjunction with drugs known to produce adequate analgesia. Where use of anesthetics would negate the results of the experiment, such procedures should be carried out in strict accordance with the NIH Guide. If the study requires the death of the animal, the animal must be killed in a humane manner at the conclusion of the observations.

The postoperative care of animals shall be such as to minimize discomfort and pain, and in any case shall be equivalent to accepted practices in schools of veterinary medicine.

When animals are used by students for their education or the advancement of science, such work shall be under the direct supervision of an experienced teacher or investigator. The rules for the care of such animals must be the same as for animals used for research.

Source: Guide for the care and use of laboratory animals. DHEW Publication No. (NIH) 80-23, Revised 1978, Reprinted 1980. Office of Science and Health Reports, DRR/NIH, Bethesda, MD, 20205.

Index

t indicates table; *f* indicates figure

C

D

E

H

I

R

S

X

Y

Z